Contemporary Issues in
LUNG CANCER
A NURSING PERSPECTIVE

SECOND EDITION

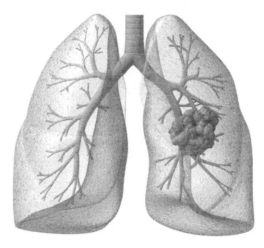

Edited by

MARILYN L. HAAS, PHD, ANP-C

Mountain Radiation Oncology
Asheville, North Carolina

JONES AND BARTLETT PUBLISHERS

Sudbury, Massachusetts

BOSTON   TORONTO   LONDON   SINGAPORE

World Headquarters

Jones and Bartlett Publishers
40 Tall Pine Drive
Sudbury, MA 01776
978-443-5000
info@jbpub.com
www.jbpub.com

Jones and Bartlett Publishers Canada
6339 Ormindale Way
Mississauga, Ontario L5V 1J2
Canada

Jones and Bartlett Publishers International
Barb House, Barb Mews
London W6 7PA
United Kingdom

Jones and Bartlett's books and products are available through most bookstores and online booksellers. To contact Jones and Bartlett Publishers directly, call 800-832-0034, fax 978-443-8000, or visit our website, www.jbpub.com.

Substantial discounts on bulk quantities of Jones and Bartlett's publications are available to corporations, professional associations, and other qualified organizations. For details and specific discount information, contact the special sales department at Jones and Bartlett via the above contact information or send an email to specialsales@jbpub.com.

ISSN: 1535-9999
ISBN: 978-0-7637-6051-9

The authors, editor, and publisher have made every effort to provide accurate information. However, they are not responsible for errors, omissions, or for any outcomes related to the use of the contents of this book and take no responsibility for the use of the products and procedures described. Treatments and side effects described in this book may not be applicable to all people; likewise, some people may require a dose or experience a side effect that is not described herein. Drugs and medical devices are discussed that may have limited availability controlled by the Food and Drug Administration (FDA) for use only in a research study or clinical trial. Research, clinical practice, and government regulations often change the accepted standard in this field. When consideration is being given to use of any drug in the clinical setting, the health care provider or reader is responsible for determining FDA status of the drug, reading the package insert, and reviewing prescribing information for the most up-to-date recommendations on dose, precautions, and contraindications, and determining the appropriate usage for the product. This is especially important in the case of drugs that are new or seldom used.

Production Credits
Publisher: Kevin Sullivan
Acquisitions Editor: Emily Ekle
Acquisitions Editor: Amy Sibley
Associate Editor: Patricia Donnelly
Editorial Assistant: Rachel Shuster
Associate Production Editor: Katie Spiegel
Senior Marketing Manager: Barb Bartoszek
V.P., Manufacturing and Inventory Control: Therese Connell
Composition: Auburn Associates, Inc.
Cover Design: Kristin E. Parker
Cover Image: © Eraxion/Dreamstime.com
Printing and Binding: Malloy, Inc.
Cover Printing: Malloy, Inc.

6048
Printed in the United States of America
13 12 11 10 09   10 9 8 7 6 5 4 3 2 1

Dedication

When our lives are busy with work, professional, and community activities, I am very fortunate to come home to my family and find refuge to renew and replenish my strength to begin new days. It is this love, support, and caring that my husband offers me every day. Although my sons, William and Kenneth, are building their own careers, they are never too far to offer words of encouragement and love.

To my returning authors, I continually learn from your clinical knowledge and expertise and thank you for your endless hours to support this project. To my new authors, I am very appreciative of your abilities to pick up where others have taken a different path or added new chapters to update the clinical practice; your time and talents are valued.

Finally, to our patients who demonstrate the courage to fight, willingness to share their feelings and concerns, and who truly live each day with optimism for a cure—may we all continue to strive for this same goal.

Contents

Preface

Being diagnosed with lung cancer is one of the greatest challenges men and women, along with their family members and friends, can ever face in their lifetimes. While there are more than 12 different kinds of lung cancer, most cases fall within two categories: small cell and non-small cell lung cancer. Although the statistics for survival are dismal, healthcare professionals can impact education and research to fight this disease. Only by becoming more knowledgeable about lung cancer can we ever make progress to lengthen survival time and quality of life.

The intent of this book is unchanged from the original first edition. It is to provide seasoned oncology nurses and other healthcare professionals the opportunity to explore in-depth issues that face lung cancer patients. Thus, this work is a launching avenue for others upon which to build more evidence-based practice in the care of lung cancer patients. *Contemporary Issues in Lung Cancer,* Second Edition, is divided into six sections. The first section, Part One, provides the latest up-to-date information about incidence, prevalence, epidemiology, risk factors, and the biology of lung cancer. Also, there is a discussion about the controversies in detecting and screening for lung cancer. Part Two presents the various treatment modalities and the issues that surround the procedures. New advances in the greater role that combined chemotherapy plays in treating this disease are discussed in depth. The chapters in Part Three address the special issues that face lung cancer patients: fatigue, end of life, nutrition, dyspnea, and radon exposure. In Part Four, the authors share their expertise in exploring psychosocial issues associated with having lung cancer. Part Five offers insight into providing assistance and resources for individuals and families who are facing this disease. A new chapter describes how navigators play an integral part of the oncology team. Finally, Part Six exposes the reality of the untold story, the unaddressed issues, and the challenges that healthcare professionals face today. Excellent resources for both the healthcare professionals and lung cancer patients are identified. Future directions and application of evidence-based research will strengthen and support the care needed to fight this cancer.

Contributors

Elisa Becze, BA
Editorial Manager
Oncology Nursing Society
Pittsburgh, Pennsylvania

Sheila Boegli, MSN, RN, CCRN, CCNS
Advanced Practice Nurse
Cardiothoracic Surgery
Bethesda North Hospital
Cincinnati, Ohio

Julie M. Bowman, RN, OCN
Staff Nurse in Radiation Oncology
Caldwell Memorial Hospital
Lenoir, North Carolina

Pamela M. Calarese, MS, RN, CS
Adult Nurse Practitioner
Thoracic Oncology
Dana Farber Cancer Institute
Boston, Massachusetts

Doris Dickerson Coward, PhD, RN
Retired Associate Professor
School of Nursing
The University of Texas at Austin
Austin, Texas

Angelina Esparza, MPH, RN
Director
ACS Patient Navigator Program
American Cancer Society, National Home Office
Atlanta, Georgia

Marilyn L. Haas, PhD, ANP-BC
Adult Nurse Practitioner
Mountain Radiation Oncology
Asheville, North Carolina

Mary Lou Heater, MSN, CNS, APRN-BC
Advanced Practice Nurse
The University of Texas
M.D. Anderson Cancer Center
Houston, Texas

Doris Howell, PhD, RN
Princess Margaret Hospital & Lawrence Bloomberg
    Faculty of Nursing
University of Toronto & Ontario Cancer Institute
Toronto, Ontario, Canada

Katherine Katen Moore, MSN, APN-C, AOCN
Nurse Practitioner, Breast and Gastrointestinal
    Cancer Groups
The Cancer Institute of New Jersey
University of Medicine and Dentistry
New Brunswick, New Jersey

Giselle J. Moore-Higgs, ARNP, PhDc, AOCN
Assistant Director, Clinical Trials Office
University of Florida Shands Cancer Center
Gainesville, Florida

Kenneth R. Olivier, MD
Associate Consultant
Radiation Oncology
Mayo Clinic
Rochester, Minnesota

Karin Olson, PhD, RN
Faculty of Nursing
University of Alberta
Edmonton, Alberta, Canada

Judy R. Prewitt, MSN, RN, ANP-BC, AOCN
Associate Chief Nurse Officer Practice
Duke University Hospital
Durham, North Carolina

Nancy J. Raymon, MN, RN, AOCN
Formerly Director of Program Development
Coordinator of Urologic Cancer Program
Hoag Cancer Center
Newport Beach, California

Amy Kuhns Roberts, MSW, LCSW
Patient Resource Navigator
Mission Hospital
Radiation Therapy
Asheville, North Carolina

Kelly M. Smallcomb, MS, RD, LDN
Clinical Dietitian
Boston Medical Center
Boston, Massachusetts

Tina M. St. John, MD
Executive Director and Medical Director
Caring Ambassadors Program, Inc.
Vancouver, Washington

Sophie Sun, MD, FRCPC
Medical Oncologist
British Columbia Cancer Agency - Vancouver
   Centre
Vancouver, British Columbia, Canada

Janelle M. Tipton, MSN, RN, AOCN
Oncology Clinical Nurse Specialist
University of Toledo Medical Center
Toledo, Ohio

**Pamela Hallquist Viale, RN, NIS, CS, ANP,
   AOCNP**
Assistant Clinical Professor
University of California, San Francisco
Department of Physiological Nursing
San Francisco, California

Deborah Lowe Volker, PhD, RN, AOCN
Associate Professor
School of Nursing
The University of Texas at Austin
Austin, Texas

Gail M. Wilkes, MS, RNC, AOCN, ANP
Oncology Educator/Nurse Practitioner
Boston Medical Center
Boston, Massachusetts

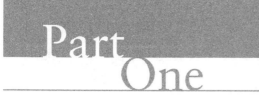

Part
One

*Overview of Small
Cell Lung Cancer
and Non-Small Cell
Lung Cancer*

Chapter 1

Separating Out the Differences Between Lung Cancers

Marilyn L. Haas

Introduction

In the United States, lung cancer has become the "unspoken" or ignored cancer. Lung cancer does not typically elicit the same emotional feelings and/or empathy from healthcare professionals and the general public as do other cancers, such as breast cancer. Lung cancer carries very real social stigmas, and it is one of the few cancers with a known carcinogen that contributes to its etiology. Although this deadly disease has become the number-one killer, national attention, research studies, and funding are lagging behind. The striking difference is very evident in Figures 1–1 and 1–2 from the National Cancer Institute (NCI). In 2002 NCI's Office of Science Planning and Assessment (OSPA) appropriated $237.5 million for lung cancer research and only increased the funding to $242.9 million for the fiscal year 2006 (NCI, 2008a). In comparison, NCI OSPA spent a larger sum of $522.6 million for breast cancer research in 2002 and $584.7 million in 2006 (NCI, 2008b). Also, NCI offers Specialized Programs of Research Excellence (SPOREs) grants that promote interdisciplinary research by mov-ing basic research findings from the laboratory environment to clinical practice settings. For 2008, there are only seven SPOREs relating to lung-cancer-specific grants as compared to the 11 SPOREs funded for breast-cancer-specific grants (NCI, 2008c).

Lung cancer education becomes the priority to increase awareness. Education unveils this deadly disease and exposes more about disease preva-lence, risk factors, disease progression, treatment options, and quality of life for the affected indi-viduals. It is our duty as health professionals to stimulate more interest in researchers and the community at large. As healthcare professionals we should advocate for more funding to eradicate this disease.

This first chapter will explore the patterns and trends in lung cancer. Recognizing the differences between small cell lung cancer and non-small cell lung cancer becomes especially important in the treatment options that will be presented in later chapters. After examining the epidemiology of lung cancer, one will begin to appreciate the risk factors involved with each type of cancer. It is only then that healthcare professionals can begin to have an impact on prevention.

Figure 1–1 NCI funding for breast cancer.

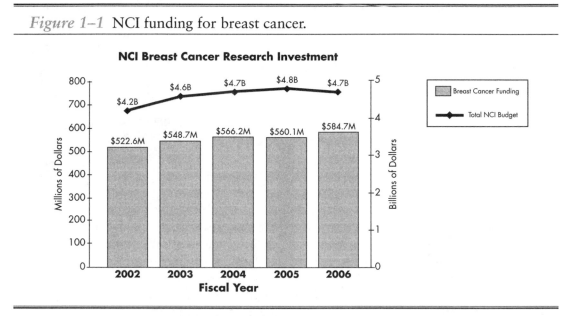

Source: National Cancer Institute (NCI). (2008b). A snapshot of lung cancer. http://planning.cancer.gov/disease/Breast-Snapshot. pdf. Accessed July 7, 2008.

Figure 1–2 NCI funding for lung cancer.

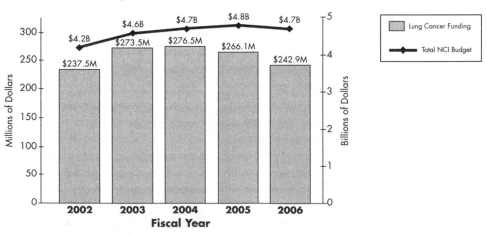

Source: National Cancer Institute (NCI). (2008a). A snapshot of lung cancer. http://planning.cancer.gov/disease/Lung-Snapshot. pdf. Accessed July 7, 2008.

Epidemiology of Lung Cancer

In the United States, lung cancer is the second most common cancer diagnosed in men and women today (Jemal, et al., 2008). The American Cancer Society estimates there will be 215,020 new cases of lung and bronchial cancers diagnosed in 2008: 114,690 new cases in males and 100,330 new cases in females (Jemal, et al., 2008). This represents approximately 15% of all newly diagnosed cancers in the United States.

Reported in the 2001–2005 Surveillance Epidemiology and End Results (SEER), African American males develop higher rates of lung cancer than other ethnic groups (Table 1–1) (Reis, et al., 2007). For every one Caucasian male, there are 13 African American males that develop lung cancer. Caucasian and African American females have the highest incidence rates of lung cancer (54.9 and 54.6 per 100,000 people, respectively), followed by Asian/Pacific Islanders, American Indians, and Hispanic women.

The risk of lung cancer goes up with age. The SEER data reports the median age at the time of diagnosis is 71 years of age (Reis, et al., 2007). There was no one under the age of 20 years diagnosed with the disease. The highest group was between 65 and 74 years of age (Table 1–2).

Although the lung is the second most common site diagnosed for cancer, lung cancer remains the leading cause of cancer death in both men and women in the United States. In 2008, there will be 161,840 estimated deaths: 90,810 men and 71,030 women (Jemal, et al., 2008). Age at the time of death is very similar to age at time of diagnosis as well (Table 1–2). The survival rates reported by SEER don't vary much among race either (Table 1–3). Overall, the 5-year survival rate for lung cancer is 15.2% (Table 1–3) (Reis, et al., 2007). This low rate is related to the fact that the majority of new cases are diagnosed at a regional or distant stage, for which survival is especially poor. Histologic cell type and anatomic extent of the disease are primary prognostic factors in lung cancer.

Table 1–1 NCI SEER Cancer Statistics (2007 Data Submission)

Incidence Rates by Race		
Race/Ethnicity	Male	Female
All races	79.4 per 100,000 men	52.6 per 100,000 women
White	79.3 per 100,000 men	54.9 per 100,000 women
Black	107.6 per 100,000 men	54.6 per 100,000 women
Asian/Pacific Islander	53.9 per 100,000 men	28.0 per 100,000 women
American Indian/Alaska Native	54.3 per 100,000 men	39.7 per 100,000 women
Hispanic	44.2 per 100,000 men	25.4 per 100,000 women

Source: SEER, data 2001–2005.

Table 1–2 Age at Time of Lung Cancer Diagnosis/Death

Age	Percentage at Diagnosis	Percentage at Death
< 20 years	0 %	0 %
20–34 years	0.2 %	0.1 %
35–44 years	1.9 %	1.6 %
45–54 years	8.8 %	7.8 %
55–64 years	21.0%	19.5%
65–74 years	31.9%	31.9%
75–84 years	28.9%	30.5%
> 85 + years	7.3%	9.0%

Source: SEER, data 2001–2005.

Types of Lung Cancer

Lung cancers arise from abnormal epithelial cells in the airways of the lung. The World Health Organization (WHO) divides lung cancer into two major types: non-small cell lung cancer (NSCLC) and small cell lung cancer (SCLC). The division is based on biology, therapy, and prognosis. Approximately 95% of all lung cancers are classified as either NSCLC or SCLC, and 5% are other cell types (Midthun, 2008). The majority of cell types are NSCLC (80–85%), and lesser amounts are SCLC (NCCN, 2008). Within NSCLC are three major subtypes: adenocarcinoma, squamous cell (epidermoid) carcinoma, and large cell carcinoma.

Table 1–3 Five-Year Survival Rates of Lung Cancer Individuals

Relative Survivor Rate (measurement of survival among cancer patients in comparison to the general population)	5-Year Survival Rate
Overall	15.2%
Caucasian males	13.4%
Caucasian females	17.9%
African American males	10.4%
African American females	14.5%

Source: SEER, data 2001–2005.

Table 1–4 Stage Distribution at Lung Cancer Diagnosis

	Time at Diagnosis	5-Year Survival Rates
Local	16%	49.5%
Regional	25%	20.6%
Distant	51%	2.8%
Unknown	8%	8.3% (unstaged)

Adenocarcinoma represents about 40% of lung cancer cases in the United States. It is the most common form of lung cancer in nonsmoking individuals, is often located peripherally to bronchi, and tends to metastasize to the brain, adrenals, and bone. Squamous cell carcinoma represents 30–35% of lung cancers. It usually occurs centrally near the main stem bronchi and is usually associated with smoking. Large cell carcinoma, representing 5–15% of lung cancers, is often located peripherally to bronchi. It grows and spreads quickly. Recently, three more subtypes of lung adenocarcinomas have been identified from gene expression profiling using DNA microarrays: bronchioid, squamoid, and magnoid (Hayes, et al., 2006). These subtypes correlate with survival and metastatic patterns. Bronchioid tumors are correlated with increased survival in early stage disease, whereas squamoid tumors are associated with increased survival in advanced disease.

SCLC is in a separate category because of its rapid proliferation, high growth fraction, and the early development of widespread metastases. SCLC starts in the hormonal cells in the lungs and multiplies rapidly. The histologic classification of SCLC has changed over time. Initially, the WHO classified SCLC into three histologic subtypes: oat cell, intermediate cell type, and a combined oat cell (SCLC combined with squamous cell or adenocarcinoma) (Hirsch et al., 1988). In 1999, the WHO and the International Association for the Study of Lung Cancer (IASLC) eliminated the intermediate cell carcinoma and added a new category of large cell neuroendocrine carcinoma (Travis et al., 1999; Junker, Wiethege, & Muller, 2000). This new category divides cell types into: classical small cell lung (SCLC), large cell neuroendocrine cancer, and a combined small cell carcinoma, consisting predominantly of SCLC with some areas of NSCLC.

Lung Cancer Staging

Before statistics can really be understood and used for analyses or decision making, it is important to distinguish between the different stages of lung cancer. The American Joint Committee on Cancer (AJCC) was formed by the American College of Surgeons and other sponsoring organizations to standardize staging of patients with cancer. In 1977, the AJCC began publication of the *AJCC Cancer Staging Manual* in hopes that it would become the standard reference for staging criteria. In the 1980s, the AJCC was able to formulate a consensus system for classifying and staging cancer in collaboration with the International Union Against Cancer. Agreement between these two organizations has enabled the application of a universal system for cancer staging to all solid cancers.

Important changes in the staging of NSCLC occurred in 1997. Tables 1–5 and 1–6 display the latest version (sixth) of the *AJCC Cancer Staging Manual* (AJCC, 2002). Specifically, stage I tumors were further subdivided into IA and IB. Survival difference based on this distinction has been noted in clinical trial analyses. Stage II disease was similarly divided into stage IIA and IIB. Again, A and B were divided to reflect survival differences. Stage IIIA remains the same except for tumors designated as T3, N0, M0 because the survival of patients with these tumors is similar to that of patients with T2, N1, M0 disease. Consequently, both of these categories are now grouped together as stage IIB disease. Stages IIIB and IV remain unchanged except for the changes made to the T4 and M1 descriptors. Specifically, malignant pericardial effusion has been added to the T4 descriptor, the presence of satellite tumors within the lobe of the lung with the primary tumor is classified as T4, and an intrapulmonary ipsilateral distant metastasis is classified as M1.

Even though the tumor-nodes-metastasis (TNM) staging classification in Table 1–6 has shown significance and has proven to be beneficial for predicting survival in patients with NSCLC, the TNM staging system does not have the same prognostic significance for individuals with SCLC. Rather, SCLC is divided into two different categories: limited and extensive. Clinically, limited is described as being confined to one side of the chest and nearby lymph nodes. Tumors of this sort can generally be encompassed in a tolerable radiation port field for treatment. Two-year survival is 15% (Scott, 2000). Extensive disease includes any pleural or pericardial effusion, lung metastases, and mas-

sive tumor that would require prohibitive radiation fields (Chao, Perez, & Brady, 2002). The 2-year survival is a dismal 2% (Scott, 2000).

There are plans for a seventh edition of the *AJCC Cancer Staging Manual* (Greene and Sobin, 2008). AJCC expects to publish their new edition in 2009, and it will be implemented for patients who are diagnosed after January 1, 2010. New anatomic markers and molecular or serum markers will be included in the staging and management strategies. In the proposed changes, there will be numerous changes in the T (tumor) descriptors, no changes to the N (nodal) descriptors, and there will be changes in the M (metastasis) descriptors (refer to Table 1–7) (Goldstraw, et al., 2007). This will change the staging as well (Table 1–8) (Goldstraw, et al., 2007).

Risk Factors

Lung cancer is one of the few cancers that have identified, specific, known carcinogens. Epidemiological studies have convincingly established that nicotine use is the major cause of lung cancer today (Reddy, 2000; Edwards, Brown, & Wingo, et al., 2005; NCI, 2008d). This causative link was well publicized in the 1960s, when national reports in the United States and Great Britain informed the public about the risks of smoking in lung cancer. Studies have shown that 87% of all lung cancers are related to smoking (American Cancer Society, 2001). Smoking is the cause of all four histological types of lung cancers. Certainly, the incidence of lung cancer is directly related to the duration of tobacco use and the daily dose of nicotine (Godtfredsen, Prescott, & Osler, 2005). The more a person smokes, the higher the risk of lung cancer. Nicotine addiction is discussed further in Chapter 16, Understanding and Treat-

---

Table 1–5 AJCC Staging of Lung Cancer

Primary Tumor (T)

TX   Primary tumor cannot be assessed, or tumor is proven by the presence of malignant cells in sputum or bronchial washings but cannot be visualized by imaging or bronchoscopy.

T0   No evidence of primary tumor.

Tis   Carcinoma in situ.

T1   Tumor 3 cm or less in greatest dimension, surrounded by lung or visceral pleura, without bronchoscopic evidence of invasion more proximal than the lobar bronchus (i.e., not in main bronchus).

T2   Tumor with any of the following features of size or extent:

   More than 3 cm in greatest dimension.

   Involves main bronchus, 2 cm or more distal to the carina.

   Invades the visceral pleura.

   Associated with atelectasis or obstructive pneumonitis that extends to the hilar region but does not involve the entire lung.

T3   Tumor of any size that directly invades any of the following: chest wall (including superior sulcus tumors), diaphragm, mediastinal pleura, parietal pericardium; tumor in the main bronchus less than 2 cm distal to the carina but without involvement of the carina; or associated atelectasis of obstructive pneumonitis of the entire lung.

T4   Tumor of any size that invades any of the following: mediastinum, heart, great vessels, trachea, esophagus, vertebral body, carina; separate tumor nodule(s) in the same lobe; or tumor with a malignant pleural effusion.

Regional Lymph Nodes (N)

NX   Regional lymph nodes cannot be assessed.

N0   No regional lymph node metastasis.

N1   Metastasis to ipsilateral peribronchial and/or ipsilateral hilar lymph nodes and intrapulmonary nodes involved by direct extension of the primary tumor.

N2   Metastasis to ipsilateral mediastinal and/or subcarinal lymph node(s).

N3   Metastasis in contralateral mediastinal, contralateral hilar, ipsilateral or contralateral scalene or supraclavicular lymph node(s).

Distant Metastasis (M)

MX   Distant metastasis cannot be assessed.

M0   No distant metastasis.

M1   Distant metastasis present (includes synchronous separate nodule(s) in a different lobe).

Source: Used with the permission of the American Joint Committee on Cancer (AJCC®), Chicago, Illinois. The original source for this material is the AJCC Cancer Staging Manual, 6th edition (2002) published by Lippincott-Raven, Philadelphia, Pennsylvania.

Table 1–6 Stage Grouping

Stage grouping of the TNM subsets has been revised as follows. TNM refers to: primary tumor (T), regional lymph node (N), and distant metastasis (M).

Occult Carcinoma	TX	N0	M0
Stage 0	Tis	N0	M0
Stage IA	T1	N0	M0
Stage IB	T2	N0	M0
Stage IIA	T1	N1	M0
Stage IIB	T2	N1	M0
	T3	N0	M0
Stage IIIA	T1	N2	M0
	T2	N2	M0
	T3	N1	M0
	T3	N2	M0
Stage IIIB	Any T	N3	M0
	T4	Any N	M0
Stage IV	Any T	Any N	M1

Source: Used with the permission of the American Joint Committee on Cancer (AJCC®), Chicago, Illinois. The original source for this material is the AJCC Cancer Staging Manual, 6th edition (2002) published by Lippincott-Raven, Philadelphia, Pennsylvania.

ing Tobacco Dependence in Adults with Lung Cancer. Also, the Registered Nurses' Association of Ontario (RNAO) developed best practice guidelines to help nurses integrate smoking cessation into daily practice. The guidelines can be found on their Web site: http://www.rnao.org/Page.asp?PageID=924& ContentID=802. Evidence, though, suggests that lung cancer has a multistep carcinogenesis, and genetic damage occurs with tobacco use (Rosewich, Adler, & Zielen, 2008; Shinozaki, Yuasa, & Takata, 2008; Krull, Bornstein, Saxer, Walter, & Ramseier, 2008).

Other air pollutants—both indoor and outdoor—are suspicious carcinogens and place individuals at high risk for developing lung cancer. One's risk is increased by radon gas, discussed more in depth in Chapter 11, Environmental Risk: Indoor Radon Exposure. Radon gas is the second leading cause of lung cancer (Ettinger, et al., 2008). It is especially risky for underground miners (Edling & Axelson, 1983; Schottenfield, 1996). Second-hand smoke (also referred to as passive smoke), household combustion devices, and building materials are among the other indoor carcinogens (Asomaning, et al.,

---

Table 1–7 Proposal TNM Staging for Seventh Edition of AJCC Manual

---

Tumor Size—The proposed N descriptors are:

- T0: No evidence of primary tumor
- Tis: Carcinoma in situ
- T1: Tumor that is ≤3 cm in its greatest dimension, does not invade the visceral pleura, and is without bronchoscopic evidence of invasion more proximal than a lobar bronchus

  T1a: Tumor is ≤ 2 cm in its greatest dimension
  T1b: Tumor is > 2 cm in its greatest dimension

- T2: Tumor with any of the following characteristics: > 3 cm but ≤ 7 cm in its greatest dimension, invades a mainstem bronchus with its proximal extent at least 2 cm from the carina, invades the visceral pleura, or is associated with either atelectasis or obstructive pneumonitis that extends to the hilar region without involving the entire lung

  T2a: Tumor is ≤ 5 cm in its greatest dimension
  T2b: Tumor is > 5 cm in its greatest dimension

- T3: Tumor with any of the following characteristics: > 7 cm in its greatest dimension; invades the chest wall (including superior sulcus tumors), diaphragm, phrenic nerve, mediastinal pleura, parietal pericardium, or a mainstem bronchus less than 2 cm from the carina without invasion of the carina; is associated with either atelectasis or obstructive pneumonitis of the entire lung; or satellite nodules are located in the same lung lobe as the primary tumor
- T4: Tumor of any size that invades the mediastinum, heart, great vessels, trachea, recurrent laryngeal nerve, esophagus, vertebral body, or carina; or metastatic nodules located in a different lobe of the ipsilateral lung

Regional lymph nodes—No changes to the N descriptors

Metastasis—The proposed M descriptors are:

- M0: No distant metastasis
- M1a: Malignant pleural effusion, pericardial effusion, pleural nodules, or metastatic nodules in the contralateral lung
- M1b: Distant metastasis

Source: Goldstraw, et al., 2007.

2008). Occupational hazards can include coal gasification, coke production, exposure to soot, and aluminum production (Schottenfield, 1996). Exposure to nickel, arsenic, uranium, and chromium are other hazards. Asbestos, a tiny airborne mineral, increases the risk of developing lung cancer (Ettinger, et al., 2008). It is estimated that 3-4% of lung cancer is related to asbestos exposure (Omenn et al., 1986). These substances, though, account for a far lower number of lung cancers than does smoking. A summary of risk factors is located in Table 1–9.

Table 1–8 Updated Proposal TNM Staging for Seventh Edition of AJCC Manual

- Stage 0: TisN0M0
- Stage IA: T1a-1bN0M0
- Stage IB: T2aN0M0
- Stage IIA: T1a-2aN1M0 or T2bN0M0
- Stage IIB: T2bN1M0 or T3N0M0
- Stage IIIA: T3N1M0 or T1a-3N2M0 or T4N0-1M0
- Stage IIIB: T4N2M0 or T1a-4N3M0
- Stage IV: Any T Any N M1a-1b

Source: Goldstraw, et al., 2007.

Tuberculosis can develop into lung cancers, particularly in the regions of scar tissue. The risk of lung cancer can be five times greater in men and 10 times greater in women who have contracted tuberculosis (Steinitz, 1965). The most common histological type is adenocarcinoma.

Table 1–9 Pollutants Associated with the Etiology of Lung Cancer

Tobacco smoke (first- and second-hand)

Coal gasification

Nickel, arsenic, and cadmium exposure

Radon gas

Coke production

Chloromethyl ethers

Household combustion devices

Soot exposure

Uranium and chromium exposure

Building materials (asbestos)

Aluminum production

Associations between diet and the development of lung cancer have not yet been established. Analysis of the role of nutrients in the etiology of lung cancer is confounded by numerous methodological problems and the conflicting data in these studies (Ginsberg, Kris, & Armstrong, 1993). It is hypothesized that carotenoids, vitamins C and E, and selenium can scavenge the free radicals produced by tobacco smoke, solvents, and pollutants. Certainly, more rigorous studies are needed in this area of prevention. Individuals who eat at least five servings of fruits and vegetables per day have a lower risk of lung cancer, although studies cannot tease out which factors provide the protection because they contain many different combinations of healthy elements, such as antioxidants (http://www.your diseaserisk.wustl.edu).

The focus for healthcare providers should be placed on prevention and reduction to exposure. More public education is needed about the risks and dangers associated with lung cancers. In the era of computers, PDQ, a service offered by the National Cancer Institute (NCI), can be a helpful educational tool. The PDQ is a computer system that gives up-to-date information on cancer and its prevention, detection, treatment, genetics, and supportive care. Patients and their families, physicians, nurses, and other healthcare professionals make up the intended audience. PDQ also provides information about new clinical trials, physicians who treat cancer, and hospitals with cancer programs. NCI's primary Web site, http://www.nci.nih.gov, contains information about the Institute and its programs. The cancer literature at NCI's Web site, http://www.cancer.gov/search/cancer_literature, contains material for healthcare professionals, patients, and the public, including information from PDQ about cancer treatment, screening, prevention, genetics, supportive care, and clinical trials, and from PubMed, a bibliographic database.

Other easily accessible Web sites offer a free screening questionnaire, fact sheet, and risk list. Harvard School of Public Health has developed their Harvard Center for Cancer Prevention Web site (http://www.diseaserisk index. harvard.edu/update), which estimates an individual's risks for lung cancer, among other types of cancers, and provides personal tips on prevention. Support groups are also found on the Internet for education and advocacy. Two popular sites for lung cancer are Caring Ambassadors Program (CAP) for Lung Cancer and Alliance for Lung Cancer Advocacy, Support, and Education (ALCASE). CAP provides state-of-the-art, user friendly information and support to lung cancer patients and their loved ones through a variety of online and printed materials. CAP Lung Cancer's commitment to people who are living with lung cancer is to help them achieve their optimal wellness throughout their journey with lung cancer (http://www.LungCancer CAP.org). CAP Lung Cancer has Ask a Doc® that provides an informational resource for people living with lung cancer and their loved ones. Questions are addressed weekly with posted responses on their site. ALCASE offers free cancer profiling for NSCLC and SCLC as well as education and research (http://www .alcase.org/). Another Web site that serves as a gateway to other sites is Lung Cancer Online (http://www.lungcancer online.org). This is a site for professionals as well as the general public that provides basic lung cancer information resources. Links to journals, references, news, alternative medicine, research, and professional and patient organizations can be located on this site. Also, information on how to use the database is located on the PDQ site. For further Internet resources, please refer to Chapter 20, When Lung Cancer Consumers Seek Evidence.

Future Directions: Conclusions

Despite an incredible amount of effort, lung cancer statistics for the 21st century are still frightening and depressing. Although there has been an explosion of knowledge about the biology of lung cancer and a better understanding of risk factors for lung cancer, improvements in the 5-year survival rates have been minimal, rising only from 8% to 15%. Nevertheless, there is some room for optimism. Accurate diagnosing and staging of lung cancer is imperative, but the challenges to the oncological community are to apply the emerging technology and new resources to detect earlier stages of the disease, learn more about the progression of various types of lung cancer, and target innovative therapeutic modalities. In other words, we should focus more on clinical research and education in regards to the process of carcinogenesis; this approach will lead us to better treatment of cancer. It is doubtful that various manipulations in the late stage of lung cancer will noticeably change the statistics, but certainly we can remain hopeful. Screening of well-delineated high-risk populations and early detection should prove to be much more effective, as is evident in cancers that affect other organs.

References

American Cancer Society. (2001). *Cancer facts and figures.* New York: Author.

American Joint Committee on Cancer. (2002). *AJCC cancer staging manual* (6th ed.). Philadelphia: Lippincott-Raven.

Asomaning, K., Miller, D., Liu, G., Wain, J., Lynch, T., Su, L., et al. (2008). Second hand smoke, age of exposure and lung cancer risk. *Lung Cancer, 61*(1), 13–20.

Chao, K., Perez, C., & Brady, L. (2002). *Radiation oncology: Management decisions* (2nd ed., pp. 303–320). Philadelphia: Lippincott Williams & Wilkins.

Edling, C., & Axelson, O. (1983). Quantitative aspects of radon daughter exposure and lung cancer in underground miners. *British Journal of Industrial Medicine, 40*(2), 182–187.

Edwards, B., Brown, M., Wingo, P., Howe, H., Ward, E., Ries, L., et al. (2005). Annual report to the nation on the status of cancer, 1975–2002, featuring population-based trends in cancer treatment. *Journal of the National Cancer Institute, 97*(19), 1407–1427.

Ettinger, D., Akerley, W., Bepler, G., Chang, A., Cheney, R., Chirieac, L., et al. (2008). Non-small cell lung cancer. *Journal of the National Comprehensive Cancer Network, 6*(3), 228–269.

Ginsberg, R., Kris, M., & Armstrong, J. (1993). Non-small cell lung cancer. In V. T. De Vita, S. Hellman, & S. Rosenberg (Eds.), *Principles and practice of oncology.* Philadelphia: JB Lippincott.

Godtfredsen, N., Prescott, E., & Osler, M. (2005). Effect of smoking reduction on lung cancer risk. *Journal of the American Medical Association, 294*(12), 1505–1510.

Goldstraw, P. L., Crowley, J., Chansky, K., Giroux, D., Groome, P., Rami-Porta, R., et al. (2007). The IASLC lung cancer staging project: Proposals for the revision of the TNM stage groups in the forthcoming (seventh) edition of the TNM classification of malignant tumors. *Journal of Thoracic Oncology, 2*(8), 706–714.

Greene, F., & Sobin, L. (2008). The staging of cancer: A retrospective and prospective appraisal. *CA: A Cancer Journal for Clinicans, 58*(3), 180–190.

Hayes, D., Monti, S., Parmigiani, G., Gilks, C., Naoki, K., Bhattacharjee, A., et al. (2006). Gene expression profiling reveals reproducible human lung adenocarcinoma subtypes in multiple independent patient cohorts. *Journal of Clinical Oncology, 24*(31), 5079–5090.

Hirsch, R., Matthews, M., Aisner, S., Campobasso, O., Elema, J., Gazdar, A., et al. (1988). Histopathologic classification of small cell lung cancer. Changing concepts and terminology. *Cancer, 62*(5), 973–977.

Jemal, A., Siegel, R., Ward, E., Hao, Y., Xu, J., Murray, T., et al. (2008). Cancer statistics, 2008. *CA: A Cancer Journal for Clinicians, 58*(2), 71–96.

Junker, K., Wiethege, T., & Muller, K. (2000). Pathology of small-cell lung cancer. *Journal of Cancer Research and Clinical Oncology, 126*(7), 361.

Krull, M., Bornstein, M., Saxer, U., Walter, C., & Ramseier, C. (2008). Effects of tobacco use on general health: Relevant information for dentistry (Part 1: Pulmonary diseases and other malignancies). *Schwiz Monatsschr Zahnmed, 118*(5), 405–420.

Midthun, D. (2008). *Overview of the initial evaluation, treatment and prognosis of lung cancer.* Retrieved August 3, 2008, from www.uptodate.com

National Cancer Institute (NCI). (2008a). *A snapshot of lung cancer.* Retrieved July 8, 2008, from http://planning.cancer.gov/disease/Lung-Snapshot.pdf

National Cancer Institute (NCI). (2008b). *A snapshot of lung cancer.* Retrieved July 8, 2008, from http://planning.cancer.gov/disease/Breast-Snapshot.pdf

National Cancer Institute (NCI). (2008c). *SPOREs: Specialized programs of research excellence.* Retrieved August 3, 2008, from http://spores.nci.nih.gov

National Cancer Institute (NCI). (2008d). *Lung cancer prevention (PDQ). Health professional version.* Retrieved July 7, 2008, from http://www.cancer.gov/cancertopics/pdq/prevention/lung/healthprofessional/allpages/print

National Comprehensive Cancer Network (NCCN). (2008). *Non-small cell lung cancer. V.2.2008.* Retrieved July 12, 2008, from http://www.nccn.org/professionals/physician_gls/PDF/nscl.pdf

Omenn, G., Merchant, J., Boatman, E., Dement, J., Kuschner, M., Nicholson, W., et al. (1986). Contribution of environmental fibers to respiratory cancer. *Environmental Health Perspectives, 70*, 51–56.

Reddy, A. (2000, October 22). *Non-small cell lung cancer: Imaging and staging.* Paper presented at the 42nd annual meeting of the American Society for Therapeutic Radiology and Oncology.

Ries, L. A. G., Melbert, D., Krapcho, M., Stinchcomb, D. G., Howlader, N., Horner, M. J., et al. (Eds.). (2007). SEER cancer statistics review, 1975–2005. Bethesda, MD: National Cancer Institute. Based on

November 2007 SEER data submission, published to the SEER Web site 2008. Retrieved July 1, 2008, from http:// seer.cancer.gov/csr/1975_2005/

Rosewich, M., Adler, S., & Zielen, S. (2008). Effects of active and passive smoking on the health of children and adolescents. *Pneumologie, 62*(7), 423–429.

Schottenfield, D. (1996). Epidemiology of lung cancer. In H. Pass, J. Mitchell, D. Johnson, & A. Turrisi (Eds.), *Lung cancer: Principles and practice.* New York: Lippincott-Raven.

Scott, W. (2000). *Lung cancer: A guide to diagnosis and treatment.* Omaha, NE: Atticas Books.

Shinozaki, N., Yuasa, T., & Takata, S. (2008). Cigarette smoking augments sympathetic nerve activity in patients with coronary artery disease. *International Heart Journal, 49*(3), 261–272.

Steinitz, R. (1965). Pulmonary tuberculosis and carcinoma of the lung: A survey from two population-based disease registers. *American Respiratory Diseases, 92*(5), 758–766.

Travis, W., Colby, T., Corrin, B., Shimosato, Y., Brambilla, E., Sobin, L., et al. (1999). *Histological typing of lung and pleural tumors* (3rd ed.). New York: Springer-Verlag.

Chapter 2

Biology of Lung Cancer

Judy R. Prewitt

Introduction

In 2008, it is estimated that there will be 215,020 new cases of lung cancer in the United States (Jemal, et al., 2008). This breaks down to 114,690 new cases of lung cancer in males and 100,330 new cases of lung cancer in females (Jemal, et al., 2008). Unfortunately, the estimated lung cancer deaths for 2008 are 161,840, with 90,810 for males and 71,030 for females. Lung cancer remains the leading cause of all cancer-related deaths in 2008 with a mortality rate of 31% in males and 26% in females (Jemal, et al., 2008). It is interesting to note that mortality rates have decreased for all four major cancer sites—female breast, colon and rectum, prostate, and lung and bronchus—except for female lung cancer, where the rates continued to increase by 0.2% per year from 1995 through 2004. With respect to race and ethnicity, it was reported that from 2000 to 2004, 82/100,000 white males and 54.6/100,000 white females developed lung cancer, while 110.6/100,000 African-American males and 53.7/100,000 African-American females developed lung cancer. Hispanic/Latino males had an incidence of 44.7/100,000, while the Hispanic/Latino females had an incidence of 25.2/100,000. Mortality rates from 2000 to 2004 for white males were 72.6/100,000, with white females being 42.1/100,000. During the same time, African-American males had a mortality rate of 95.8/100,000, and African-American females' mortality rate was 39.8/100,000. Hispanic/Latino males had a mortality rate of 36/100,000, and the Hispanic/Latino female mortality rate was 14.6/100,000 (Jemal, et al., 2008).

It is important for us to examine the biology of lung cancer to explore potential avenues of intervention. With new technology and insight into pathobiology of lung cancer, it is important to examine the potential gene and genome approaches for early detection of lung cancer, as well as potential new therapies. Over the past years, it has become clinically evident that there are numerous clonal genetic and epigenetic alternations that lead to lung cancer development. Early clonal genetic lesions resulting from smoking are being identified, as well as molecular differences between small cell and non-small cell lung cancer. There is also emerging distinction at the cellular level between types of cancer in regards to the clinical outcomes.

Recent molecular developments are leading to increasing knowledge about the development of cancer. With the new technology, such as precise laser capture microdissection, we can now begin to examine the small number of preneoplastic cells in smoking-damaged respiratory epithelium. This same technology is enabling researchers to examine the thousands of genes in individual lung cancers, which has demonstrated congruence between the histological and clinical presentation (Fong, et al., 2003).

It has been accepted for years that smoking is a major cause of lung cancer (Fong, et al., 2003). Recently, it has been demonstrated that genetic damage to the smoking-exposed respiratory epithelium remains decades after smoking cessation. In addition, it is known that about 50% of all lung cancer occurs in former smokers. With this knowledge, it is postulated that genetic damage may occur with smoking but continues to accumulate in bronchial epithelial cells. These cellular changes may continue to eventually develop into an overt lung cancer. These genetic and cellular targets of the carcinogenic process are noted to consist of the hallmarks of cancer (Hanahan & Weinberg, 2000):

- Abnormalities in self-sufficiency of growth signals
- Evading apoptosis
- Insensitivity to antigrowth signals
- Limitless replicative potential
- Sustained angiogenesis
- Tissue invasion and metastases

Given that current therapies have had limited impact upon survival rates for lung cancer, it is imperative that we search for other options. With this new knowledge, lung cancer biology has become an area of intense exploration in an effort to find new and innovative treatments for lung cancer.

Hallmarks of Cancer

Molecular advances have augmented the knowledge of changes acquired by lung cancers. New techniques, such as precision laser capture microdissection, allow for exact testing to localize DNA lesions as well as aberrant gene expression. Additionally, gene microarrays allow the review of thousands of genes compromising lung cancer. The ability to examine DNA alternations has led to the outlining of genetic damage and development of genetic and cellular targets of carcinogenesis. These have been termed the "Hallmarks of Cancer" (Fong, et al., 2003).

Self-Sufficiency of Growth Signals: Proto-Oncogenes and Growth Stimulation by Autocrine and Paracrine Factors

The growth factors and respective receptors are produced by the lung cancer or proximal stromal cells, thus leading to the autocrine and paracrine loops. Autocrine stimulation is directly on the tumor cells and is self-stimulatory. It may secrete a ligand, which acts like a growth factor and increases proliferation or tumor growth. Paracrine stimulation is a result of tumor growth factors that stimulate adjacent cells. The activation of these receptors can lead to stimulation of cell division and survival (Onn, et al., 2007; Fidler, 2008).

Proto-oncogenes are encoded genes that influence cellular proliferation and differentiation. Additionally, mutations in these genes can lead to the development of cancer (Works &

Gallucci, 1996). If a single gene is mutated, every protein molecule encoded by that gene will be altered which can lead to altered cell proliferation and eventual dysplasia (Onn, et al., 2006). Growth factors, growth factor receptors (GFRs), signal transducing proteins, and nuclear regulatory proteins are proto-oncogenes. Damage to these genes can lead to point mutations, chromosomal translocations, and gene amplification. Point mutations are specific areas of alteration in the DNA molecule, such as replacement of cytosine for tyrosine. Chromosomal translocations occur when part of a gene is physically moved to another part of the gene. This new location will influence the genetic behavior. Amplification is duplication of the gene multiple times, often hundreds of times, so that the effect of this genetic material is overexpressed or more evident. With damage to these genes, cellular proliferation can occur, leading to tumorigenesis (Works & Gallucci, 1996; Sekido, Fong, & Minna, 2005).

Tyrosine kinases are important mediators of the signaling cascade, governing processes, such as growth, differentiation, metabolism, and apoptosis, which comprise a group of potentially stimulatory regulators of lung cancer (Paul & Mukhopadhyay, 2004) (see Figure 2–1). The family of epidermal growth factor receptors (EGFR) is noted to be present in approximately 70% of non-small cell lung cancers (NSCLC) (Sekido, et al., 2005). This receptor is noted to be a poor prognostic factor for survival for many cancers, although this is not confirmed for lung cancer. The EGFR family is made of EGFR HER1, HER2, HER3, and HER4. Their activation results in several tumorigenic processes. EGFR also activates the mitogen-activated protein kinase pathway, which eventually mediates cell survival (Onn, et al., 2006) (see Figure 2–2).

HER2 (ERBB2) is a member of the EGFR family and is expressed in more than one-third of NSCLCs, especially noted in adenocarcinoma. The expression of HER2 correlates with a shorter survival in adenocarcinoma and may be a marker for drug resistance (Graziano, et al., 2001; Sekido, et al., 2005). KIT proto-oncogene, another tyrosine kinases receptor, and its ligand are found in many small cell lung cancers (SCLC); however, targeted therapy for these receptors has not demonstrated any objective response (Wistuba, Gazdar, & Minna, 2001; Sekido, et al., 2005).

The RAS gene family, another tyrosine kinases receptor, has been implicated in the development of lung cancer. RAS family (KRAS, HRAS, and NRAS) can be activated by point mutations codons 12, 13, or 61. In this family, mutations of at least one member have been noted approximately 20–30% of the time, especially with adenocarcinomas, but rarely in SCLC. KRAS accounts for 90% of the RAS mutations in adenocarcinoma. About 70% of KRAS mutations are $G \rightarrow T$ transposition with the substitution of the normal glycine with cysteine or valine. The $G \rightarrow T$ transposition also affects the p53 (TP53) gene in lung cancer and is associated with DNA damage seen with smoking. Thus, the detrimental effect of smoking is felt to be evidenced in the lungs by the correlation of smoking tobacco products and the KRAS mutation. The presence of KRAS suggests a poorer prognosis in early- and late-stage NSCLC, although more research is necessary (Sekido, et al., 2005).

The MYC family is a proto-oncogene that activates downstream genes that regulate cellular division. This family of genes includes MYC, MYCN, and MYCL. MYC is frequently activated in both SCLC and NSCLC with MYCN

Figure 2–1 Tyrosine kinase (receptor tyrosine kinase signaling pathway PKC, protein kinase C; EGFR, epidermal growth factor receptor; EGF, epidermal growth factor; TGF, transforming growth factor; RTKI, receptor tyrosine kinase inhibitor; STAT, signal transducers and activators of transcription; PI3K, phosphatidylinositol 3"-kinase; MEK mitogen-activated protein kinase; MAPK, mitogen-activated protein kinase).

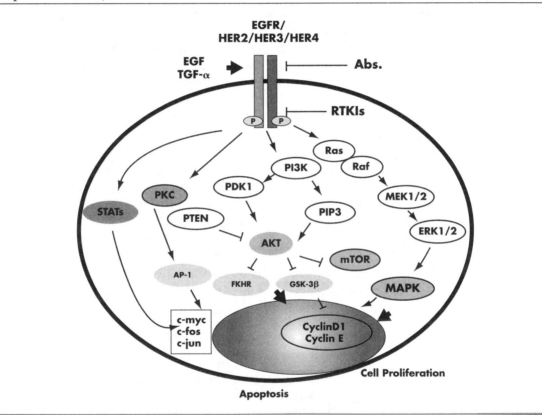

Source: Scagliotti, N., & Hirsch, F. (2004). The biology of epidermal growth factor receptor in lung cancer. *Clinical Cancer Research,* *10*(Suppl. 2), 4227–4332.

and MYCL usually occurring only in SCLC. MYC activation is usually by gene amplification or transcriptional dysregulation with each of these leading to protein overexpression. In SCLC, MYC amplification is associated with decreased survival (Sekido, et al., 2005). In about 36% of SCLC, increased MYC mRNA levels were detected in resected metastatic tumors from people who had a recurrence following chemotherapy, thus suggesting that amplification of MYC is a poor prognostic factor (Onn, et al., 2006).

Figure 2–2 Epidermal growth factor receptor signaling.

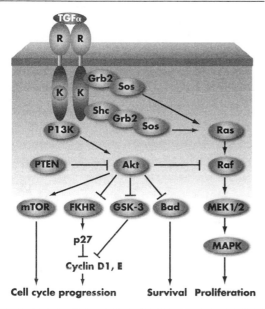

Source: Mendelsohn, J., et al. (2003). *J Clin Oncol* 21, 2787-2799. Accessed May 26, 2008. Copyright © American Society of Clinical Oncology.

The expression of several growth factors has been identified in lung cancer or in the surrounding tissue, leading to a series of autocrine and paracrine growth stimulation for the development of lung cancer (Wistuba, et al., 2001). Gastrin-releasing peptide bombesin (GRP/BN) plays a role in lung development and repair, as well as the promotion of lung cancer (Sekido, et al., 2005). Studies have demonstrated that GRP is expressed in 20–60% of SCLC but less frequently in NSCLC (Sekido, et al., 2005).

A signaling pathway that may be relevant to lung carcinogenesis is the Sonic Hedgehog (SHH). The Sonic Hedgehog pathway mediated epithelial–mesenchymal interactions by effecting or signaling adjacent lung mesenchyme. This pathway is activated in repair of acute airway injury, as well as in a subset of SCLC (Sekido, et al., 2005).

An emerging pathway is the insulin-like growth factor (IGF) signaling system. It is known that this system plays a key role in the growth and development of normal tissues and regulates overall growth of organisms. Within this system there are three ligands: IGF-I, IGF-II, and insulin itself (Ryan & Goss, 2008). These ligands interact with at least four receptors: type I IGF receptor (IGF-IR), the type II IGF receptor (IGF-IIR), insulin receptor (IGR-IR), and hybrid receptors of IGF and insulin. Thus far, increased expression of IGF-I and IGF-II has been discovered in tumor growth. It is increasingly evident that IGFs play a role in promoting tumor growth (Ryan & Goss, 2008). This is a target area for potential cancer treatment (see Table 2–1).

Evading Apoptosis

Apoptosis is programmed cell death, usually due to a physiologic process. Cancer cells have acquired a mechanism to avoid apoptosis. The impact of avoiding apoptosis affects tumor pathogenesis by allowing cancer cells to survive beyond their normal life span; subverting the need for exogenous survival factors, such as tolerance to hypoxia; and allowing time to accumulate genetic alternations. It is noted that avoiding apoptosis is an important complement to proto-oncogene activation because many deregulated oncoproteins that drive cell division also activate apoptosis, such as MYC, E1a, and cyclin D1. There is also a referred benefit to avoid apoptosis in that there is an increased threshold for cell death, leading to chemoresistance and radioresistance (Reed, 2006).

Table 2–1 Major Genetic Aberrations in NSCLC and SCLC

		NSCLC	SCLC
MYC	Amplifications	5–20%	20–35%
RAS	Mutations	15.20%	< 1%
EGFR	Mutations	20%	
INK4a	LOH	70%	50%
P16^{INK4A}	Mutations	20–50%	< 5%
P14^{ARF}	Mutations	20%	65%
p53	LOH	60%	75–100%
	Mutations	50%	75%
RB	LOH	30%	70%
	Mutations	15–30%	90%
FHIT	Mutations	40%	80%
TSG101	Mutations		90%
DMBT1	Mutations	40–50%	100%
LOH in various regions	3p	70–80%	90–100%
	P	10–20%	50%
	4q	30%	80%
	8p	80–100%	80–90%
Promoter hypermethylation			
RASSFIA		30–40%	90–100%
INK4a	p16	25–40%	ND
	p14^{ARF}	8%	ND
RAR		40%	70%
TIMP-3		25%	ND
CDH1		55%	ND
DAPK		19%	ND
GSTP1		1%	ND
MGMT		20–40%	ND

NSCLC, non-small cell lung cancer; SCLC, small cell lung cancer; LOH, loss of heterozygosity; DMBT1, deleted in malignant brain tumor; ND, not determined; TIMP-3, tissue inhibitors of metalloproteinase-3; CDH1, E-cadherin; DAPK, death-associated protein kinase; GSTP1, glutathione S.

Source: Modified from Meuwissen, R., & Berns, A., 2005. Mouse models for human lung career. *Genes & Development*, 643–664.

In lung cancer, there are many molecules in the apoptotic pathway that are abnormal, with the most prominent alternation being p53. BLC2 is an antiapoptotic gene that is overexpressed in SCLC (75–95%) and in NSCLC (25–35% in squamous cells carcinoma and 10% in adenocarcinoma) (Sekido, et al., 2005). Another potential pathway to avoid apoptosis is through β1 integrin-stimulated tyrosine kinase activation. Also, Fas (CD95) and its ligand (FasL) are implicated in avoiding apoptosis (Sekido, et al., 2005).

Insensitivity to Antigrowth Signals: Tumor Suppressor Genes (TSGs)

Tumor suppressor genes (TSGs) exert a negative effect on regulation. TSGs are genes that regulate normal cellular growth. Their expression leads to normal cellular regulation. The inactivation of these leads to loss of function, which contributes to the development of a malignancy. The loss of function may be manifested by the inability to receive signals or the inability to accurately process the signals that are received (Onn, et al., 2006; Sekido, et al., 2005).

The TSG p53 maintains the integrity of the gene when presented with cellular stress from DNA damage, such as from gamma or ultraviolet irradiation and carcinogens (Wistuba, et al., 2001; Sekido, et al., 2005). The p53 gene acts as a transcription factor to regulate downstream genes, including cell-cycle checkpoints (i.e., P21), apoptosis (BAX), DNA repair (GADD45), and angiogenesis (thrombospondin) (Sekido, et al., 2005). Loss of p53 functions leads to mutations and deletions that result in continuance of replication of genetically damaged cells and accumulation of multiple mutations and subse-

quent development of cancer (Wistuba, et al., 2001). The p53 gene, located at chromosome 17p13, is the most frequently mutated TSG in human malignancies. Mutations of p53 affect about 90% of NSCLC, with occurrence of 51% in squamous cell, 54% in large cell carcinomas, and 39% in adenocarcinomas. In SCLC the occurrence of p53 is 50% (Sekido, et al., 2005). Mutations of p53 are correlated with tobacco smoke carcinogens (Wistuba, et al., 2001). About 15% of lung cancers develop antibodies to the TP53 protein. This suggests that mutant TP53 protein overexpression can lead to a humoral immune response. Currently there is ongoing research targeting p53, such as introducing a wild-type p53 gene using retroviral or adenoviral vectors (Sekido, et al., 2005).

Other components of the p53 pathway may also contribute to the development of lung cancer. Upstream regulators of p53 are the HDM2 oncogene product and p14ARF TSG product. Overexpression of HDM2 is found in lung cancer and impacts the function of p53. The p14ARF TSG controls cell growth by interfering with HDM2 inhibition of p53. Both HDM2 overexpression and p14ARF inactivation may be restricted events to human lung cancers (Sekido, et al., 2005).

The p16-cyclin D1-CDK4 retinoblastoma (RB) pathway is a key cell cycle regulator at the G_1/S phase, and many cancers demonstrate this mutation (Wistuba, et al., 2001; Minna, 1993). The p16INK4A gene is an inhibitor of CDK4 or CDK7. The normal role of p16INK4A is to maintain a cycle by keeping RB unphosphorylated. Thus, if mutation of p16INK4A occurs, the cycle cannot be restrained. Often p16INK4A is abnormal in human malignancy (Sekido, et al., 2005). In NSCLC, p16INK4A is mutated in about 14% of primary tumors; however, there can be other activity, such as homozygous deletions of aberrant promoter methylation, that lead to downregulation of p16INK4A. Given this interaction, p16INK4A is absent in about 40% of NSCLC and is the most common component of the p16INK4A-cyclin D1-CDK4-RB pathway inactivation in NSCLC. There is also an interaction between p16INK4A and p14ARF through altered reading of the same DNA locus. These changes may also impact upon the p53 pathway through p14ARF by means of the ability of p14ARF to stabilize p53. Thus, the p16 INK4A/p14ARF site can affect the RB and p53 TSG pathways (Sekido, et al., 2005).

Cyclin D1 is overexpressed in 12–47% of NSCLCs. It has been noted that overexpression of cyclin D1 is associated with a poor prognosis. Overexpression of cyclin D1 or CDK4 can disrupt the p16INK4A-cyclin D1-CDK4-RB pathway (Sekido, et al., 2005). Cyclin D1 is a protein that is required for cell cycle progression from $G_1 \rightarrow$ S phase (Scagliotti, Selvaggi, Novello, & Hirsch, 2004).

The function of the RB gene, located on chromosomal region 13q14, is to block the progression from G_1 to S. RB mutations are noted in 90% of SCLC and 15–30% of primary NSCLC. In NSCLC, cyclin D1, CDK4, and p16 abnormalities are common, but they are rare in SCLC. The infrequency of RB alternations is expected as the p16INK4A-cyclin D1-CDK4-RB pathway is already altered due to other components in NSCLC (Sekido, et al., 2005). An interesting note is that a person with retinoblastoma, or his or her relative who carries the RB in the germ line, has an excess risk of developing SCLC if he or she survives to adulthood. Other RB-related genes that have been implicated in the development of lung cancer are p107 and RB1/p130 (Sekido, et al., 2005).

Chromosome 10 (PTEN), located at 10q23, helps regulate cell cycle division. The PTEN enzyme communicates to stop dividing and initiates cells to undergo programmed cell death or apoptosis. PTEN mutations were identified in only 10–25% of NSCLC. Given this, it is postulated that PTEN may play a limited role in lung cancer. Other potential targets are TSLC1, which is located at 11q23, and MYO18B at 22q12 (Sekido, et al., 2005).

The frequent loss of alleles has been identified on chromosomes in lung cancer. This chromosome-acquired loss of heterozygosity (LOH) is a traditional feature of TSG inactivation that suggests loss at multiple chromosome regions. One area of particular study is chromosome 3p. Chromosome 3p has been shown to have multiple areas of allele loss, including 3p25-26, 3p21.3-22, 3p14, and 3p12. Allele loss on 3p has been demonstrated to be lost in more than 90% of SCLC and 80% of NSCLC, which strongly suggests one or more TSGs on this chromosome (Wistuba, et al., 2001; Sekido, et al., 2005). This location is noted as a frequent and early event in the development of lung cancer. Thus far, 3p is the earliest genetic change found in lung cancer development, with noted occurrence in patches of normal epithelium accompanying lung cancer as well as in the morphologically normal tissue in smokers (Sekido, et al., 2005).

Several distinct 3p regions have been identified as potential areas in the development or promotion of lung cancer. One area identified, 3p21.3, has been noted to have multiple TSGs located in one small region. These TSGs for potential study are: RASSF1A, FUS1, SEMA3B, and BLU. It has been demonstrated that RASSF1A is one TSG that has been inactivated in 90% of SCLC and 40–50% of NSCLC (Sekido, et al., 2005).

The fragile histidine triad (FHIT) gene maps to 3p14.2 region. FHIT is a protein that is absent in many lung cancers, especially squamous cell (87%) and adenocarcinoma (57%). FHIT gene is active in regulating cell activity, including DNA activity. Loss of the FHIT protein is strongly associated with smoking (Sekido, et al., 2005). It is postulated that FHIT is active in the apoptosis pathway and cell-cycle control (Sekido, et al., 2005; Onn, et al., 2006). Another TSG, located at 3p12-13, is the *DUTT1/ ROBO1* gene. This is a point of research as in mice models; it demonstrated inadequate lung development and bronchial hyperplasia (Sekido, et al., 2005).

Evidence supports the retinoic acid receptor beta (RAB-β) mapped at 3p24 as being important in the resistance of lung cancer cells to retinoids and being a candidate for 3p TSG. Loss of RAB-β is noted in about 50% of lung cancers and is postulated to be the reason that prevention trials using retinoids failed (Winterhalder, Hirsch, Kotantoulas, Franklin, & Bunn, 2004; Sekido, et al., 2005).

To date, using genomics and biological pathways remains investigational in lung cancers. However, novel applications are being trialed. Currently, DNA microarray is being used to examine specific genetic profiles with the goal to determine the impact of certain chemotherapy upon the cancer (Potti, et al., 2006). With this knowledge, researchers are hoping to identify the best drug to treat an individual's cancer (Hsu, et al., 2008).

Limitless Replicative Potential: Telomerase

While the genetics of lung cancer are being defined, other areas also are important in consid-ering the development and progression of lung cancer. Telomerase activity is believed to play a critical role in lung cancer. Telomerase is a ribonucleocomplex that is critical for cellular mortality. With abnormal expression, telomerase leads to the immortality of the cancer cells. Recently, it has been demonstrated that telomere maintenance and cellular response to telomere dysfunction is critical to the genomic instability, organ homeostasis, chronic disease, aging, and tumorigenesis. Through this work, it has provided insight into how advancing age can lead to epithelial cancers, as well as how chronic inflammation and degeneration may lead to an increased cancer risk (Wong & Depinho, 2005). In human cells, a loss of RB or p53 pathway functions can trigger progressive telomere erosion leading to loss of "capping" function. This capping feature loss can result in increased chromosomal instability, leading to progressive loss of cell viability and proliferation capacity in the cell population resulting in "cellular crisis" or mortality (Wong and Depinho, 2005).

Additionally, it has been demonstrated that high levels of telomerase activity are present in 100% of SCLC and 80–85% of NSCLC (Sekido, et al., 2005). Increased telomerase activity is associated with increased cellular proliferation and advanced stage NSCLC. It has been demonstrated that human telomerase reverse transcriptase (hTERT) messenger RNA, an expression of telomerase, is indicative of poor survival in patients with stage 1 NSCLC (Sekido, et al., 2005).

Sustained Angiogenesis

Angiogenesis continues to be an active area of research. Tumor angiogenesis is necessary for cancer cells to continue to grow beyond a few millimeters in size and provides regulation of inducers and inhibitors released by the tumor cells and host cells. Vascular endothelial growth factor (VEGF), basic fibroblast growth factor, and angiogenic CXC chemokines, such as interleukin-8, are areas associated with the induction of lung cancer. Presently, clinical trials for anti-VEGF monoclonal antibody with chemotherapy are ongoing (Liao, Wang, Zhenqiong, Feng, & Zhu, 2001; Sekido, et al., 2005; Onn, et al., 2006).

Tissue Invasion and Metastases

Another area of exploration in the development and progression of lung cancer is cell adhesion. Cellular adhesion is the ability of the cells to adhere to each other. Tumor cells have been demonstrated to downregulate E-cadherin, thus increasing their ability to break off from the primary tumor and metastasize (Gribbon & Loescher, 2000; Sekido, et al., 2005). E-cadherin expression is associated with tumor dedifferentiation, increased lymph node involvement, and poor survival in patients with NSCLC. Decreased expression of α_3 is associated with a poorer prognosis in adenocarcinoma. Matrix metalloproteinases (MMP) are active in stromal degradation, which is felt to be a factor with metastasis. Gelatinase A expression, an MMP, has been noted in about 50% of SCLC and 65% of NSCLC. Additional stromelysin 3 overexpression has been detected in stromal elements of NSCLC (Sekido, et al., 2005). This remains an active area for clinical research.

Genetic Predisposition

The majority of lung cancers arise from smoking and tobacco smoke, which contains many substances, including carcinogens, cocarcinogens, and tumor promoters. Ten carcinogens that have led to lung cancer promotion have

been identified in animal models. However, it is known that not all people who smoke develop lung cancer; in fact, only about 11% of those who use tobacco products develop lung cancer. This suggests that there are genetic factors that may influence the risk of lung cancer among those who smoke. It is suspected that the genetic factors modify the risk. The genetic areas that have received the most scrutiny thus far have been P450 genes CYP1A1, CYP2Dy, and CYP3E1, as well as the enzyme glutathione S-transferase (GSTM1) (Fong, et al., 2003; Sekido, et al., 2005).

Cellular Characteristics

Evidence supports the development of lung cancer from a pluripotent stem cell with the ability to differentiate into different histological subtypes. In normal differentiation, the stem cell will develop into the cells found in the tracheobronchial tree, including pseudostratified reserved cells, ciliated goblet columnar cells, neuroendocrine cells, and type I and II pneumocytes, which line the alveoli. Lung cancer arises from the epithelium of the respiratory tract. It is accepted that a series of morphological changes occur before lung cancer can be recognized (Ingle, 2000; Andreeff, Goodrich, & Koeffler, 2006).

As in most cancers, there are a series of morphological changes, hyperplasia, metaplasia, dysplasia, and carcinoma in situ. These are felt to represent the preneoplastic or precancerous changes. Lung cancer is thought to arise like other epithelial malignancies, although it is not clearly understood. It is postulated that metaplastic changes occur in bronchial mucosal cells due to chronic exposure and repeated injury by inhaled agents, along with compensatory inflammatory process (Onn, et al., 2006). The process progresses as mucosal basal cells proliferate and generate mucus-secreting goblet cells. The normal columnal epithelium is replaced with stratified squamous epithelium. As this process continues, neoplasia is noted as cellular atypia, and mitotic activity leads to mucosal dysplasia. Eventually, this process continues until there is invasion of malignant cells into the underlying stroma, showing the first signs of invasive cancer. This process can take from 5 to 20 years (Onn, et al., 2006).

Small Cell Lung Cancer

SCLC accounts for 10–15% of all lung cancers (Onn, et al., 2006). SCLC can be further stratified to an occurrence of lung cancer in men between 10% and 20% and in women between 10% and 30%. The major risk factor is tobacco exposure, with up to 90% of those with SCLC having tobacco exposure. It is noted that the incidence of SCLC has paralleled the use of cigarette smoking with a 20- to 50-year lag (Murren, Turrisi, & Pass, 2005).

SCLC typically arises from the large central airways, usually presenting in the main stem or lobular bronchi. Histologically, SCLC is usually arranged in clusters, sheets, or trabecular separated by fibrovascular stroma. They have small cells with scanty cytoplasm and are round or oval, occasionally lymphocyte-like, although about twice the size of a lymphocyte (Kobzik, 1999; Fretz & Hughes, 2001; Murren, et al., 2005). Frequently, necrosis and areas of hemorrhage are seen (Ingle, 2000). The nuclei are often in the shape of the cell and may show dense homogenous chromatin. The nucleoli may be difficult to identify. Due to the fact that the cells are fragile, "crush artifact" may be identified (Fretz & Hughes, 2001; Murren, et al., 2005).

SCLC is an aggressive cancer that frequently metastasizes early to hilar, mediastinal, and distant sites (Thomas, Williams, Cobos, & Turrisi, 2001). The goal of staging of SCLC is to establish the prognosis, to identify those with disease limited to the chest that would benefit from combined modality therapy, and to assess risk of mortality from aggressive chemotherapy. Given that surgery plays a minor role in SCLC, a two-stage system was developed by the Veterans Administration Lung Study Group (VALSG). This two-stage system uses limited stage to define disease confined to one hemithorax that can be encompassed in a reasonable radiation field. These people are candidates for combined modality therapy. All other people are considered to have extensive stage disease. At presentation, about 60–70% of people have extensive stage SCLC, and 30–40% present with limited-stage disease (Murren, et al., 2005).

SCLC is subdivided into pure small cell, mixed small cell/large cell carcinoma, and a combination small cell carcinoma. The mixed small cell/large cell SCLC is distinguished by the presence of prominent, frequent nucleoli and a coarse nuclear chromatin pattern. In the mixed small cell/large cell, this typically coexists with squamous carcinoma, although other types, such as adenocarcinoma, may be present (Murren, et al., 2005).

The frequency of mixed small cell/large cell SCLC is between 3% and 6%, and for combined SCLC, the frequency is between 1% and 3%. However, it is unclear at this time if these histological differences have a different prognosis or response rate to treatment (Murren, et al., 2005).

While the diagnosis of SCLC is dependent primarily on morphologic assessment, immunocytochemistry plays a vital role, and electron microscopy is useful in difficult cases. SCLC is immunoreactive for keratin and epithelial membrane antigen. If the tumor does not stain for these, other diagnoses must be considered (Murren, et al., 2005).

About 75% of SCLC are associated with paraneoplastic syndromes. SCLC is the most common type of cancer to result in a clinical hormone syndrome (Fretz & Hughes, 2001; Murren, et al., 2005). Paraneoplastic syndromes that may occur are: ectopic adrenocorticotropic hormone (ACTH) production causing symptoms of Cushing syndrome; syndrome of inappropriate antidiuretic hormone (SIADH), Eaton-Lambert syndrome, also known as myasthenia syndrome (Kobzik, 1999). Additionally, SCLC is commonly associated with superior vena cava syndrome (Murren, et al., 2005).

Non-Small Cell Lung Cancer

The majority of NSCLC are a result of tobacco exposure, with about 80% of lung cancer deaths attributable to tobacco use. In addition to tobacco abuse, there are environmental and occupational risk factors. The most prevalent exposures are asbestos and silica fibers; organic compounds, such as chloromethyl ether and polycyclic aromatic hydrocarbons (PAHs); diesel fumes and air pollution; metals, such as chromium and nickel; arsenic; and ionizing radiation (Schrump, et al., 2005).

NSCLC refers to a group of pulmonary neoplasms that are often associated with tobacco abuse and share common propriety of not being responsive to the treatments of SCLC. The majority of NSCLC are histologically heterogeneous, which impacts the diagnosis. This can

lead to disparity of diagnosis, thus most diagnoses are with resected specimens rather than a bronchial sample. Lung cancers are generally classified by the best differentiated region in the specimen and graded by the most poorly differentiated component (Onn, et al., 2006; Schrump, et al., 2005).

Squamous Cell Lung Cancer

At one time, squamous cell carcinoma was the most prevalent type of lung cancer. In the past 30 years, there has been a decline in its incidence with an increase in the incidence of adenocarcinoma. It is postulated that this is related to the increased use of filtered cigarettes, leading to deeper inhalation with deposits of the carcinogens accumulating in the peripheral airways of the lung, where adenocarcinomas arise (Ginsberg, Vokes, & Rosenweig, 2001; Thomas, et al., 2001; Schrump, et al., 2005).

Squamous cell carcinomas compose about one-third of all lung cancers. They usually originate in the large, more central bronchi and are associated with squamous metaplasia. Central cavitation from necrosis is a common finding from pathologic review, as well as radiograph evidence. The well-differentiated squamous cell cancers tend to grow slowly with less chance of metastasis than the poorly differentiated type. With continued progression, changes progress leading to a mild, moderate, and severe dysplasia with eventual carcinoma in situ. When the carcinoma in situ penetrates the basement membrane and involves the lamina propria, it is invasive and demonstrates the ability to metastasize (Brashers & Davey, 1998; Fretz & Hughes, 2001; Onn, et al., 2006).

This malignancy may be tested with cytologic examination early on due to the fact that these cells exfoliate or shed (Ginsberg, et al.,

2001). As the tumor grows, it can invade into the bronchial lumen, producing obstruction, atelectasis, or pneumonia (Ginsberg, et al., 2001; Schrump, et al., 2005). These tumors can necrose and cavitate in approximately 10% of cases (Thomas, et al., 2001; Fretz & Hughes, 2001).

Histologically, these cells are composed of sheets of epithelial cells ranging from well differentiated to poorly differentiated. The nuclei tend to be irregular with coarsely clumped chromatin. Three histological features are key to the diagnosis: keratin formation, seen as increased eosinophilia of cells; keratin pearl formation, which is laminated whorls of eosinophilic cells; and intercellular bridges, which are fine paralleled lines between cells (Fretz & Hughes, 2001). These tumors tend to be slow growing with progression from an in situ to an invasive cancer taking between 3 and 4 years (Strauss, 1998; Ginsberg, et al., 2001; Thomas, et al., 2001).

Adenocarcinoma

Adenocarcinoma is currently the most common lung cancer, accounting for about 45% of all lung cancers (Onn, et al., 2006). This subtype is the most common cause of lung cancer in women and nonsmokers and is most commonly associated with lung scarring related to other causes (Valanis, 1996; Fretz & Hughes, 2001). Most tumors are shown in the periphery of the lung radiographically but are located in the smaller airways histologically (Schrump, et al., 2005). Due to the peripheral location, they are associated with less pulmonary symptoms than other more centrally located cancers. These cancers are also less likely to be discovered through sputum cytology or other types of cytology (Schrump, et al., 2005). Adenocarcinomas may arise as solitary pulmonary lesions; however, they may be multicentric (Strauss, 1998). Adenocarcinomas grow more slowly than squamous cell carcinomas (Kobzik, 1999). However, they invade lymphatic and blood vessels relatively early and for this reason have a higher rate of distant metastasis than squamous cell carcinoma with an associated poorer survival rate (Strauss, 1998).

Histologically, these tumors form glands and produce mucin. Well-differentiated tumors are characterized by acinar formation with poorly differentiated adenocarcinomas appearing as solid sheets of tumor cells that may exhibit a tendency to form small acini and less prominent glandular differentiation. Immunohistochemistry and electron microscopy have been used with increasing frequency by pathologists. Adenocarcinomas stain positive for carcinoembryonic antigen and mucin (Strauss, 1998; Ginsberg, et al., 2001; Thomas, et al., 2001; Onn, et al., 2006).

Bronchoalveolar Carcinoma

Bronchoalveolar carcinoma (BAC) is a rare subtype of adenocarcinoma that represents about 2% of all lung cancer. There are two variants: mucinous and nonmucinous. The mucinous type is noted by the growth of malignant mucus-containing goblet cells on the surface of alveolar walls. This variant tends to be multifocal and fatal. The nonmucinous BAC is composed of type II pneumocytes showing nuclear anaplasia and pleomorphism. The malignant cells grow over the alveolar walls in a monolayer, eventually inhibiting gas exchange in the affected alveolar sac leading to right-to-left intrapulmonary shunt (Schrump, et al., 2005). Nonmucinous BAC is more likely to be a solitary tumor. People with a solitary nonmucinous BAC that is well differentiated have a much better prognosis than those with the other forms (Onn, et al., 2006).

Large Cell Carcinoma

Large cell carcinoma represents about 9–15% of all lung cancers. These tumors are less well differentiated than adenocarcinoma or squamous cell carcinoma and do not express glandular or squamous differentiation on light microscopy (Thomas, et al., 2001). With the advent of immunohistochemical staining, electron microscopy, and monoclonal antibodies, tumors previously diagnosed as undifferentiated large cell carcinoma are now being classified as poorly differentiated adenocarcinoma or squamous cell carcinoma (Ginsberg, et al., 2001). The World Health Organization has delineated five variants of large cell carcinoma. Of these variants, the large cell neuroendocrine carcinoma and basaloid carcinoma have the most dismal prognosis (Brambilla, Travis, Colby, Corrin, & Shimosato, 2001).

Large cell carcinoma tends to develop in the periphery of the lung, invading subsegmental bronchi or larger airways (Thomas, et al., 2001). Central necrosis is common, although cavitation is rare (Fretz & Hughes, 2001). Large cell carcinomas are made of large cells without cytoplasmic differentiation. The prognosis of large cell undifferentiated carcinoma is similar to that of adenocarcinoma. When the tumor demonstrates necrosis and high mitotic rate, they are noted to have a poorer prognosis (Schrump, et al., 2005).

Conclusion

The search for molecular and biological targets for NSCLC and SCLC continues as a goal to assist in the determination of outcomes and assessing the need for adjuvant chemotherapy (Bunn, Soriano, Johnson, & Heasley, 2000). The exploration of the biology of lung cancer is an exciting and evolving area of study; more research is necessary to completely understand the issues that influence the development, progression, and treatment of lung cancer. As the frontier of genetic alterations and molecular complexity is defined, it is hoped that new areas for prevention, detection, and treatment will evolve.

References

Andreeff, M., Goodrich, D., & Koeffler, H. (2006). Cancer of the lung. In D. Kufe, R. Bast, W. Hail, W. Hong, R. Pollack, R. Weichselbaum, et al. (Eds.), *Holland-Frei cancer 7 medicine* (7th ed., pp. 27–40). Hamilton, Ontario: B.C. Decker.

Brambilla, E., Travis, W., Colby, T., Corrin, B., & Shimosato, Y. (2001). The new World Health Organization classification of lung tumours. *European Respiratory Journal, 18*(6), 1059–1068.

Brashers, V., & Davey, S. (1998). Alternations in pulmonary function. In K. McCance & S. Huether (Eds.), *Pathophysiology: The biological basis for disease in adults and children* (3rd ed., pp. 1158–1200). Baltimore: Mosby.

Bunn, P., Soriano, A., Johnson, G., & Heasley, L. (2000). New therapeutic strategies for lung cancer: Biology and molecular biology come of age. *Chest, 117*(4) (Suppl. 1), 163–168.

Fidler, I. (2008). University of Texas, MD Anderson Cancer Center, Department of Cancer Biology. *Overview by the chairman*. Retrieved on May 24, 2008, from http://www.mdanderson.org/departments/cancerbiology/

Fong, K., Sekido, Y., Gazdar, A., & Minna, J. (2003). Lung cancer. 9: Molecular biology of lung cancer: Clinical implications. *Thorax, 58*(10), 892–900.

Fretz, P., & Hughes, J. (2001). In J. Galvin & M. Petterson. University of Iowa: Health Care. *Lung tumors: A multidisciplinary database: Pathologic types*. Retrieved on May

24, 2008, from http://www.vh.org/Providers/ Texbooks LungTumors/TitlePage.htm

Ginsberg, R., Vokes, E., & Rosenweig, K. (2001). Non-small cell lung cancer in cancer. In V. DeVita, S. Hellman, & S. Rosenberg (Eds.), *Cancer: Principles and practice of oncology* (6th ed., pp. 925–983). Philadelphia: Lippincott Williams & Wilkins.

Graziano, S., Tatum, A., Herndon, J., Box, J., Memoli, V., Green, M., et al. (2001). Use of neuroendocrine markers, p53, and HER2 to predict response to chemotherapy in patients with stage III non-small cell lung cancer: A Cancer and Leukemia Group B study. *Lung Cancer, 33*, 115–123.

Gribbon, J., & Loescher, L. (2000). Biology of cancer. In C. Yarbro, M. Frogge, M. Goodman, & S. Groenwald, *Cancer nursing: Principles and practice* (5th ed., pp. 17–34). Sudbury, MA: Jones and Bartlett.

Hanahan, D., & Weinberg, R. (2000). The hallmarks of cancer. *Cell, 100*(1), 57–70.

Hsu, S. D., Acharya, C. R., Riedel, R. F., Redman, R. C., Garman, K. S., Dressman, H. K., et al. (2008, June 1). *Use of co-activation of lung cancer specific developmental pathway genes, TTF-1, NKX2-8 and PAX9, to predict prognosis and guide therapeutic strategies.* Oral session presented at the 44th Annual Meeting of the American Society of Clinical Oncology, Chicago, IL.

Ingle, R. (2000). Lung cancers. In C. Yarbro, M. Frogge, M. Goodman, & S. Groenwald, *Cancer nursing: Principles and practice* (5th ed., pp. 1298–1328). Sudbury, MA: Jones and Bartlett.

Jemal, A., Siegel, R., Ward, E., Hao, Y., Xu, J., Murray, T., et al. (2008). Cancer statistics, 2008. *CA: A Cancer Journal for Clinicians, 58*(2), 71–96.

Kobzik, L. (1999). The lung. In R. Cotran, V. Kumar, & T. Collins (Eds.), *Pathologic basis of disease* (6th ed., pp. 697–755). Philadelphia: W.B. Saunders.

Liao, M., Wang, H., Zhenqiong, L., Feng, F., & Zhu, D. (2001). Vascular endothelial growth factor and other biological predictors related to the postoperative survival rate on non-small lung cancer. *Lung Cancer, 33*, 125–132.

Minna, J. (1993). The molecular biology of lung cancer pathogenesis. *Chest, 103*(4), 4494–4502.

Murren, J., Turrisi, A., & Pass, H. (2005). Small cell lung cancer. In V. DeVita, S. Hellman, & S. Rosenberg (Eds.), *Cancer: Principles and practice of oncology* (7th ed., pp. 810–843). Philadelphia: Lippincott Williams & Wilkins.

Onn, A., Vaporciyan, A., Chang, J., Komaki, R., Roth, J., & Herbst, R. (2006). Cancer of the lung. In D. Kufe, R. Bast, W. Hail, W. Hong, R. Pollack, R. Weichselbaum, et al. (Eds.), *Holland-Frei cancer 7 medicine* (7th ed., pp. 1179–1224). Hamilton, Ontario: B.C. Decker.

Paul, M., & Mukhopadhyay, A. (2004). Tryosine kinase-role and significance in cancer. *International Journal of Medical Science, 1*(2), 101–115.

Potti, A., Dressman, H. K., Bild, A., Riedel, R. F., Chan, G., Sayer, R., et al. (2006). Genomic signatures to guide the use of chemotherapeutics. *Nature Medicine, 12*(11), 1294–1300.

Reed, J. (2006). Cancer of the lung. In D. Kufe, R. Bast, W. Hail, W. Hong, R. Pollack, R. Weichselbaum, et al. (Eds.), *Holland-Frei cancer 7 medicine* (7th ed., pp. 41–52). Hamilton, Ontario: B.C. Decker.

Ryan, P., & Goss, P. (2008). The emerging role of the insulin-like growth factor pathway as a therapeutic target in cancer. *The Oncologist, 13*(1), 16–24.

Scagliotti, G., Selvaggi, G., Novello, S., & Hirsch, F. (2004). The biology of epidermal growth factor receptor in lung cancer. *Clinical Cancer Research, 10*(12 Pt 2), 4227–4232.

Schrump, D., Altorki, N., Henschke, C., Carter, D., Turrisi, A., & Gutierrez, M. (2005). Non-small cell lung cancer. In V. DeVita, S. Hellman, & S. Rosenberg (Eds.), *Cancer: Principles and practice of oncology* (7th ed., pp. 753–810). Philadelphia: Lippincott Williams & Wilkins.

Sekido, Y., Fong, K., & Minna, J. (2005). Cancer of the lung. In V. DeVita, S. Hellman, & S. Rosenberg (Eds.), *Cancer: Principles and practice of oncology* (7th ed., pp. 745–752). Philadelphia: Lippincott Williams & Wilkins.

Strauss, G. (1998). Neoplastic disease. In G. Baum, J. Crapo, B. Celli, & J. Karlinsky (Eds.), *Textbook of pulmonary disease* (6th ed., pp. 1329–1382). Philadelphia: Lippincott-Raven.

Thomas, C., Williams, T., Cobos, E., & Turrisi, A. (2001). Lung cancer. In R. Lenhard, R. Osteen, & T. Gansler (Eds.), *American Cancer Society's clinical oncology* (3rd ed., pp. 269–298). Philadelphia: American Cancer Society.

Valanis, B. (1996). Epidemiology of lung cancer: A worldwide epidemic. *Seminars in Oncology Nursing, 12*(4), 251–259.

Winterhalder, R., Hirsch, F., Kotantoulas, G., Franklin, W., & Bunn, P. (2004). Chemoprevention of lung cancer: From biology to clinical reality. *European Society for Medical Oncology, 15*(2), 185–196.

Wistuba, I., Gazdar, A., & Minna, J. (2001). Molecular genetics of small cell lung carcinoma. *Seminars in Oncology, 28*(2)(Suppl. 4), 3–13.

Wong, K., & Depinho, R. (2005). Telomerase. In V. DeVita, S. Hellman, & S. Rosenberg (Eds.), *Cancer: Principles and practice of oncology* (7th ed., pp. 105–112). Philadelphia: Lippincott Williams & Wilkins.

Works, C., & Gallucci, B. (1996). Biology of lung cancer. *Seminars in Oncology Nursing, 12*(4), 276–284.

Chapter 3

Controversies in Detection and Screening

Marilyn L. Haas

Introduction

Lung cancer, the number-one killer of males and females, has no definitive guidelines established for detection and screening (American Cancer Society, 2008; NCI, 2007). Therefore, researchers still continue to search for better technology for earlier diagnosis and treatment. However, it is the continued responsibility of healthcare providers to watch for potential warning signs in high-risk patients and follow up with appropriate diagnostic tests.

This chapter discusses the issues surrounding early detection, screening, and several diagnostic tests. The discussion will explain the pros and cons of screening and its impact on detecting lung cancer. Although one can find the specific steps of any of these diagnostic tests in procedure textbooks, the focus of this section is on the practicality, sensitivity, and specificity of the diagnostic tests that are discussed.

Early Detection/Patient Screening

Based on the high lung cancer incidence and mortality rates cited in preceding chapters and the facts associating current and former tobacco users with lung cancer, there has been a persistent, ongoing debate concerning the need for and the usefulness of screening for lung cancer (NCI, 2007; Alberg & Samet, 2003; Ettinger, 2001; Lee, et al., 2001; Reddy, 2000). To date, prospective studies of lung cancer screening have not demonstrated persuasively that screening for lung cancer with chest radiography alone or in combination with sputum cytology or other diagnostic tests saves lives. Currently, there are no official recommendations for screening for lung cancer, even in high-risk populations. There is agreement to enroll high-risk individuals into clinical trials (NCCN, 2008a). To date, there are six clinical trials listed on the National Cancer Institute's Web site that are designed to help determine the issue of lung cancer screening (NCI, 2008a). Generally speaking, it is certainly interesting that lung cancer has no published recommendation/guidelines when other common cancers have screening tests and recommendations.

As practitioners have become aware of the alarming facts and numerous research screening studies (Henschke, et al., 2006; Bach, et al., 2007), staging has become very important in detecting lung cancer and determining treatment.

Table 3–1 Randomized Controlled Trials of Chest X-Rays

Study Site	Sample Size	Study Arms	Number of Lung Cancers Found During Study	Characteristics of Lung Cancers Found During Study		Deaths from Lung Cancer Over period of follow-Up	
				Early-Stage	Late-Stage	No. of Deaths	Lung Cancer Mortality Rate (Per 1000 Person-Years)
London	29,723	CXR every 6 mos. for 3 yrs.	132	44	57	62	NR
	25,311	Single CXR at end of 3 yrs.	97	22	54	59	NR
Mayo	4618	CXR, and sputum cytology every 4 mos. for 6 yrs.	206	99	107	122	3.2
	4593	Advised to have CXR and sputum cytology annually	160	51	109	115	3.0
Czechoslovakia	3172	CXR annually	39	20	19	247	NR
	3174	CXR and sputum cytology at end of 3 yrs.	27	10	17	216	NR

Abbreviations: CXR, chest radiography; NR, not reported.
Source: Bach, 2008.

Current technologies that aid in detecting early-stage lung cancer are presented and evaluated here. Although the decisions to order and utilize certain diagnostic studies are still in the realm of the physician or midlevel practitioners, it is imperative that every healthcare professional understands the specificity and sensitivity of each test and the advantages and disadvantages to each diagnostic test. This knowledge will enable healthcare providers to discuss the procedures and results with the patient. Healthcare professionals can direct interested individuals to a professionally managed Web site—National Cancer Institute, http://nci.nih.gov/cancertopics/types/lung—that provides details on lung cancer preventions, screening, clinical trials, and research. This site might aid in patients' understanding and in subsequent discussions with healthcare providers. The following is a discussion of the diagnostic tests used to assist in the detection of lung cancer.

Diagnostic Test: Chest X-Ray

The primary advantages of chest X-rays are related to the low cost and availability. Chest X-rays are obtained for various reasons, whether part of annual history and physicals, preoperative workups, or for following other comorbidity diseases. Films can be utilized as baselines and for comparisons. Randomized studies between 1950 and the 1980s demonstrated that chest X-rays were beneficial in detecting early-stage cancers (see Table 3–1).

While chest radiography is probably one of the most valuable tools in the diagnosis of lung cancer, the sensitivity of chest X-rays for lung cancer detection is dependent on the size and lo-

cation of the lesion, quality assurance factors related to image quality, and the skill of the interpreting physician (Ginsberg, Vokes, & Rosenzweig, 2001). Failure to detect lesions at a favorable size, or even at a larger size, can occur because the mediastinum, ribs, and other aspects of chest structure may obstruct them. Errors in perception on the part of the interpreter are also common. Detection of mediastinal lymph node metastases, invasion of the chest wall, or invasion of mediastinal structures cannot be assessed accurately and need further diagnostic testing.

Past screening trials in the early 1980s did not show a reduction of lung cancer mortality in the screened populations (see Table 3–1). Conclusions were not supportive of annual chest X-rays because they were not sensitive at detecting lesions < 2 cm in size, and patients with chronic obstructive pulmonary disease had a four- to six-fold increased risk of lung cancer independent of their smoking history (Jett, 2000).

Supporting the position that chest X-rays do not save lives is reported in a study by Dr. Marcus (2006) in the Mayo Lung Project. Marcus and colleagues reviewed cases from 1971 to 1983 and found that tumors identified in chest X-rays never caused serious illnesses or death (Marcus, et al., 2006). In fact, 46 of the cases in the interventional arm suggested overdiagnosis. Even after 16 additional years after follow-up, there is evidence to suggest that overdiagnosing occurs with chest X-rays.

A later study reported by Whitworth (2005) differs in opinion and suggests that chest X-rays can detect early lung cancers, although it cautions that false-positive results can occur, causing needless extra tests. It was in this preliminary report of 1992 that the National Cancer Institute (NCI) launched the largest screening trial involving four cancer types, including lung cancer. The large sample size of 154,942 men and women were randomly assigned to a control group and a screening group that received a single-view, posterior-anterior chest X-ray. Of the 67,038 individuals who received chest X-rays, 8.9% had abnormal results that required more testing. The chest X-rays detected 6.3 lung cancers per 1000 current smokers, 4.9 lung cancers per 1000 former smokers, and 0.4 lung cancers per 1000 individuals who never smoked. Men had higher rates than women on chest X-rays (Oken, et al. 2005).

Another NCI-supported study was the National Lung Screening Trial (NLST), which compared standard chest X-ray and computed tomography (CT). Discussed in further detail under the CT section, both chest X-rays and spiral CT scans have found lung cancers early (Gierada, et al., 2008; NCI, 2008b).

Sputum Cytology

Sputum cytology was believed to have potential for the early detection of lung cancer, but it showed little added advantage over chest X-rays in the National Cancer Institute cooperative trials; it was also not associated with any reduction in deaths from lung cancer (Berlin, Buncher, Fontana, Frost, & Melaned, 1984). In those trials, approximately one in four cancers was detected by sputum cytology alone, and the majority of these were squamous cell carcinomas that were diagnosed at a favorable stage. Although sputum cytology is the least invasive means of obtaining a specific diagnosis in a patient who is suspected of having lung cancer, this method is not necessarily the easiest because it depends on rigorous specimen sampling and preservation techniques. The average overall sensitivity is 64%, but it drops to 40% for pe-

ripheral lesions (Detterbeck, 2000). Attempts to refine the use of sputum cytology, however, are continuing. Earlier randomized, controlled studies in the United States tested whether a combination of chest X-rays and sputum examination could be more effective than either alone or by utilizing practice guidelines in detecting early lung cancer (persistent cough, shortness of breath, hoarseness, hemoptysis, and so on). These studies found that prospective screening practice guideline programs for lung cancer did not have any significant improvement in overall survival rates compared with using chest X-rays and sputum (Minna, Sekido, Fong, & Gazdar, 1997).

Low-Radiation-Dose Computed Tomography (Spiral or Helical CT)

With the introduction of computed tomography (CT) scanning in the late 1970s, a giant step was taken in the ability to diagnose and stage lung cancer by employing noninvasive imaging techniques. It is probably the most promising tool for early lung cancer detection. Adding intravenous contrast material is useful in distinguishing mediastinal structures and assessing potential vascular invasion. It has the potential to detect 75–80% of lung cancers in stage I (Jett, 2000). The newer low-radiation spiral CT is a diagnostic test that scans the entire chest in 15 seconds, during a single breath hold. The spiral CT provides 5 mm multiplanar slices of the chest and is more sensitive than a chest X-ray in the detection of small pulmonary nodules, mediastinum adenopathy, small pleural effusions, and the ability to detect abnormalities below the diaphragm (Schoepf, 2001).

The Early Lung Cancer Project (ELCAP) was a nonrandomized trial designed to evaluate screening with low-radiation-dose CT. Low-dose CT was ordered for 1,000 volunteers, aged 60 years and older, who had a smoking history of at least 10 pack years and who were acceptable candidates for thoracic surgery. The CT significantly outperformed conventional chest X-ray in the detection of small pulmonary nodules (Henschke, et al., 2001). Noncalcified pulmonary nodules were detected three times as commonly (23% versus 7%), malignancies four times as commonly (2.7% versus 0.7%), and stage I malignancies six times as commonly (2.3% versus 0.4%). These researchers believed that obtaining a CT of the chest was more cost effective for curable stages of lung cancers. In a later report by Henschke and colleagues on ELCAP data (2008), repeat screenings were reviewed to evaluate lung cancer. Of the 1184 patients having repeat CT screenings, only 2.5% (30 patients) were positive.

Despite the recent data from the ELCAP, which demonstrate that lung cancer screening can detect early stage (stage I) lung cancer, translating into increased survival rates, the National Comprehensive Cancer Network (NCCN) Lung Cancer Panel does not recommend the use of routine screening spiral CT as standard clinical protocol (NCCN, 2008b). Dr. Ettinger, who is the chairperson for the NCCN committee, is waiting for the 2009 results from the national study before making a final determination. Certainly spiral CT spurs optimism; however, without more conclusive data, patients who receive screening spiral CTs should be enrolled in clinical trials. Hopefully then and only then can a definitive answer be obtained and the potential benefits and risks be identified.

Other organizations do not support the use of screening CTs. Please refer to Table 3–2 for their lung cancer screening recommendations.

Table 3–2 CT Screening Recommendations for Lung Cancer

Professional Organization	Year	Recommendations
American Cancer Society (ACS)	2008	ACS does not recommend testing for early detection of lung cancer in asymptomatic individuals. However, the ACS historically has recognized that patients at high risk of lung cancer due to significant exposure to tobacco smoke or occupational exposures may decide to undergo testing for early lung cancer detection on an individual basis after consultation with their physicians.
American College of Surgeons	2007	The panel does not recommend low-dose helical CT for screening of lung cancer except in the context of a well-designed clinical trial. The panel also recommends against the use of serial chest radiographs to screen for the presence of lung cancer. Additionally, the panel recommends against the use of single or serial sputum cytologic evaluation to screen for the presence of lung cancer.

continues

Table 3–2 CT Screening Recommendations for Lung Cancer (continued)

Professional Organization	Year	Recommendations
National Cancer Institute (NCI)	2008	The NCI states that there is no good evidence that screening for lung cancer using chest X-ray or sputum cytology can reduce lung cancer mortality. The evidence is inadequate to determine whether low-dose helical computed tomography screening reduces mortality from lung cancer. Currently, NCI is conducting the National Lung Screening Trial (NLST), a randomized controlled trial designed to determine whether annual screening with low-dose computed tomography (LDCT) can reduce lung cancer mortality among persons who are at elevated risk for that disease. (More than 50,000 persons aged 55 to 74 years with a history of heavy or long-term smoking have been enrolled in NLST, and the trial is now closed to further recruitment. Participants in NLST have been randomly assigned to receive either three annual LDCTs or three annual chest X-rays. Data collection and analysis in NLST are scheduled to continue for 8 years.)
National Comprehensive Cancer Network (NCCN)	2008	The NCCN panel does not recommend the routine use of Network (NCCN) screening CT as standard clinical practice despite the recent data from ELCAP demonstrating that lung cancer screening can detect stage I lung cancer, which could translate to an increase in survival of lung cancer patients.
Society of Thoracic Radiology	2001	It is the consensus of this committee that mass screening for lung cancer with CT is not currently advocated.

Adapted from: Aberle, D., Gamsu, G., Henschke, C., Naidich, D., & Swensen, S. (2001). Consensus statement of the Society of Thoracic Radiology: Screening for lung cancer with helical computed tomography. Cardiac imaging, Part II. *Journal of Thoracic Imaging, 16*(1), 65–68.

National Comprehensive Cancer Network. (2008). *NCCN clinical practice guidelines in oncology: Non-small cell lung cancer*. Retrieved August 2008, from www.nccn.org

National Cancer Institute. (2008). *Lung cancer screening (PDQ)*. Retrieved August 2008, from http://www.cancer.gov/cancertopics/pdq/screening/lung/HealthProfessional/page2#Section_88

Bach, P., Silvestri, G., Hanger, M., & Jett, J. (2007, September). American College of Chest Physicians. Screening for lung cancer: ACCP evidence-based clinical practice guidelines (2nd ed.). *Chest, 132*(Suppl. 3), 69S–77S.

Smith, R., Cokkinides, V., & Brawley, O. (2008). Cancer screening in the United States, 2008¡ A review of current American Cancer Society guidelines and cancer screening issues. *CA: A Cancer Journal for Clinicians, 58*, 161–179.

Source: Bach, 2008.

Positron Emission Tomography (PET)

Positron emission tomography (PET) scanning differs from CT and magnetic resonance imaging (MRI) scanning in that it can discriminate between cells that are rapidly dividing, that is, hypermetabolic sites (neoplasia as well as inflammation). PET scans detect tumor physiology, as opposed to anatomy, and are thought to be potentially more sensitive than CT scans (Patz & Erasmus, 1999; Gould, Maclean, Kuschner, Rydzak, & Owens, 2001; van Tinteren et al., 2002).

PET scans are becoming a part of initial workups, even though the scans are not recommended by NCCN for that purpose (NCCN, 2008a). NCCN does recommend PET scans for stage I and II disease to ensure the patient does not have possible metastatic disease. PET scans may often delineate a tumor from adjacent atelectasis, which is critical in limiting treatment fields for radiation therapy.

Studies have reported that PET scans mediastinal node sampling sensitivity is 88%, and the average specificity is 94% (Detterbeck, 2000). This is probably why there has been more interest in using PET scanning, especially to evaluate mediastinal nodes, because CT scanning has known limitations for evaluating these lymph nodes. Even though the sensitivity and specificity of PET scanning is high, its limitation is in its poor anatomic location of the tumor, its high cost, and its limited availability.

Sometimes it is difficult to differentiate hilar nodes from mediastinal nodes. Also, there are false positives with infectious and inflammatory lesions. False negatives may occur with tumors of low metabolic activity, small tumors, and in hyperglycemic states. A comparison study evaluated by Pieterman and colleagues (2000) between the sensitivity and specificity of CT versus PET for the detection of mediastinal metastases in patients with NSCLC showed higher rates for PET scanning. (PET sensitivity was 91% and specificity was 86%, as compared to CT, which was 75% and 66%, respectively.)

As mentioned, NCCN does not yet recommend PET scanning as part of the routine initial evaluation of NSCLC. It does recognize the promising value it can add in pretreatment and posttreatment to follow up chest X-rays, CT, or MRI scans. While PET improves the detection rate of malignancy compared to conventional diagnostic studies, treatment decisions are unclear. Van Tinteren and colleagues (2002) reported that patients who underwent PET scans were more likely to have unnecessary surgery (21%) versus those who did not receive the scan (41%).

Although Medicare does not set standards, it has expanded its coverage for PET scans. Effective July 1, 2001, PET scans were covered for diagnosis, initial staging, and restaging of NSCLC (Medicare, 2001). The Medicare Bulletin also contains further explanation as to whether PET scans are to be used for staging and/or restaging when the stage of cancer is "in doubt" after a standard diagnostic workup is completed by CT or MRI. PET scans are helpful in picking up occult metastases, and they do have some prognostic abilities.

Combining PET and CT may better improve metastatic detection of the intrathoracic lymph nodes. Two studies supporting integrating PET/CT are observational studies. Antoch et al. (2003) compared PET/CT with MRI, focusing on the nodal disease. Ninety-eight patients were reviewed, and PET/CT was found to be 98% accurate in predicting tumor stage as compared to magnetic resonance imaging (79%). Pozo-Rodriguez and colleagues (2005) reviewed potentially respectable NSCLC patients. While mediastinoscopy does prove pathology through an invasive procedure, PET/CT proved to have 98% sensitivity, followed by PET (94%) and CT alone (86%).

Magnetic Resonance Imaging (MRI)

Magnetic resonance imaging (MRI) investigation of pulmonary lesions has been disappointing and has offered no improvement over CT scanning, except to evaluate the extent of tumor invasion or destruction of peripheral structures, such as the brachial plexus, vertebral body, and spinal canal (Miller, Gorenstein, & Patterson, 1992; Shaffer, 1997). MRIs may be of value in clinical stage III disease if combined-modality therapy is being considered (Scott, 2000). Therefore, MRI is considered to be an adjunct to CT scans. In the setting of lung cancer, though, MRIs are the most effective modality for detecting brain metastases and evaluation of adrenal lesions (Schellinger, Meinck, & Thron, 1999).

Bronchoscopies

Image-guided transthoracic bronchoscopy fine-needle aspirations (FNA) have revolutionized lung cancer staging. This procedure facilitates precise biopsy of lung lesions and virtually all mediastinal lymph node areas (Harrow, et al., 2000; Savage & Zwischenberger, 2000). Because chest X-rays, CT, and PET scanning identify suspicious lesions, they cannot make a tissue differential. Transthoracic bronchoscopies have allowed for less invasive and costly diagnostic testing, offering high yields.

In 1996, the FDA approved an even newer device, known as autofluorescence bronchoscopy (Xillix LIFE-Lung), which allows physicians to observe whether cells fluoresce or reflect light normally. A fluorescent dye is injected into and taken up by the tumor cells; the dye causes the cells to fluoresce under blue light. If the cells do not fluoresce normally, a sample is taken to determine whether they are cancerous. This technique is used in special circumstances when ordinary bronchoscopy fails to reveal a tumor detected by sputum cytology. One multicentered trial reported a higher sensitivity (2.7 times) in detecting carcinomas utilizing LIFE-Lung bronchoscopies as compared to the normal use of white light bronchoscopies (Jett, 2000). Currently, there is an open Phase II NIH trial (NCT00260598) to evaluate the usefulness and accuracy of the "LIFE-Lung bronchosopy in patients at risk for developing lung cancer" (ClinicalTrials.gov).

Genetic Markers

Researchers are continuing their investigation of genetic markers or fingerprints to detect the presence of cancer cells. These markers are found in blood samples utilizing highly sophisticated laboratory tests. Unfortunately, there are no genetic markers available on the market to detect and diagnose early-stage lung cancer.

Recently, there is excitement and emphasis on the identification of the p53 tumor suppressor gene. Scientists have been investigating the p53 tumor suppressor gene in both NSCLC and SCLC. This gene influences DNA repair and cell death. Gene p53 slows down DNA destruction. Studies are being conducted to inject normal p53 genes into tumors, thus deterring cancer growth. Other markers are beginning to validate markers for lung cancer: FHIT and microsatellite alterations at loci on chromosome 3 (Andriani, et al., 2003), as well as p16, H-cadherin, APC, and RASSF1A (Belinsky, et al., 1998).

Conclusions

Numerous years have been devoted to evaluating diagnostic tests to screen lung cancer. Hopefully, new insights will emerge to diagnose lung cancer earlier. Certainly, there are intensive efforts to improve lung cancer screening with advanced technologies—low-radiation-dose computed tomography and/or molecular techniques—but large controlled trials have not been funded. Definitive trials are desperately needed to determine if diagnostic tests, such as spiral CTs, can be used as screening tools to reduce lung cancer mortality. Only then will the National Cancer Institute, American Cancer Society, and National Comprehensive Cancer Network be able to recommend screening guidelines. Therefore, because lung cancer affects a vital organ and has debilitating symptoms (dyspnea, cough, hemoptysis, chest discomfort, and a low quality of life), it is imperative that healthcare providers become aggressive in identifying the etiology of its symptoms. The earlier lung cancer is diagnosed, the better the outcome for the individual. For a lung cancer screening to be beneficial, it not only needs to detect early cancers but needs to alter the natural pathway that rapidly causes deaths.

References

Alberg, A. J., & Samet, J. M. (2003). Epidemiology of lung cancer [Abstract]. *Chest, 123*(Suppl. 1), 21s–49s.

American Cancer Society. (2008). *Cancer facts and figures 2008*. Atlanta, GA: Author. Retrieved May 30, 2008, from http://www.cancer.org/downloads/STT/2008 CAFF finalsecured.pdf

Andriani, F., Conte, D., Mastrangelo, T., Leo, M., Racliffe, C., Roz, L., et al. (2003). Predictive markers and cancer prevention. *International Journal of Cancer, 108*(1), 91–96.

Antoch, G., Vogt, F., Freudenbery, L., Nazaradeh, F., Goehde, S., Barkhausen, J., et al. (2003). Whole-body dual-modality PET/CT and whole-body MRI for tumor staging in oncology. *Journal of the American Medical Association, 290*(24), 3199–3206.

Bach, P. (2008). Lung cancer screening. *Journal of the National Comprehensive Cancer Network, 6*(3), 271–275.

Bach, P., Jett, J., Pastorino, U., Tockman, M., Swensen, S., & Begg, C. (2007). Computed tomography screening and lung cancer outcomes. *Journal of the American Medical Association, 297*(9), 953–961.

Belinsky, S., Nikula, K., Palmisano,W., Michels, R., Saccomanno, G., Gabrielson, E., et al. (1998). Aberrant methylation of p16 INK4a is an early event in lung cancer and a potential biomarker for early diagnosis. *Proceedings of the National Academy of Sciences of United States of American, 95*(20), 11891–11896.

Berlin, N., Buncher, C., Fontana, R., Frost, J., & Meland, M. (1984). The National Cancer Institute cooperative early lung cancer detection program. *American Reference Respiratory Disease, 130*(4), 545–549.

Detterbeck, F. (2000). Diagnosis and staging of non-small cell lung cancer. Diagnosis and treatment of lung cancer: An evidence-based guide for the practicing clinician. *Chest, 1*(2), 1–13.

Ettinger, D. (2001). New NCCN recommendations for non-small cell lung cancer. *Oncology News International, 10*(4), 1, 39.

Gierada, D., Pilgram, T., Ford, M., Fagerstrom, R., Church, T., Nath, H., et al. (2008). Lung cancer: Interobserver agreement on interpretation of pulmonary findings at low-dose CT screening. *Radiology, 246*(1), 265–272.

Ginsberg, R., Vokes, E., & Rosenzweig, K. (2001). *Non-small cell lung cancer. Principles and practice of oncology* (6th ed.). Philadelphia: Lippincott Williams & Wilkins.

Gould, M., Maclean, C., Kuschner, W., Rydzak, C., & Owens, D. (2001). Accuracy of positron emission tomography for diagnosis of pulmonary nodules and mass lesions. *Journal of the American Medical Association, 285*(7), 914–924.

Harrow, E., Abi-Salch, W., Blum, J., Harkin, T., Gasparini, S., Addrizzo, B., et al. (2000). The utility of transbronchial needle aspiration in the staging of bronchogenic carcinoma. *American Journal of Respiratory Critical Care Medicine, 161*(2 Pt 1), 601–607.

Henschke, C., McCauley, D., Yankelevitz, D., Naidich, D., McGuinnes, G., Olli, S., et al. (2001). Early lung cancer action project: A summary of the findings on baseline screening. *The Oncologist, 6*(2), 147–152.

Henschke, C., Naidich, D., Yankelevitz, D., McGuinness, G., McCauley, D., Smith, J., et al. (2008). Early lung cancer action project: Initial findings on repeat screenings. *Cancer, 112*(10), 2329–2330.

Henschke, C., Yankelevitz, D., Libby, D., Pasmantier, M., & Smith, J. (2006). Survival of patients with stage I lung cancer detected on CT screening. *The New England Journal of Medicine, 355*(17), 1763–1771.

Jett, J. (2000). Screening for lung cancer in high-risk groups: Current status of low-dose spiral CT scanning and sputum markers. *Seminars in Respiratory and Critical Care Medicine, 21*(5), 385–392.

Lee, J., Kiu, D., Lee, J., Kurie, J., Khuri, F., Ibarguen, H., et al. (2001). Long-term impact of smoking on lung epithelial proliferation in current and former smokers. *Journal of the National Cancer Institute, 93*(14), 1042–1043.

MacManus, M. (2000). PET scans predict survival in non-small cell lung cancer patients. *Oncology News International, 9*(11), 14.

Marcus, P., Bergstralh, E., Zweig, M., Harris, A., Offord, K., & Fontana, R. (2006). Extended lung cancer incidence follow-up in the Mayo lung project and overdiagnosis. *Journal of the National Cancer Institute, 98*(11), 748–756.

Medicare. (2001). *Medicare bulletin* (GR 2001-4, pp. 18–19).

Miller, J., Gorenstein, L., & Patterson, G. (1992). Staging: The key to rational management of lung cancer. *The Annals of Thoracic Surgery, 53*(1), 170–178.

Minna, J., Sekido, Y., Fong, K., & Gazdar, A. (1997). Cancer of the lung: Molecular biology of lung cancer. In D. Hellman & M. Rosenberg (Eds.), *Principles and practice of oncology* (5th ed.). Philadelphia: Lippincott-Raven.

National Cancer Institute (NCI). (2007, March 6). *Study finds lung cancer screening may not reduce deaths*. NCI cancer bulletin. Retrieved July 18, 2008, from http:// nci.nih.gov/cancertopics/screening/lung-ct0307/ print?page=&keyword=

National Cancer Institute (NCI). (2008a). *Clinical trials search results*. Retrieved July 18, 2008, from http://nci. nih.gov/search/ResultsClinicalTrials.aspx?protocol searchid=4861070

National Cancer Institute (NCI). (2008b). *Clinical trials (PDQ). National lung screening trial (NLST)*. Retrieved July 18, 2008, from http://www.cancer.gov/clinical trials/view_clinicaltrials.aspx?version=health professional&cdrid=257938&protocolsearchid= 451616

National Comprehensive Cancer Network (NCCN). (2008a). *Non-small cell lung cancer. V.2.2008*. Retrieved July 18, 2008, from www.nccn.org

National Comprehensive Cancer Network (NCCN). (2008b). *NSCLC: Highlights of Updated Guidelines*. Highlights of the 13th Annual Conference: Clinical Practice Guidelines & Quality Cancer Care, Elsevier Oncology, Huntington, NY, p. 33.

Oken, M., Marcus, P., Hu, P., Beck, T., Hocking, W., Kvale, P., et al. (2005). Baseline chest radiograph for lung cancer detection in the randomized prostate, lung, colorectal and ovarian cancer screening trial. *Journal of the National Cancer Institute, 97*(24), 1832–1839.

Patz, E., & Erasmus, J. (1999). Positron emission tomography imaging in lung cancer. *Clinical Lung Cancer, 1*(1), 42–48.

Pieterman, R., van Putten, J., Meuzelaar, J., Mooyaart, E., Vaalburg, W., Koeter, G., et al. (2000). Preoperative staging of non-small cell lung cancer with positron-emission tomography. *New England Journal of Medicine, 343*(4), 254–261.

Pozo-Rodriguez, F., Martin de Nicolas, J., Sanchez-Nistal, M., Maldonado, A., Garcia de Barajas, S., Calero-Garcia, R., et al. (2005). Accuracy of helical computed tomography and (18) fluorodeoxyglucose positron emission tomography for identifying lymph node mediastinal metastases in potentially respectable non-small-cell lung cancer. *Journal of Clinical Oncology, 23*(33), 8348–8356.

Reddy, A. (2000, October 22). *Non-Small Cell Lung Cancer: Imaging and Staging*. American Society for Therapeutic Radiology and Oncology, 42nd Annual Meeting.

Savage, C., & Zwischenberger, J. (2000). Image-guided fine needle aspirate strategies for staging of lung cancer. *Clinical Lung Cancer, 2*(2), 101–110.

Schellinger, P., Meinck, H., & Thron, A. (1999). Diagnostic accuracy of MRI compared to CCT in patients with brain metastases. *The Journal of Neurooncology, 44*(3), 275.

Schoepf, J. (2001). Lung cancer screening with 1mm multislice CT scans. *Oncology News International, 10*(1), 10.

Scott, W. (2000). *Lung cancer: A guide to diagnosis and treatment*. Omaha, NE: Atticus Books.

Shaffer, K. (1997). Radiologic evaluation in lung cancer: Diagnosis and staging. *Chest,* 112(Suppl. 4), 235S–238S.

van Tinteren, H., Hoekstra, O., Smit, E., van den Bergh, J., Schreurs, A., Stallaert, R., et al. (2002). Effectiveness of positron emission tomography in the preoperative assessment of patients with suspected non-small cell lung cancer. *Lancet,* 359(9315), 1388–1392.

Whitworth, A. (2005). Screening chest x-ray detects early-stage lung cancers at high rates, study results show. *JNCI Journal of the National Cancer Institute* 97(24), 1795–1799.

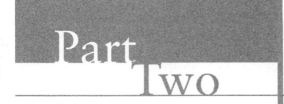

Part Two

Oncology Treatment Modalities

Chapter 4

Managing Patients Through Thoracic Surgery

Sheila Boegli

Introduction

The history of thoracic surgery originated with the first successful pneumonectomy by Graham and Singer, which was reported in 1933 (Shields, 2000). As time evolved, advances led to smaller resections while reducing mortality in the 1940s. These surgical improvements included sleeve resection, bronchoplastic procedures, segmentectomy, and lobectomy. With the introduction of surgical stapling, lung resections are now safer, faster, and less traumatic to the patient. This chapter will present surgical techniques and procedures, along with nursing care postoperative. Also, selected complementary alternative medicine modalities that could be applicable to the postoperative patient will be discussed.

Goal of Surgical Therapy

The ultimate goal of surgical therapy is complete resection, leading to a cure. It is the goal of the healthcare provider and the goal sought by the patient. Additionally, it is important to preserve remaining lung function to the maximum extent possible. For primary lung cancer, stage I disease, the treatment of choice is surgery. Every patient with locoregional non-small cell lung cancer should be approached as a potential candidate for resection (LoCicero, Ponn, & Daly, 2000).

Surgery for lung cancer has three parts. The components are:

1. Establishment or confirmation of the diagnosis. This is done by radiographic studies and biopsies, specifically chest X-rays, chest CT scans, and biopsies of the thoracic mass.
2. Complete resection of the tumor.
3. Systematic sampling or complete dissection of lymph nodes draining the primary tumor. This is achieved by a pulmonary resection but can be done by mediastinoscopy.

Prior to having surgery, the patient must first be deemed resectable and operable. A resectable patient is one who has disease that is still local or local—regional in scope and that can be removed with surgery (Johnston, 1997). Only a few patients with stage III and especially stage IV disease are ever considered for surgery. When the disease has invaded other vital structures, such as the mediastinal vessels or surrounding lymph nodes, the course of therapy changes significantly.

Patients may also present with malignant pleural effusions. Malignant pleural effusions occur as an inflammatory response to a pleural tumor that results in increased microvascular permeability. This, in turn, produces small volumes of pleural effusions. The causative pathology needs to be identified and corrected. In this case, the tumor is the inflammatory agent, and surgery may not be an option. The pleural effusion needs to be drained and sent to pathology. The patient will require other medical-oncological therapy, such as chemotherapy and radiation therapy.

Conversely, operability describes someone who can tolerate, with acceptable risk, the surgical procedure that is necessary to remove the cancer. A patient who presents at the initial consult with notable shortness of breath, poor pulmonary function tests, and supplemental oxygen may not be a candidate for a complete pulmonary resection. However, the thoracic surgeon may be able to offer a wedge resection.

All components of the patient's medical and surgical history combined with the initial examination need to be considered carefully when thoracic surgery is being considered. If both the resectable and operable criteria are met, then surgery is scheduled and performed (Johnston, 1997).

Diagnostic Assessment

Accurate diagnosis and staging of lung cancer is essential for determining which patients would benefit from surgery. Assessment follows a logical progression from radiographic studies to invasive techniques. Radiographic studies would include a computed tomography (CT) scan of the thorax, positron emission tomography (PET) scan, and possibly magnetic resonance imaging

(MRI). Invasive assessment includes biopsy and/or surgery.

Usually, a pulmonary nodule is identified on chest X-ray. The CT scan is then used to evaluate the pulmonary nodule. A CT scan of the thorax relies on the fact that malignant tumors are highly vascularized and therefore are enhanced by intravenous contrast material (Reed & Silvestri, 2000). This type of radiographic assessment is the standard. Other types of radiographic evaluations have been implemented, such as the PET scan, which is controversial. Although the PET scan can help to evaluate indeterminate pulmonary lesions, it can present false positives. Most times these false positives can be the result of active infectious or inflammatory lesions (Reed & Silvestri, 2000). On occasion there have been false negatives that are related to low metabolic activity. Carcinoid tumors are a type of malignancy that may yield a false negative result. The PET scan can help the thoracic surgeon in the recommendation of further invasive testing or resection options, particularly when clinical pretest probability and CT results are discordant (Gould, et al., 2003). Integrated PET/CT has fewer false negative results but an increase in false positive results (Lee, et al., 2007). However, it yields significantly improved results when contrast uptake is increased (Lee, et al., 2008). Positive PET scan findings need pathologic or radiologic confirmation. If the PET scan is positive in the mediastinum, lymph node status needs pathologic confirmation (NCCN, 2008).

When a node has been determined to be suspicious for cancer, a definitive diagnosis must be made. This is done through CT-guided transthoracic fine-needle aspiration (TTNA) biopsy, bronchoscopy, or thoracoscopy. A fine-needle biopsy has been the procedure of choice for the diagnosis of peripheral pulmonary nodules. In a study done in 1993 by Salazar and Westcott, there was a reported accuracy of between 80–90%. A repeat fine-needle biopsy was diagnostic in 35–65% of these patients. A nondiagnostic fine-needle biopsy usually indicates the need for bronchoscopy or mediastinoscopy. Improvements in fine-needle biopsy stem from needle guidance and positioning technologies, resulting in increased diagnostic accuracy (Yoshimatsu, et al., 2008).

A bronchoscopy can diagnose, stage, and in some cases, treat lung cancer. It is the procedure of choice in patients with centrally located masses. The diagnostic yield of fiber optic bronchoscopy for centrally located lung masses presumed to be cancer is approximately 70% and increases to greater than 90% when the lesion is visualized in the airway (Reed & Silvestri, 2000). A bronchoscopy is also used to rule out endobronchial lesions because they do not show up well on the CT scan. Endobronchial ultrasound (EBUS) guided fine-needle biopsy seems to be an improvement over bronchoscopy (Paone, et al., 2005).

Thoracoscopy is commonly used to diagnose peripheral nodules or masses located in the peripheral third of the lung, with a sensitivity and specificity approaching 100% (Gould, et al., 2007). It is also used when the transthoracic biopsy is negative. With thoracoscopy, the excised tissue is sent for pathological evaluation, and, if it is positive, definitive surgery, including mediastinal staging, is indicated.

When a diagnosis has been made, the next step is staging of the lung cancer. Diagnosis and staging may occur simultaneously. Both can be done through mediastinoscopy, endobronchial ultrasound, or endoscopic ultrasound (EUS) fine-needle biopsy. Mediastinoscopy remains the gold standard for the staging of lung cancer and the diagnosis of thoracic disease (Gould, et al., 2007). In a retrospective review of all mediastinoscopies performed at the Washington University School of Medicine, St. Louis, Missouri, from January 1988 through September 1998 on 1,745 of 2,137 patients known or suspected to have lung cancer, it was determined that a mediastinoscopy is a safe and highly effective procedure (Hammoud, et al., 1999). Of the 422 patients with N2 or N3 disease, only 28 of these patients underwent resection (Hammoud, et al., 1999). The remaining 1,323 patients in this study had no evidence of metastatic disease. In this group, 947 patients had lung cancer. It was also found that the mediastinoscopy established a definitive diagnosis in 93.6% of the patients, further supporting the efficacy and safety of this procedure (Hammoud, et al., 1999). For a patient with stage III or stage IV disease, a mediastinoscopy will provide the necessary information to help plan the necessary adjuvant therapy.

Mediastinoscopy can be a controversial procedure, and some would argue that it is unnecessary, especially if the patient will undergo pulmonary resection. Resection may take place despite the results of the mediastinoscopy. Because mediastinoscopy requires anesthetic sedation, which has its own risk factors, it should be sensibly combined with other procedures whenever possible. If one is trying to determine what medical/surgical options are available, a mediastinoscopy may or may not offer helpful information. A mediastinoscopy is typically done on patients with an undiagnosed pulmonary nodule or nodules that are greater than 1 cm.

Newer techniques have been used to avoid the need for mediastinoscopy. These include endobronchial ultrasound and endoscopic ultrasound biopsy, used independently or together, to sample mediastinal nodes. Both are invasive but do not require anesthesia. The locations of nodes to be biopsied usually determine the choice of technique.

Operative Criteria for Surgical Resection

When the staging of a lung cancer has confirmed resectability, the patient's suitability as an operative candidate is addressed. Healthcare professionals must address the mental preparedness of the patient who has been diagnosed with lung cancer and now faces surgical resection. Patients can become preoccupied with their illness. They may begin to focus on their disease and the potential for a poor outcome. This, in turn, can lead to depression. Depression is not uncommon in cancer patients, and many patients can experience this as a clinical disease. Left untreated, it may lead to a poor surgical outcome. Medications are available that can help combat some of the symptoms that a depressed patient may be experiencing. Clinicians need to be aware of a patient's emotional stability prior to undergoing surgery. Conversely, an attitude that is positive will generally improve how a patient feels about the potential prognosis and disease process. Involvement of family or a significant other will generally lead to better patient understanding of the disease, better compliance, and a better outcome. Support groups can help to decrease anxieties that may be associated with treatment, prognosis, or the unknown. Discussing events about the surgery with other members of the healthcare team may provide insight into the actual surgical procedure and what may

occur postoperatively. Being prepared for surgery will usually have a positive effect on the surgical outcome.

Physiological barriers can also have an adverse effect on a patient's postoperative course. In the assessment of patients who are being considered for thoracotomy, two major assessments are made: cardiac and pulmonary function.

General thoracic procedures can have a profound effect on the cardiopulmonary system. A lung resection decreases the pulmonary vascular bed and can result in an acute increase in right ventricular and pulmonary artery pressure leading to right ventricular failure. Decreased lung compliance and diffusion capacity, with a resultant increase in the work of breathing, may aggravate a preexisting cardiac disease or lead to new onset ischemia. These comorbidities may have an impact on the patient's postoperative course.

Although cardiac morbidity is rare, those patients that suffered a myocardial infarction just 3 months prior to having surgery have a disproportionately increased risk of surgical mortality. The risk of perioperative infarction is inversely related to the time interval between the original myocardial infarction and the surgical procedure (Alexander & Anderson, 2000). This particular patient group should be sent for a cardiology workup prior to having thoracic surgery. Patients who have major factors (unstable coronary syndrome, decompensated heart failure, significant arrhythmias, or severe valvular disease) also should undergo preoperative cardiological evaluations (Colice, et al., 2007).

Unique to patients having a thoracotomy is the effect of pulmonary parenchymal resection on postoperative pulmonary function. All patients who are being considered for thoracotomy should have pulmonary function tests (PFTs) performed. PFTs are used to assess a patient's pulmonary reserve (Reilly, 1999). Specifically, the forced vital capacity (FEV1) and the diffusion lung capacity (DLCO) are assessed. The FEV1 measures a patient's forced expiratory volume. Patients who are considered to be high risk are those with an FEV1 less than 0.7 L and/or 40% predicted. The DLCO measures carbon monoxide and reflects the efficiency of gas exchange (Reilly, 1999). A patient's DLCO should measure greater than 60% predicted. Any patient with values less than those mentioned here should not receive surgery until further workup is performed by a pulmonologist.

Age can have a poor outcome on a hospital course. As a patient increases in age, so does the surgical risk. Surgical risks are 55% higher in patients that are 65 years and older (United States Department of Health and Human Services, 1999). Patients over 70 years of age are considered to be high risk. These patients typically have existing comorbidities, such as cardiac disease, diabetes, and chronic obstructive pulmonary disease (COPD). The elderly patient population does not tolerate anesthesia very well. Conversely, in a patient population under 40 years old, it is anticipated that this age group would have a lower morbidity and mortality than its elders. In 1998, 24 pneumonectomies were performed in patients over 70 years old. It revealed a 12.5% mortality (Ginsberg, et al., 1983). In another study, increasing age was a significant predictor for a prolonged length of stay (Wright, et al., 2008). In a 2003 study by Birim and colleagues, for 126 patients greater than 70 years of age who underwent curative intent surgical resection, the overall 30-day mortality rate was 3.2%, with comorbid disease having the greatest influence on mortality. A retrospective analysis from Johns

Hopkins Hospital reported that 17% of the octogenarians who were diagnosed with lung cancer between 1980 and 2002 underwent surgical resection for curative intent. They reported a 30-day mortality rate of 8.8%. Port and colleagues (2004) reported a 30-day mortality rate of 1.6%. Fukuse, Satoda, and Hijiiya (2005) found that dependence for performing activities of daily living and impaired cognition were important predictors of complications following pulmonary surgery. Therefore, age alone should not preclude curative intent resection.

In evaluating a patient for surgery, it is imperative that the surgeon and the surgical team evaluate all associated comorbidities to determine if the patient is a candidate for surgery.

Thoracic Incisions

The most common incision for open general thoracic surgical procedures is the lateral thoracotomy, sometimes called the axillary thoracotomy. For many years, the posterolateral thoracotomy was considered to be the incision of choice for most operations involving the esophagus and lung. With increased use of double-lumen endotracheal tubes and refinement of the instrumentation, especially stapling techniques, the posterolateral thoracotomy is reserved for more difficult cases (Fry, 2000). Although there are several other thoracic incisions utilized in thoracic surgery, for the purpose of this chapter, only the posterolateral and axillary thoracotomy will be discussed.

The posterolateral thoracotomy incision is made with the patient in a left lateral decubitus position with padding to the elbows, knees, and dependent axilla (see Figure 4–1). The incision starts in front of the anterior axillary line, curves 4 cm under the tip of the scapula, and takes a

Figure 4–1 The incision curves in an S shape, passing 4 cm under the tip of the scapula, over in the fifth interspace anteriorly.

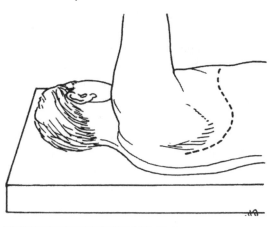

Source: Shields, et al., 2000.

vertical direction between the posterior midline over the vertebral column and medial edge of the scapula. The incision curves in an S shape. Rib resection is recommended for patients over 40 years of age to decrease the incidence of rib fracture. The main advantage to this technique is the superb exposure for most thoracic procedures. The disadvantage is the length of the incision and amount of muscle and soft tissue transected.

The axillary thoracotomy was originally developed for operations on the upper thoracic sympathetic nerve system. The incision is useful when a double-lumen endotracheal tube is used, such as in an uncomplicated pulmonary resection. Additionally, the only muscle transected with this incision is the intercostal muscle group. The chief advantages of this incision are the speed of opening and closing, the reduced blood loss from minimal muscle transection, and the resulting reduced postoperative discomfort (Fry, 2000).

In preparation for the procedure, the patient is positioned in a lateral decubitus position with the arm abducted at 90 degrees and positioned on an armrest (see Figure 4–2). A sequential compression device is applied on the legs and an axillary roll is placed. Due to the limited expo-

Figure 4–2 (A) The arm is abducted 90 degrees on a rest and padded with care. Note the sequential compression device on the legs and the axillary roll. (B) An incision is made in line with the desired interspace. It is not necessary to raise skin flaps.

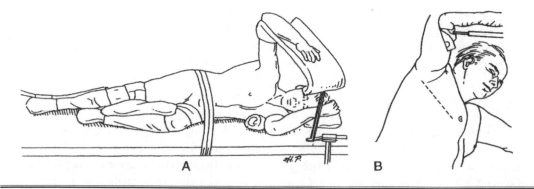

Source: Shields, et al., 2000.

sure of the axillary thoracotomy incision, it should only be performed by an experienced thoracic surgeon. It is a useful incision that deserves wider application than it has received, and it is associated with less postoperative discomfort than a posterolateral thoracotomy or median sternotomy (Fry, 2000).

Operative Procedure

The type of operative procedure that is performed depends upon the tumor location, the ability to perform the surgery, and the need to preserve functional, uninvolved lung tissue whenever possible. Performing a compromised operation for the sake of minimizing morbidity or decreasing a hospital stay is a mistake and should not be done. Although there are several other types of thoracic surgical procedures, the more common ones will be mentioned here. The more common types of thoracic surgery performed are lobectomy, pulmonary wedge resection, sleeve resection, and pneumonectomy.

The lobectomy is an ideal resection of lung cancer that is confined to a single lobe that permits removal of the tumor along with associated pleural and drainage pathways (Shields, 2000). This surgery is typically reserved for tumors of stage I and is the standard surgical resection. Due to such a high success rate with surgery, adjuvant therapy is not done outside clinical trials. Several studies are now being done to determine whether chemotherapy administered before or after surgery is beneficial in reducing the number of recurrences.

Recurrence rates are significant, with a 5-year survival rate for T1N0M0 patients at 80%; the 5-year survival rate for T2N0M0 patients is 85% (Martini, et al., 1999). The benefit of adjuvant therapy in this population is dually dependent on the availability of effective therapies

and methods to follow patients for response or failure (Harwood, 1996). To date, no additional adjuvant therapy is recommended or performed.

A pulmonary wedge resection is a nonanatomic operation that should be definitive therapy in poor-surgical-risk patients or patients with metastatic lesions from sites such as the gastrointestinal tract, head and neck, breast, and genitourinary tract. This operation is reserved for patients for limited lung reserve as well as for small peripheral tumors. The physiologic effect following this surgery is minimal, as is the morbidity and mortality. The disadvantage of this operation is a 10–15% recurrence in the lobe left behind (LoCicero, et al., 2000).

A sleeve resection is done for those tumors that protrude into the main bronchus. If a tumor is at the origin of the right upper lobe bronchus and a lobectomy cannot be performed, a resection of the right main and intermediate bronchial sleeve allows for adequate margins around the tumor. Bronchial reanastomosis preserves uninvolved right lower and middle lobes. This is the most popular type of sleeve resection, but there are variations of the procedure (see Figure 4–3). In the hands of skilled thoracic surgeons, the sleeve resection is becoming more common, thereby preventing pneumonectomy, which can be compromising.

Generally, the best operation is the least resection that removes the primary tumor and its involved lymphatics (Goldstraw, 2000). The conservative resection was introduced as a compromise for the patient who was unable to tolerate a more extensive resection. Each approach, be it a lobectomy, sleeve resection, or segmentectomy, has been shown to be an adequate cancer operation, with survival at least as good as with more extensive resections. The basic goal of resecting all of the primary tumor and its involved lymphatics must be achieved. In some

Figure 4–3 Indications for sleeve resection of right- and left-sided bronchial carcinoma in relation to tumor stage. Tumor and involved lymph nodes are given in black. The extent of resection is indicated by gray. (A) Indications for upper lobe sleeve resection of right- and left-sided tumors, respectively. (B) Indications for lower right-sided bilobectomy and left-sided resection of the lower lobe and main bronchus (reverse or Y-sleeve resection). Arrows point to hilar or peribronchial lymph node metastases from a peripherally located tumor.

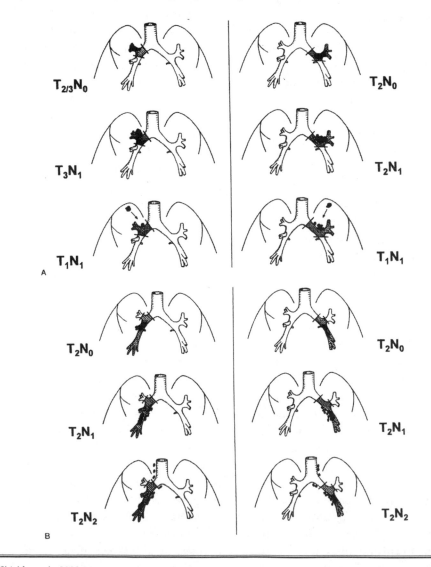

Source: Shields, et al., 2000.

cases it may still be only possible with a pneumonectomy (Goldstraw, 2000). A pneumonectomy is required when a lobectomy or one of its modifications is not sufficient to remove all local–regional disease. The majority of pneumonectomies are still performed for lung cancer. It is occasionally performed for pulmonary metastases and rare thoracic tumors. The extent of resection is rarely known before surgery, and all patients who undergo thoracotomy for lung cancer should be assessed for suitability for pneumonectomy (Goldstraw, 2000). Typically, a cost–benefit assessment is made. The cost of the operation is the patient's risk of death and the likely reduction in exercise capacity. The benefit offered by the penumonectomy is the possibility of cure or extended survival. Typically, this surgery is associated with more than twice the mortality rate of a lobectomy, as well as more long-term respiratory complications. Whether this procedure is performed or not, it is imperative that lung function is preserved. All aspects of an initial assessment—including quality of life, comorbidities, and potential for cure—need to be explored. If it has been determined that performing a pneumonectomy would not offer a significant benefit to a patient's life, then other treatment modalities need to be considered.

Postoperative Nursing Care

Postoperative nursing care for the thoracotomy patient should focus on two major areas: pain and pulmonary management.

Although a variety of different interventions have been employed to reduce the pain that a patient is experiencing, significant pain frequently follows a thoracotomy. Immediately postoperative, these patients are given intravenous (IV) or epidural patient-controlled analgesia (PCA). Frequently patients are left on PCA until the chest tube is removed, and when they are able to take pain medication by mouth, the PCA pump is discontinued. The IV pain medication that is usually used is of an opioid derivative, such as morphine. A small number of patients are placed on intravenous ketorolac tromethamine (Toradol) (Hoffman-LaRoche, Inc., 2000). Patients can have spasms that occur due to the resection of the intercostal muscle. The intercostal muscles become irritated and actually undergo spastic movements as mobility increases. Ketorolac tromethamine, a nonsteroidal anti-inflammatory, helps to relieve these symptoms. Combined with the narcotic analgesic, pain is reduced to a manageable limit. (Ketorolac tromethamine is contraindicated in patients with renal disease and should not be given for greater than 7–10 days.)

Other adjunct therapies are instituted, such as sitting up in a chair to reduce tension along the suture site and early ambulation to reduce muscle spasms and to promote good pulmonary management.

Pulmonary management is crucial to a patient's recovery following thoracotomy. After the pain has been reduced, the patient is then allowed to take deep breaths, and early ambulation is promoted. These measures are employed to decrease pulmonary complications, such as pneumonia and atelectasis. Postoperative patients are given an incentive spirometer and are instructed to cough and deep breathe at least 10 times an hour. This allows the functional parenchyma, the alveoli, to expand and decrease the incidence of pulmonary secretions. These measures decrease the likelihood of developing postoperative pneumonia.

It is not uncommon for a patient to return for the first postoperative visit several weeks after the initial surgery complaining of shortness of breath. Shortness of breath can be attributed to the thoracotomy incision and diminished lung capacity secondary to removal of the involved portion of the lung. This symptom can occur following a pulmonary resection, and over a few months' time, it will slowly resolve. Reassurance to the patient, increased mobility, and adequate pain control will help reduce this unpleasant side effect. Conversely, if the shortness of breath progressively worsens and a fever develops, accompanied with a lack of appetite, then the appropriate pulmonary workup for pneumonia should be performed. Identifying complications early in the postoperative course will enable the patient to have a quicker recovery period.

All patients who have a pulmonary resection may be at risk for atrial arrhythmias, such as atrial fibrillation. Atrial fibrillation occurs in up to 19% of patients following lung cancer resection (Roselli, et al., 2005). Prophylactic use of either calcium channel blockers or β-blockers will significantly reduce the risk of atrial tachyarrhythmias after thoracic surgery (Sedrakyan, et al., 2005). Due to the close proximity of the vagus nerve during the intraoperative period, irritation may cause atrial fibrillation to occur. Patients therefore are monitored early in the postoperative course for such arrhythmias. If atrial fibrillation should occur, patients are started on the appropriate β-blocker to control for rapid ventricular response and to assist the patient to return to sinus rhythm. In rare instances, cardioversion may be required.

Atrial fibrillation can potentiate the risk for developing a stroke. For this reason, anticoagulation therapy with heparin (Celsus Laboratories, Inc., 1987) and then warfarin sodium (Coumadin) (DuPont Pharmaceuticals Company, 1999) may be indicated if the atrial fibrillation is of new onset or if there is an alternating pattern of atrial fibrillation and sinus rhythm. Typically, a short course of therapy for atrial fibrillation upon discharge is indicated and is usually discontinued at the patient's first postoperative visit.

Any time an incision is made, the patient is at risk for a wound infection. Although every precaution is taken to prevent wound infections from occurring, the thoracotomy incision must be carefully monitored. It is not unusual to have a slightly elevated temperature in the first 24 hours postoperative. However, should this temperature continue into postoperative day two or three, then the source of infection must be explored. The patient is cultured appropriately from sputum, urine, and blood. The surgical incision is inspected for any overt signs of infection, and the appropriate blood work is obtained. If an organism is identified, then the appropriate antibiotic is prescribed. If the wound requires drainage, then an incision and drainage are performed, and the wound is packed lightly and monitored closely over the patient's hospital course and at the time of discharge. Home care nursing may need to be arranged to provide additional wound care.

Emotional support is often neglected in the postoperative management of a patient who has undergone surgery for lung cancer. All too often nursing and medical staff become focused on the medical and surgical tasks that are necessary to care for a patient. As stated earlier, a patient's preoperative emotional state can have a great impact on the entire surgical course. Following through with a program of adequate, healthy emotional support is beneficial to the recovery process. If necessary, support groups or other patients should be made readily available to assist with questions or concerns that may arise during this emotional time. Healthcare personnel should take the time to explain what is involved with the procedure, what to expect postoperatively, and at the time of discharge, what the patient may experience. Combined with a supportive family, caring healthcare personnel, and an excellent surgeon, a patient should be able to have a comfortable hospital course.

Results Following Surgical Resection

A successful surgical operation can be measured by observing its complications. Typical major complications seen with lung resection procedures are pulmonary and cardiovascular in origin. Pulmonary complications may include pneumonia, emphysema, bronchopulmonary fistulas, and prolonged air leaks. These may require long-term oxygen therapy, ventilatory support, and a long-term hospital stay. As previously mentioned, many medical interventions are done to prevent these pulmonary complications.

Cardiovascular complications may include tachyarrhythmias, such as atrial fibrillation, that require medical therapy or cardioversion. A myocardial infarction (MI) is likely to occur if the patient has had an MI within 3 months of surgery (Yang, personal communication, May 15, 2001). Cardiac failure, as well as MI, is usually seen in the older patient population group. The 30-day mortality following surgical resection revealed that, as the age of the patient increased, the mortality increased. A 70-year-old patient had a mortality rate of 7.1%. The rate is 4.1% for the 60–69-year-old group and 1.3% for the less than 60-year-old group following a surgical resection (Ginsberg, et al., 1983).

Figure 4–4 depicts the survival rates after surgical resection by the stage of disease. Fifty percent of the patients had stage IV disease, 30% had stage III disease, and 10% had stage I and stage II disease (Mountain, 1986). The 5-year survival rates after surgical resection show that surgery accounts for nearly all of the 13–14% of lung cancer patients who are long-term survivors. Furthermore, chemotherapy and radiation therapy are curative in some patients, but the vast majority of cure rates can be attributed to surgery alone.

Figure 4–4 Survival rates after surgical resection by stage of disease [P < .001].

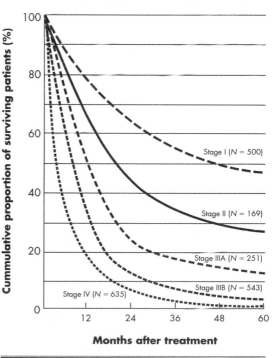

Source: Adapted from Mountain, 1986.

Photodynamic Therapy

Photodynamic therapy (PDT) is a compelling and cost-effective therapy that is an alternative to surgery for lung cancer patients. It is a two-step process that involves injecting a light-activated drug that targets cancer cells. Several days later, the cancerous cells are exposed to a spectrum of light by way of a laser. The light "switches on" the drug, destroying the cancer cells (Bruce, 2000). A typical example is porfimer sodium (Photofrin) (Sanofi Pharmaceuticals, Inc., 1996), which can selectively concentrate in cancer cells while largely clearing from healthy tissue (Bruce, 2000).

In one study involving 18 men and three women ranging in age from 53 to 81 years who underwent therapy at the Mayo clinic, it was found that at first 71% of the lung cancer disappeared in the patients and, after one year, 52% still had no detectable lung cancers (Mayo Clinic, 1997). Two to 10 years later, 43% have been spared surgery. Studies in Japan have shown that PDT completely eradicated 90% of small superficial tumors (Lam, 1994).

Many new techniques and photochemical agents are emerging because PDT is the topic of much new research. For example, when coupled with photodynamic diagnosis (PDD), complete remission rates of 92.1% (35 of 38 lesions) have been reported with centrally located, early stage lung cancer in 29 patients (Usuda, et al., 2007). In another study, 40 patients with NSCLC were treated with PDT, with a 72% (36 of 50 treated lesions) overall controlled rate (Corti, et al., 2007). PDT appears to be particularly effective for early inoperable or recurrent NSCLC. It should be considered as a treatment option in patients who are ineligible for resection (Moghissi, et al., 2007).

There are three main contraindications to PDT. These are known allergies to the photochemical agent, existing tracheoesophageal or bronchoesophageal fistulas, and patients with tumors that are eroding into a major vessel (Bruce, 2000). Precautionary measures should be exercised in patients with endobronchial tumors in which inflammation from the therapy itself can cause obstruction of the patient's airway. Esophageal varices are at high risk due to increased incidence of bleeding if PDT is given directly to the varices.

Interactions with PDT drugs and other drugs are understudied. An increased photosensitivity reaction could occur with the concomitant use of drugs considered to be photosensitizing agents, such as tetracycline, phenothiazines, and thiazide diuretics, to name a few (Bruce, 2000). There are agents that enhance the effects of PDT drugs, such as porfimer sodium, and there are agents, such as vitamin A compounds, vitamin E, ethanol, aspirin, and betacarotene that decrease their effects.

Postoperative PDT patients must be instructed to protect their skin from the effects of photosensitivity and ocular sensitivity. They must protect their exposed skin from any source of UV light because second- and third-degree burns have been reported (Bruce, 2000). They should wear clothing such as long-sleeved shirts, slacks, gloves, shoes, and socks. Dark sunglasses and a wide-brimmed hat are also recommended as protection from the sun's ultraviolet rays. The photosensitivity begins as soon as the injection occurs and will last for approximately 4 to 6 weeks (Bruce, 2000). At home, these patients should avoid exposure to strong indoor lighting and close proximity to unshaded light bulbs. The use of helmet-type hair dryers should be discouraged. Patients are usually also told to remain at least 6 feet from unshielded windows, including automobile windows, unless fully protected.

PDT is less invasive than conventional surgery. It shrinks and eliminates tumors, alleviates symptoms, and offers hope to patients for better quality of life. The patient satisfaction rate is high (based on 200 patients) (Moghissi, 2007). PDT is a compelling course of treatment for the elderly patient with a cardiac history who is not a surgical candidate. It is a good nonsurgical option that significantly reduces surgical and anesthesia risks.

Improving Postoperative Care: Other New Surgical Techniques, Enhancements, and Diagnostic Tools

Video-assisted thoracic surgery (VATS) improves patient care by decreasing the recovery period. Many surgeries can be done using the VATS technique. A VATS procedure enables a surgeon to make two to four tiny openings between the ribs while viewing the patient's internal organs on a television monitor (United States Surgical Corporation, 1999). Blebs can be treated, diagnoses and treatments around the lung and heart can be done, and mediastinal tumors can be evaluated. Additionally, a VATS procedure can be used to treat myasthenia gravis, nervous system disorders, and esophageal achalasia. Patients who have had previous thoracic surgery may not be candidates for a VATS procedure due to the potential of adhesions. The thoracic surgeon will need to make that assessment.

A VATS procedure has the benefit of reduced pain due to a smaller incision. Because ribs are not spread or cut, bone pain is reduced as compared to an open procedure. This generally allows

for a shorter hospital stay and, in many cases, a quicker return to work. The typical hospital length of stay is 1 to 3 days. Most patients are instructed to rest for about a week and then gradually increase their activity as they feel better.

VATS for lobectomy and segmentectomy is becoming increasingly popular. A study by Daniels and colleagues (2002) found VATS resection to be safe, with complication rates similar to that of open lobectomy. McKenna, reporting on 1100 VATS lobectomies performed at Cedar Sinai Medical Center between 1992 and 2004, confirmed that VATS lobectomies can achieve cure rates similar to those performed via thoracotomy (McKenna, Houck, & Fuller, 2006). Cattaneo and colleagues (2008) reported that VATS approach in the elderly patient resulted in a significantly lower rate of complications compared with thoracotomy (28% versus 45%) and a shorter median length of stay (5 days versus 6 days). There were no perioperative deaths in the VATS patients, compared with an in-hospital mortality rate of 3.6% of thoracotomy patients.

Robot-assisted surgery is being evaluated in many facilities for lobectomy. To date, it has not been shown to improve patient outcomes or reduce postoperative complications. Presently, robot surgical time requirements exceed conventional surgical times.

A surgical lung sealant is an acrylic-based surgical adhesive (superglue) used to reduce air leaks at the time of surgery. In a multihospital study done in 1998, the studies showed that there was a reduction in the number of air leaks following a pulmonary resection (Wain, et al., 2001). The sealant is applied intraoperatively with a syringe to the stapled area, and a light source is applied to polymerize the glue, sealing the treated area. The application of sealant resulted in control of air leaks in 92% of the patients who were treated (Wain, et al., 2001). This lung sealant has been shown to reduce hospital stays due to fewer postoperative air leaks and is now in common use.

Prolonged air leaks are a complication of thoracic surgery. A patient with minimal leakage or drainage can usually be discharged from the hospital with a Heimlich Chest Drain Valve. An improvement to the Heimlich valve is the Pneumostat Chest Drain Valve.

Currently there is no practical or definitive screening method for lung cancer, as there is for prostate and breast cancer (ACS, 2008). Chest X-rays may detect lung cancers too late, often when a cure may be difficult to achieve. Molecular detection of lung cancer is currently being researched in an attempt to detect the presence of lung cancer through blood and sputum samples. Using a polymerase chain reaction (PCR) based nucleotide acid analysis, lung cancer may be detected through blood and sputum samples as a screening tool to diagnose lung cancers. This type of screening is the focus of significant research and may one day become part of a routine screening physical examination.

Low-dose CT (LDCT) scanning remains the most promising of new lung cancer screening techniques, but the results of ongoing randomized trials are not expected for at least 2 to 3 years. Using relatively low radiation exposure to create a low-resolution image of the entire thorax, LDCT screening is capable of detecting very small, early stage cancers so that their growth can be observed noninvasively. Previous research has demonstrated that compared with chest X-ray (CXR), LDCT detects approximately three times as many small lung nodules; of those that are subsequently diagnosed as cancer, the overwhelming majority are stage I (Jett & Midthun, 2004). For more discussion regarding

screening, refer to Chapter 3, Controversies in Detection and Screening.

Clinical care pathways have been developed for a wide variety of disease processes that require medical and surgical intervention and are now mainstay. Clinical pathways were developed in an attempt to contain costs in an era of rising healthcare costs and limited resources (Zehr, Dawson, Yang, & Heitmiller, 1998). Pathway implementation has been shown to reduce hospital length of stay without compromising early or late outcome (Vigneswaran, Bhorade, Wolfe, Pelletiere, & Garrity, 2007) and significantly reduce diagnostic testing (Zehr, et al., 1998). An added benefit is that patients and their families are given clear expectations of what they may expect during the hospital course.

In one study done at the Johns Hopkins Hospital (JHH), it was shown that by utilizing clinical pathways, there was a marked reduction of length of stay for all major thoracic surgical procedures (Zehr, et al., 1998). Anatomic lung resections, such as segmentectomies, lobectomies, and pneumonectomies, were retrospectively analyzed for length of stay, hospital charges, and outcome (Zehr, et al., 1998). JHH found that lung resection patients had a decreased postoperative length of stay that was partly attributed to early discontinuation of a patient's chest tube (Zehr, et al., 1998). The thoracotomy clinical pathway emphasized operating room extubation and 12- to 24-hour intensive care unit care (Zehr, et al., 1998). In a retrospective examination of 183 isolated lung transplant patients, the length of stay (LOS) was 7 days, with an operative mortality of 6.5% and 1- and 3-year survival rates of 82% and 73%, respectively (Vigneswaran, et al., 2007). It was determined that the overall total charges for lung resections were reduced by 21%, with the greatest reduction in pharmaceuticals at 38%, followed by supplies at 34%, miscellaneous charges (physical therapy) at 25%, and lastly, routine charges (patient length of stay) at 22% (Zehr, et al., 1998). It was determined from this study that physicians have the greatest impact on what tests are ordered and what equipment is used. The physician becomes the utilization manager in reducing costs in all areas of patient care. The study also pointed out that patient care was not compromised (Zehr, et al., 1998).

Clinical care pathways are a method that has proven to effectively reduce cost in a high-volume surgical patient population. These pathways are a dynamic process that is revised and adjusted annually. Changes are made based upon physician and patient input. Quality of care has not been compromised, and by providing consistency in patient care in clinical care pathways, it is believed that the quality of care has improved.

Complementary and Alternative Therapies

Complementary therapies are showing increasing promise as useful and beneficial adjuncts to mainstream care. They provide supportive measures that can reduce symptoms and enhance patient well-being. Complementary therapies have been proven safe and effective over time. (Conversely, "alternative therapies" are usually unproved and unsupported and may lessen outcome, particularly when they lead to delay of regular oncology treatment.) Healthcare professionals should be able to provide evidence-based, patient-centered advice to patients regarding appropriate complementary therapies. Professionals should also be aware of popular alternative therapies, such as magnetic field therapy, counterproductive herbal treatments, and

energy field therapies, because these therapies are often promoted as viable options to mainstream care and can be very attractive to patients, particularly those in poor-outlook situations (Cassileth, et al., 2007).

Mind–body modalities are effective for the reduction of anxiety, mood disturbance, or chronic pain. These modalities include meditation, hypnosis, relaxation techniques, cognitive-behavioral therapy, biofeedback, and guided imagery. A meta-analysis of 116 studies found that mind–body therapies could reduce anxiety, depression, and mood disturbances in cancer patients and assist with their coping skills (Devine & Westlake, 1995). Mind–body techniques also may help reduce chronic low back pain, joint pain, headache, and procedural pain (Astin, 2004)

Massage therapy, when carefully applied by trained professionals, can also be beneficial for cancer patients or patients facing surgery. In one study, 87 hospitalized cancer patients were randomized to receive foot massage or control. Pain and anxiety scores decreased with massage (Grealish, Lomasney, & Whiteman, 2000). The application of deep massage or intense pressure should be avoided near lesions or anatomic distortions, such as postoperative changes. Patients with bleeding tendencies should receive only gentle, light-touch massage (Vigneswaran, et al., 2007).

Acupuncture and electroacupuncture are recommended for the reduction of nausea and vomiting (Lee & Done, 2004; Shen, Wenger, & Glaspy, 2000). Acupuncture appears to be effective in the control of cancer-related pain. In a study of 90 patients who received correct or sham acupuncture treatment, those who were treated correctly reported a 36% decrease in pain intensity 2 months from baseline, where the control group saw little reduction (Alimi, et al., 2003). While earlier smoking cessation studies are conflicting (White, Rampes, & Ernst, 2002), a recent randomized trial of 141 subjects showed that acupuncture could significantly reduce smoking, particularly when combined with education (Bier, et al., 2002).

In a randomized study of 739 patients, wearing acupressure wristbands on the day of chemotherapy significantly reduced nausea (Roscoe, Morrow, & Hickok, 2003). Conversely, the use of electrostimulation wristbands had no benefit and seemed, in some instances, to be counterproductive (Roscoe, et al., 2003).

Dietary supplements, in particular herbal products, must be used with care because they may interfere with or be antagonistic to mainstream treatment. Products that may interact should not be used concurrently during surgery, chemotherapy, or radiation (Kumar, Allen, & Bell, 2005).

Conclusion

Managing patients through thoracic surgery can be a challenging process best managed by a coordinated team approach utilizing the best available technology within the context of a physician-induced clinical care pathway. Continuing improvements in diagnostic methodology, surgical technique, and medical tools have made thoracic surgery increasingly safer and more effective. In those patients for whom surgery is not an option, several other effective treatment modalities exist, such as photodynamic therapy, chemotherapy, and radiation therapy. Useful complementary therapies exist for the improvement of patient comfort and psychological outlook. Promising molecular-level studies hold forth the possibility of still earlier and more accurate detection.

References

Alexander, J., & Anderson, R. (2000). Preoperative cardiac evaluation of the thoracic surgical patient and management of perioperative cardiac events. In T. W. Shields, J. LoCicero, & R. Ponn (Eds.), *General thoracic surgery* (5th ed., pp. 305–313). Philadelphia: Lippincott Williams & Wilkins.

Alimi, D., Rubino, C., Pichard-Leandri, E., Fermand-Brule, S., Dubreuil-Lemaire, M. L., & Hill, C. (2003). Analgesic effect of auricular acupuncture for cancer pain: A randomized, blinded, controlled trial. *Journal of Clinical Oncology, 21*(22), 4120–4126.

American Cancer Society. (2008). *Cancer facts & figures 2008*. Retrieved May 30, 2008, from http://www.cancer.org/downloads/stt/2008cafffinalsecured.pdf

Astin, J. A. (2004). Mind–body therapies for the management of pain. *Clinical Journal of Pain, 20*(1), 27–32.

Bier, I. D., Wilson, J., Studt, P., & Shakleton, M. (2002). Auricular acupuncture, education, and smoking cessation: A randomized sham-controlled trial. *American Journal of Public Health, 92*(10), 1642–1647.

Birim, O., Zuydendorp, M., Matt, A. P. W. M., Kappetin, A. P., Eijkemans, M. J. C., & Bogers, A. J. J. C. (2003). Lung resection for non-small-cell lung cancer in patients older than 70. *Annals of Thoracic Surgery, 76*(6), 1796–1801.

Bruce, S. (2000). Photodynamic therapy: Another option in cancer treatment. *Clinical Journal of Oncology Nursing, 5*(3), 95–99.

Cassileth, B., Deng, G., Gomez, J., Johnstone, P., Kumar, N., & Vickers, A. (2007). Complementary therapies and integrative oncology in lung cancer: ACCP evidence-based clinical practice guidelines (2nd ed.). *Chest, 132* (Suppl. 3), 340S-354S.

Cattaneo, S. M., Park, B. J., Wilton, A. S., Seshan, V. E., Bains, M. S., Downey, R. J., et al. (2008). Use of video-assisted thoracic surgery for lobectomy in the elderly results in fewer complications. *Annals of Thoracic Surgery, 85*(1), 231–236.

Celsus Laboratories, Inc. (1987). Heparin [Product insert]. Cincinnati, OH.

Colice, G. L., Shafazand, S., Griffin, J. P., Keenan, R., Bolliger, C. T., & American College of Chest Physicians. (2007). Physiologic evaluation of the patient with lung cancer being considered for resectional surgery: ACCP evidence-based clinical practice guidelines (2nd ed.). *Chest, 132*(Suppl. 3), 161S-177S.

Corti, L., Toniolo, L., Boso, C., Colaut, F., Fiore, D., Muzzio, P. C., et al. (2007). Long-term survival of patients treated with photodynamic therapy for carcinoma in situ and early non-small-cell lung carcinoma. *Lasers in Surgery and Medicine, 39*(5), 394–402.

Daniels, L. J., Balderson, S. S., Onaitis, M. W., & D'Amico, T. A. (2002). Thorascopic lobectomy: A safe and effective strategy for patients with stage I lung cancer. *Annals of Thoracic Surgery, 74*(3), 860–864.

Devine, E. C., & Westlake, S. K. (1995). The effects of psychoeducational care provided to adults with cancer: Metaanalysis of 116 studies. *Oncology Nursing Forum, 22*(9), 1369–1381.

DuPont Pharmaceuticals Company. (1999). Coumadin [Product insert]. Wilmington, DE.

Fry, W. (2000). Thoracic incisions. In T. W. Shields, J. LoCicero, & R. Ponn (Eds.), *General thoracic surgery* (5th ed., pp. 367–374). Philadelphia: Lippincott Williams & Wilkins.

Fukuse, T., Satoda, N., & Hijiiya, K. (2005). Importance of a comprehensive geriatric assessment in prediction of complications following thoracic surgery in elderly patients. *Chest, 127*(3), 886–891.

Ginsberg, R., Hill, L., Eagan, R., Thomas, P., Mountain, C., Deslauriers, J., et al. (1983). Modern thirty-day operative mortality for surgical resections in lung cancer. *The Journal of Thoracic and Cardiovascular Surgery, 86*(5), 654–658.

Goldstraw, P. (2000). Pneumonectomy and its modifications. In T. W. Shields, J. LoCicero, & R. Ponn (Eds.), *General thoracic surgery* (5th ed., pp. 411–421). Philadelphia: Lippincott Williams & Wilkins.

Gould, M. K., Fletcher, J., Iannettoni, M. D., Lynch, W. R., Midthun, D. E., Naidich, D. P., et al. (2007). Evaluation of patients with pulmonary nodules: When is it lung cancer? AACP evidence-based clinical practice guidelines (2nd ed.). *Chest, 132*, 108S–130S.

Gould, M. K., Sanders, G. D., Barnett, P. G., Rydzak, C. E., Maclean, C. C. McClellan, M. B., et al. (2003). Cost-effectiveness of alternative management strategies for patients with solitary pulmonary nodules. *Annals of Internal Medicine, 138*(9), 724–735.

Grealish, L., Lomasney, A., & Whiteman, B. (2000). Foot massage: A nursing intervention to modifying the distressing symptoms of pain and nausea in patients hospitalized with cancer [Abstract]. *Cancer Nurse, 23,* 237–243.

Hammoud, Z., Anderson, R., Meyers, B., Guthrie, T., Roper, C., Cooper, J., et al. (1999). The current role of mediastinoscopy in the evaluation of thoracic disease. *The Journal of Thoracic and Cardiovascular Surgery, 118*(5), 894–899.

Harwood, K. (1996). Non-small cell lung cancer: An overview of diagnosis, staging and treatment. *Seminars in Oncology Nursing, 12*(4), 285–294.

Hoffman-LaRoche, Inc. (2000). Toradol [Product insert]. Nutley, NJ.

Hong, W. (1998). *Molecular screening for lung cancer on the way.* Retrieved May 14, 2001, from www.3.mdanderson .org/~conquest/spring1998/lung.htm

Jett, J. R., & Midthun, D. E. (2004). Screening for lung cancer: Current status and future directions; Thomas A. Neff lecture. *Chest, 125,* 158s–162s.

Johnston, M. (1997). Curable lung cancer: How to find it and treat it. *Postgraduate Medicine, 101*(3), 155–163.

Kumar, N. B., Allen, K., & Bell, H. (2005). Perioperative herbal supplement use in cancer patients: Potential implications and recommendations for presurgical screening. *Cancer Control, 12*(3), 149–157.

Lam, S. (1994). Photodynamic therapy of lung cancer. *Seminars in Oncology, 21*(6, Suppl. 5), 15–16.

Lee, A., & Done, M. L. (2004). Stimulation of the wrist acupuncture point P6 for preventing postoperative nausea and vomiting. Cochrane Database System Review (CD003281).

Lee, B. E., Redwine, J., Foster, C., Abella, E., Lown, T., Lau, D., et al. (2008). Mediastinoscopy might not be necessary in patients with non-small cell lung cancer with mediastinal lymph nodes having a maximum standardized uptake value of less than 5.3. *Journal of Thoracic and Cardiovascular Surgery, 135*(3), 615–619.

Lee, B. E., von Haag, D., Lown, T., Lau, D., Calhoun, R., & Follette, D. (2007). Advances in positron emission tomography technology have increased the need for surgical staging in non-small-cell lung cancer. *Journal of Thoracic and Cardiovascular Surgery, 133*(3), 746–752.

LoCicero, J., Ponn, R., & Daly, B. (2000). Surgical treatment of non-small cell lung cancer. In T. Shields, J. LoCicero, & R. Ponn (Eds.), *General thoracic surgery* (5th ed., pp. 1311–1341). Philadelphia: Lippincott Williams & Wilkins.

Martini, N., Rusch, V., Bains, M., Kris, M., Downey, R., Flehinger, B., et al. (1999). Factors influencing ten-year survival in resected stages I to IIIA non-small cell lung cancer. *The Journal of Thoracic and Cardiovascular Surgery, 117*(1), 32–38.

Mayo Clinic. (1997). *Photodynamic therapy effective for early-stage lung cancer.* Retrieved May 10, 2001, from www.doguide.com

McKenna, R. J., Houck, W., & Fuller, C. B. (2006). Video-assisted thoracic surgery lobectomy: Experience with 1,100 cases. *Annals of Thoracic Surgery, 81*(2), 421–426.

Moghissi, K., Dixon, K., Thorpe, J. A. C., Stringer, M., & Oxtoby, C. (2007). Photodynamic therapy (PDT) in early central lung cancer: A treatment option for patients ineligible for surgical resection. *Thorax, 62*(5), 391–395.

Mountain, C. (1986). A new international staging system for lung cancer. *Chest, 89,* 225S–233S.

National Comprehensive Cancer Network (NCCN). (2008). *NCCN clinical practice guidelines in oncology. V.2.2008.* Retrieved July 17, 2008, from http://www.nccn.org.

Paone, G., Nicastri, E., Lucantoni, G., Dello Iacono, R., Battistoni, P., D'Angeli, A. L., et al. (2005). Endobronchial ultrasound-driven biopsy in the diagnosis of peripheral lung lesions. *Chest, 128*(5), 3551–3557.

Port, J., Kent, M., Korst, R., Lee, P. C., Levin, M. A., Flieder, D., et al. (2004). Surgical resection for lung cancer in the octogenarian. *Chest, 126*(3), 733–738.

Reed, C., & Silvestri, G. (2000). Diagnosis and staging of lung cancer. In T. Shields, J. LoCicero, & R. Ponn (Eds.), *General thoracic surgery* (5th ed., pp. 1297–1309). Philadelphia: Lippincott Williams & Wilkins.

Reilly, J. (1999). Evidence-based preoperative evaluation of candidates for thoracotomy. *Chest, 116*(Suppl. 6), 474S–476S.

Roscoe, J. A., Morrow, G. R., & Hickok, J. T. (2003). The efficacy of acupressure and accustimulation wrist bands for the relief of chemotherapy-induced nausea and vomiting: A University of Rochester Cancer Center Community Clinical Oncology Program multi-center study. *Journal of Pain Symptom Management, 26*(2), 731–742.

Roselli, E. E., Murthy, S. C., Rice, T. W., Houghtaling, P. L., Pierce, C. D., Karchmer, D. P., et al. (2005). Atrial fibrillation complicating lung cancer resection. *Journal of Thoracic and Cardiovascular Surgery, 130*(2), 438–444.

Salazar, A., & Westcott, J. (1993). The role of transthoracic needle biopsy for the diagnosis and staging of lung cancer. *Clinical Chest Medicine, 14*(1), 99–110.

Sanofi Pharmaceuticals, Inc. (1996). Photofrin [Product insert]. New York.

Sedrakyan, A., Treasure, T., Browne, J., Krumholz, H., Sharpin, C., & van der Meulen, J. (2005). Pharmacologic prophylaxis for postoperative atrial tachyarrhythmia in general thoracic surgery. *Journal of Thoracic and Cardiovascular Surgery, 129*(5), 997–1005.

Shen, J., Wenger, N., & Glaspy, J. (2000). Electroacupuncture for control of myeloablative chemotherapy-induced emesis: A randomized controlled trial. *Journal of the American Medical Association, 284*(21), 2755–2761.

Shields, T. W. (2000). General features of pulmonary resections. In T. Shields, J. LoCicero, & R. Ponn (Eds.), *General thoracic surgery* (5th ed., pp. 375–384). Philadelphia: Lippincott Williams & Wilkins.

United States Department of Health and Human Services. (1999). *Surgery.* Washington, DC: Author.

United States Surgical Corporation. (1999). *Video assisted lung surgery.* Retrieved August 12, 2001, from www.ussurg.com/health-care/patients/v-a-t-s/

Usuda, J., Tsutsui, H., Honda, H., Ichinose, S., Ishizumi, T., Hirata, T., et al. (2007). Photodynamic therapy for lung cancers based on novel photodynamic analysis using talaporfin sodium (NPe6) and antifluorescence bronchosopy. *Lung Cancer, 58*(3), 317–323.

Vigneswaran, W. T., Bhorade, S., Wolfe, M., Pelletiere, K., & Garrity, E. R., Jr. (2007). Clinical pathway after lung transplantation shortens hospital stay without affecting outcome. *International Surgery, 92*(2), 92–98.

Wain, J., Kaiser, L., Johnstone, D., Yang, S., Wright, C., Friedberg, J., et al. (2001). Trial of a novel synthetic sealant in preventing air leaks after lung resection. *The Annals of Thoracic Surgery, 71*(5), 1623–1629.

White, A. R., Rampes, H., & Ernst, E. (2002). Acupuncture for smoking cessation. Cochrane Database System Review (CD000009).

Wright, C. D., Gaissert, H. A., Grab, J. D., O'Brien, S. M., Peterson, E. D., & Allen, M. S. (2008). Predictors of prolonged length of stay after lobectomy for lung cancer: A Society of Thoracic Surgeons General Thoracic Surgery Database risk-adjustment model. *Annals of Thoracic Surgery, 85*(6), 1857–1865.

Yoshimatsu, R., Yamagami, T., Kato, T., Hirota, T., Matsumoto, J., Shimada, J., et al. (2008). Percutaneous needle biopsy of lung nodules under CT fluoroscopic guidance with use of the "I-I" device. *British Journal of Radiology, 81*(962), 107–112.

Zehr, K., Dawson, P., Yang, S., & Heitmiller, R. (1998). Standardized clinical care pathways for major thoracic cases reduce hospital costs. *Annals of Thoracic Surgery, 66*(3), 914–919.

Chapter 5

Chemotherapy and Lung Cancer

Pamela Hallquist Viale

Introduction

Lung cancer has not only become a common cancer, but it remains a lethal one because this type of tumor is the most frequent cause of cancer death in many countries around the world (Onn, et al., 2006; Molina, Adjei, & Jett, 2006). The death rate for this disease has declined gradually for men, but it continues to increase in women (Ramalingam & Belani, 2008). Unfortunately, almost 70% of patients with lung cancer present with advanced or metastatic disease at diagnosis (Molina, et al., 2006). Therefore, there is intense interest in changing the outcome of this disease. Despite improvements in the therapies for both general types of lung cancer, non-small cell lung cancer (NSCLC) and small cell lung cancer (SCLC), the survival rates for 5 years are still very low; however, there are new approaches in the treatment of this tumor type. Conventional chemotherapy has become an integral component of treatment in conjunction with surgery and radiation therapy for most stages of disease, but newer targeted therapies are gaining ground and have a significant role in the treatment of lung cancer. Antiangiogenesis agents are also becoming an important part of the armamentarium of treatments for lung can-

cer as well. Understanding the biology of the disease and the differences in certain subsets of lung cancer has helped to define specific targets for therapy and agents directed toward these targets (Onn, et al., 2006). Although some trial results have reported longer survivals for specific sets of patients, therapy is still not optimal for lung cancer. Therefore, prevention of this common but often deadly disease is paramount, and smoking cessation efforts along with reduction of environmental causes is crucial (Onn, et al., 2006). This chapter will review current and historical treatments for NSCLC and SCLC. Combined modality and neoadjuvant therapy will be discussed. New targeted therapies will be reviewed. Although lung cancer remains a lethal tumor for many patients, median survival times and survival rates have been improved for some patients with the use of improved, conventional chemotherapy and targeted therapy agents.

Non-Small Cell Lung Cancer

The role of conventional chemotherapy is now well established in the treatment of patients with NSCLC. Non-small cell lung cancer represents approximately 80% of all lung cancers and includes squamous cell carcinoma, adenocarcinoma, and large cell carcinoma, with most patients presenting with late-stage disease leading to a poor prognosis (Bunn & Thatcher, 2008). The American Society of Clinical Oncology (ASCO) treatment of unresectable non-small cell lung cancer guideline notes that traditional chemotherapy has a role for patients with both locally advanced and metastatic disease (Pisters, et al., 2007b; Pfister, et al., 2004). The treatment for this disease is based on staging (Ramalingam & Belani, 2008). Therefore, accurate staging is essential in the workup of the patient with newly diagnosed non-small cell lung cancer and determines the appropriate role of surgery and radiation therapy for this disease, as well as chemotherapy. Despite the significant and historical role of surgery in the treatment of certain stages of NSCLC, survival rates remained poor, with frequent relapse of disease noted at distant sites (Pisters, et al., 2007b). Both radiation therapy and chemotherapy have been used to improve the survival of patients with both resectable and nonresectable disease (Pisters, et al., 2007b).

Unresectable Non-Small Cell Lung Cancer

Almost 40% of patients with NSCLC are diagnosed with advanced-stage disease, which includes both metastatic disease or those patients who present with locally advanced disease with malignant pleural or pericardial effusion (Ramalingam & Belani, 2008). Historically, chemotherapy treatments for NSCLC began with stage IV or advanced disease, and single agent therapies were tested for efficacy in the 1980s

(Onn, et al., 2006). Of these single agent therapies, several were found to be active against lung cancer, including cisplatin, ifosfamide, mitomycin C, etoposide, vindesine, and vinblastine (Onn, et al., 2006). Although these single therapies had activity, the most progress with a demonstrated survival benefit was noted with platinum-based chemotherapy, showing improvement in stage II–IV NSCLC, as well as some data with stage IB disease (Bunn & Thatcher, 2008).

Chemotherapy options are usually chosen based on the patient's performance status (PS), because it helps to determine the ultimate outcome for the patient (Albain, Crowley, LeBlanc, & Livingston, 1991). In a retrospective analysis of 2,531 patients with extensive-stage NSCLC, Albain et al. noted that good performance status, female gender, and age greater than 70 years were significant independent predictors; hemoglobin levels greater than 11.0 g/dl, normal lactate dehydrogenase, normal calcium, and a single metastatic site also predicted more favorable status (1991).

First-Line Therapies for Advanced Non-Small Cell Lung Cancer

Cisplatin-based chemotherapy was shown to produce a small benefit clinically in patients with advanced NSCLC in a meta-analysis from 1995, and although newer therapies have shown activity in this disease as well, the platinum combination is considered the standard regimen (Hotta et al. 2007). A review of important trials discussing platinum combinations in advanced NSCLC follows.

The Role of Platinum-Based Therapies

Combination chemotherapy regimens based on platinum agents were found to be superior to best supportive care (BSC) regimens in the first-line setting with advanced NSCLC (Ramalingam & Belani, 2008). Previously considered somewhat controversial, the benefit of this combination was first published in a report of a Canadian multicenter randomized trial in 1988 (Rapp, et al.). The authors discussed the results of a prospective randomized trial that compared BSC to two chemotherapy regimens, vindesine and cisplatin (VP) and cyclophosphamide, doxorubicin, and cisplatin (CAP). Out of the 251 patients evaluated for the study, 233 were deemed eligible (Rapp, et al., 1988). Most of the patients (82.5%) had distant metastases or were ineligible for radiation or surgery due to their stage of disease. Patients in the chemotherapy arms achieved an overall response rate of 15.3% on the CAP arm and 25.3% on the VP arm. The median survival of patients treated with VP was 32.6 weeks versus 24.7 weeks with CAP and 17 weeks with BSC, although toxicity on the chemotherapy arms was significant, with higher rates of leukopenia, vomiting, and neurotoxicity (with VP) (Rapp, et al., 1988) In a large meta-analysis that examined data on individual patients ($n = 9387$) from 52 randomized clinical trials, the use of platinum-based chemotherapy was further validated (Non-Small Cell Lung Cancer Collaborative Group, 1995). This large trial showed results of a consistent benefit of as much as 10% for cisplatin-based chemotherapy in all comparisons, particularly when used with radiotherapy and supportive care. The 10% improvement was considered to be significant due to the fact that lung cancer affects so many patients (Non-Small Cell Lung Cancer Collaborative Group, 1995). Therefore, despite a modest benefit, the meta-analysis did show a statistically significant improvement in survival, with the 10% gained in survival translating to approximately 6 weeks for 1 year of survival.

Comparison of Carboplatin versus Cisplatin

The benefits of carboplatin-based chemotherapy regimens are easier administration and decreased toxicities as compared to cisplatin-based regimens (Ramalingam & Belani, 2008). More hematologic (neutropenia, thrombocytopenia, and anemia) toxicities are seen in patients who receive cisplatin regimens (Ramalingam & Belani, 2008). In fact, because of the decreased toxicities, some researchers favor carboplatin regimens despite the small advantages seen with cisplatin regimens. Researchers have directly compared the two regimens in several trials. Rosell et al. examined carboplatin with paclitaxel to cisplatin and paclitaxel in a trial of 618 patients (2002). This was a phase III study of chemotherapy-naïve patients with advanced NSCLC. The response rate was 25% for the paclitaxel–carboplatin patients versus 28% in the paclitaxel–cisplatin patients (Rosell, et al., 2002). The median survival was 8.2 months for the paclitaxel–carboplatin patients and 9.8 months for the paclitaxel–cisplatin patients. The researchers concluded that the response rates were similar, but the cisplatin arm had a significantly longer median survival, and the researchers believed that cisplatin-based chemotherapy should be the first option (Rosell, et al., 2002). However, many clinicians note that there is similar efficacy in several regimens for this tumor type and that perhaps the choice of therapy should take into account ease of administration (cisplatin requires extensive hydration, which translates into longer infusion times), toxicity profile (cisplatin is more emetogenic than carboplatin and has significant hematologic toxicity), and cost (Ramalingam & Belani, 2008). Carboplatin is also dosed differently than cisplatin. Carboplatin's method of dosing is by the area under the curve (AUC; see Table 5–1).

These data cemented the role of platinum as the standard agent used in most of our modern chemotherapy regimens. Other single agents were then combined with platinum agents in hopes of increasing efficacy (Onn, et al., 2006). These agents include topoisomerase I inhibitors, taxanes, and other analog therapies, such as gemcitabine, vinorelbine, and irinotecan. When combined with platinum, response rates have been significant for specific agents.

The Role of Platinum in Combination

The efficacy of platinum in the treatment of advanced NSCLC has been established; however, researchers have combined this agent with several other chemotherapy drugs in an attempt to improve the treatment of NSCLC. Different platinum combinations will be discussed.

Platinum and Vinorelbine Combination

Wozniak et al. studied 415 NSCLC patients with advanced-stage disease in a randomized trial to receive either cisplatin or cisplatin and vinorelbine in combination (1998). The patients who received single-agent cisplatin had a 12% partial response rate, but the patients on the cisplatin–vinorelbine arm had a 26% rate (2%

Table 5–1 Area Under the Curve Measurement (AUC)

Non-Small Cell Lung Cancer

Table 8-1. Carboplatin Dose Calculation

Calvert's formula	Dose (mg) = (target AUCa mg/ml/min)^3 (GFR ml/min + 25)
GFR determination	
Cockcroft and Gault formula	Estimated GFR = $\dfrac{\text{ABW in kg } (140 - \text{age})}{\text{Cr} \times 72} \begin{matrix} \times 1.0 \text{ in males} \\ \times 0.85 \text{ in females} \end{matrix}$
Jelliffe's formula	Estimated GFR:
	1) E (males) = ABW 3 (29.305 2[0.203 3 (age)])
	E (females) = ABW 3 (25.3 2 [0.18 3 (age)])
	2) CrCl = E/(SCr 3 14.4)
	3) CrCl/1.73 m2 = CrCl 3 1.73/BSA

[a]Most 3- to 4-week schedules employ an AUC of 5.0 to 7.5, whereas weekly schedules typically employ an AUC of < = 2.0. AUC = area under time vs. concentration curve; GFR = glomerular filtration rate; ABW = adjusted body weight; SCr = serum creatinine; E = urinary creatinine excretion rate; CrCl = creatinine clearance

complete response and 24% partial responses), although there were significantly more hematological toxicities on the combination arm (Wozniak, et al., 1998). The toxicities observed were grades 3 and 4 granulocytopenia in 81% of the patients on the combination arm versus 5% on the single agent arm. Both arms had observed toxicities of renal insufficiency, ototoxicity, and nausea and vomiting, as well as neuropathy (Wozniak, et al., 1998). Vinorelbine was approved by the Food and Drug Administration (FDA) for the treatment of NSCLC in 1994.

Platinum and Taxanes Combination

Taxanes have been found to be effective when combined with a platinum agent, and several studies have examined their efficacy in NSCLC (Ramalingam & Belani, 2008). A randomized phase III trial comparing cisplatin–etoposide to carboplatin–paclitaxel in advanced or metastatic NSCLC was reported in 2005 by Belani et al. There were 369 patients enrolled in the study, of whom 179 received cisplatin and etoposide (arm A) and 190 received carboplatin and paclitaxel (arm B). Although there were significantly more women randomized to receive cisplatin–etoposide, both arms were otherwise well balanced. The objective response rate (ORR) was 15% on arm A with 23% observed on arm B, and the median survival time for arm A was 274 days versus 233 days for arm B. The 1-year survival rate for arm B was 37% versus 32% on arm B, and there were more toxicities on arm A versus arm B (predominantly neutropenia). The researchers concluded that there was no statistically significant survival advantage for arm A versus arm B, although the carboplatin–paclitaxel patients had a higher quality of life than those who received cisplatin and etoposide (Belani, et al., 2005).

Another randomized trial looked at paclitaxel plus carboplatin (PC) over vinorelbine with cisplatin (VC) in NSCLC (Kelley, et al., 2001). With 202 patients on the VC arm versus 206 patients in the PC arm, the objective response rate was 28% for the VC patients and 25% for the PC patients, with median survival of 8 months for both arms. However, more patients on the VC discontinued their therapy due to toxicity (grade 3 and 4 leukopenia and neutropenia, with grade 3 nausea and vomiting versus grade 3 peripheral neuropathy on the PC arm), although quality of life (QOL) was similar for both arms (Kelley, et al., 2001).

An Eastern Cooperative Oncology Group (ECOG) trial studied paclitaxel in a multi-institutional trial for stage IIIB to IV NSCLC patients who were randomized to receive either paclitaxel at two different dose levels (135 mg/m2 and 250 mg/m2) with cisplatin or etoposide with cisplatin (Bonomi, et al., 2000). The 599 patients were well balanced among the three arms of the studies, and superior survival was noted with the combined paclitaxel arms (with a median survival time of 9.9 months and a 1-year survival rate of 38.9%) compared with the etoposide and cisplatin. The combination of paclitaxel (at the 135 mg/m2 dose) with cisplatin was found to be efficacious. The toxicity was fairly similar across all three arms, except for increased myalgias, neurotoxicity, and possibly treatment-related cardiac events with the higher dose of paclitaxel.

Shepherd and colleagues studied single-agent docetaxel versus BSC in NSCLC patients to determine if this therapy could result in longer survival (2000). Time to progression was significantly longer for the patients on the docetaxel arm (10.6 versus 6.7 weeks) as well as median survival (7.0 versus 4.6 months), although there were more hematological toxicities noted for the chemotherapy group (Shepherd, et al., 2000). Their conclusion was that the benefits outweighed the risk of therapy for this tumor type. Interest in the combination of docetaxel with platinum generated new trials for this agent in combination. A randomized, multinational phase III trial examined two combinations of docetaxel plus platinum in advanced NSCLC versus vinorelbine plus cisplatin as first-line therapy for this disease. Patients ($n = 1218$) were assigned to receive docetaxel at a dose of 75 mg/m2 and cisplatin 75 mg/m2 (DC) every three weeks versus docetaxel 75 mg/m2 and carboplatin (DCb) area under the curve (AUC) (see Table 5–1) of 6 every 3 weeks versus vinorelbine 25 mg/m2/week and cisplatin (VC) 100 mg/m2 every 4 weeks (Fossella, et al., 2003). The patients on the DC arm had a better overall response and survival rate versus those who received VC, and both of the docetaxel arms were better tolerated and showed better QOL scores compared to VC. The researchers concluded that platinum combined with docetaxel was both effective and better tolerated in this study (Fossella, et al., 2003).

Both paclitaxel and docetaxel are approved by the FDA in the treatment of NSCLC. Docetaxel is currently approved as a single agent second-line therapy for this disease after failure of prior platinum-based chemotherapy or in combination with cisplatin for patients with unresectable, locally advanced NSCLC who have not previously received chemotherapy for this condition (Taxotere prescribing information, 2007). Paclitaxel is approved in combination with cisplatin for first-line therapy of NSCLC

patients who are not candidates for potential curative surgery and/or radiation therapy (Taxol prescribing information, 2007).

Platinum and Irinotecan Combination

The combination of irinotecan and cisplatin has also been studied in NSCLC. A small group of 42 patients was enrolled in the study. They received irinotecan on days 1, 8, and 15, with cisplatin on day 1 for four cycles (Mok, et al., 2007). Sequential docetaxel was given to the patients no matter what clinical response was achieved. There was a response rate of 45.2% at the end of the cisplatin and irinotecan chemotherapy. The progression-free survival (PFS) was 8.0 months, with an overall median survival of 14.6 months. The researchers concluded that sequential administration of cisplatin and irinotecan followed by docetaxel is feasible, with a prolonged PFS, but the improvement in outcome via sequential treatment is not confirmed (Mok, et al., 2007). Irinotecan and cisplatin in conjunction with concurrent-split-course radiotherapy in locally advanced NSCLC was also evaluated in a phase II study, showing an overall response rate of 83% (Fukuda, et al., 2007). The researchers concluded that this combined modality is active and needs further investigation (Fukuda, et al., 2007). Irinotecan is not approved in the United States for the treatment of NSCLC.

Platinum and Ifosfamide Combination

Cisplatin, ifosfamide, and gemcitabine (GIP) has been studied in patients with NSCLC. Results from a phase II study were reported in which 60 patients received the combination of three drugs (Planchard, et al., 2006). The median survival for all patients was 9 months, with a median time to progression of 6.3 months and a PFS at 1 and 2 years for all patients of 22% and 8%, respectively (Planchard, et al., 2006). The conclusion was that the GIP combination is comparable to other triplet drug combinations, with an acceptable toxicity profile. Although ifosfamide is used in the treatment of multiple cancers, it is not specifically indicated for the treatment of NSCLC.

Platinum and Gemcitabine Combination

Gemcitabine is also approved by the FDA for the treatment of NSCLC. The drug is indicated in combination with cisplatin for the first-line treatment of patients with inoperable, locally advanced (stage IIIA or IIIB), or metastatic (stage IV) NSCLC (Gemzar prescribing information, 2007). There are several positive phase III studies that show the benefit of this combination of drug therapy for this disease. One trial compared gemcitabine–cisplatin with etoposide–cisplatin in advanced NSCLC with a primary end point of response rate (Cardenal, et al., 1999). A group of 135 chemotherapy-naïve patients were randomized to the combination of either gemcitabine or etoposide along with cisplatin given in 21 day cycles. The combination of gemcitabine–cisplatin was superior to the etoposide–cisplatin regimen, with a response rate of 40.6% versus 21.9% and a significant delay in time to disease progression (6.0 months versus 4.3 months was also noted for the gemcitabine patients). However, no significant difference was noted in survival time between the two arms (8.7 months for the gemcitabine combination patients versus 7.2 months for the etoposide patients), and the toxicities

were generally similar. Crino and colleagues studied gemcitabine and cisplatin (GC) with mitomycin, ifosfamide, and cisplatin (MIC) in patients with stage IIIB or stage IV NSCLC with QOL, response rates, survival, and toxicity as the study end points (1999). A group of 307 patients was randomized to either study arm, and the results showed that the objective response rate was 38% in the GC arm compared to 26% in the MIC arm, with a median survival time of 8.6 months for the patients on GC versus 9.6 months for patients on MIC. Hematological toxicity (namely grade 3 and 4 thrombocytopenia) was higher with GC, and the researchers concluded that GC had a similar overall survival and increased response rate for patients on GC compared to MIC (Crino, et al., 1999).

Another phase III trial of 522 assessable patients with advanced or metastatic NSCLC received either single agent cisplatin or cisplatin plus gemcitabine in combination in a randomized trial (Sandler, et al., 2000). The combination patients had a 30.4% response rate compared to 11.1% ($p < 0.0001$) in the cisplatin single-agent arm, with median time to progress disease 5.6 months compared to 3.7 months and overall survival of 9.1 months compared to 7.6 months (Sandler, et al., 2000). However, the combination arm had more toxicity than single-agent therapy, with patients showing grade 4 thrombocytopenia occurring in 25.4% versus 0.8% in the patients on the single-agent cisplatin arm. The incidence of neutropenic fevers was less than 5% in both arms, although grade 4 neutropenia occurred in 35.3% of the patients in the combination arm versus 1.2% on the cisplatin arm (Sandler, et al., 2000).

Schiller et al. compared four different chemotherapy regimens for advanced NSCLC in a randomized trial to determine which of the therapies would prove to be superior to cisplatin and paclitaxel versus cisplatin–gemcitabine, cisplatin–docetaxel, or carboplatin–paclitaxel (2002). This large study enrolled 1155 eligible patients, and the response rate for all patients was 19%, with a median survival of 7.9 months and a 1-year survival rate of 33% (Schiller, et al., 2002). Response rates and survival times were significantly different between the cisplatin–paclitaxel arm and the three other regimens; however, there was a significantly longer time to progression of disease in the cisplatin–gemcitabine arm compared to cisplatin–paclitaxel treatment. Renal toxicity was also higher in the cisplatin–gemcitabine arm. The toxicities seen included the expected myelosuppression and aforementioned renal toxicity, as well as nausea and vomiting, diarrhea, hypersensitivity reactions, weakness, and neuropathy. The researchers concluded that none of the four different chemotherapy regimens that were studied showed a significant advantage over the others for the treatment of this disease, and some of the combinations had higher toxicity (Schiller, et al., 2002). For this study, patients with a poor performance status (2) were excluded from the study after the early data suggested that these patients were more likely to suffer adverse events, including death within 30 days from any cause, leading the researchers to conclude that routine use of platinum-based combination chemotherapy in patients with a poor performance status should not be recommended (Schiller, et al., 2002).

The currently available data suggests that there is a clear role for platinum-based therapy and that platinum in combination achieves a survival benefit versus platinum alone. Choosing the appropriate starting therapy in the first-line setting requires the clinician to take into account quality of life concerns and potential toxicities of selected chemotherapy combinations (Onn, et al., 2006). Oncology nurses should be aware of possible treatment strategies for this disease as well as the common side effect profiles of these agents.

Combined Modality Therapy for Non-Small Cell Lung Cancer

Combined modality therapy is an important part of therapy for this disease. Many patients will experience recurrent and/or metastatic disease despite surgical treatment and chemotherapy. Therefore, the addition of radiotherapy has gained support, and the development of new treatment strategies is needed. In fact, combined modality with chemotherapy and radiotherapy in stage III NSCLC is considered to be the standard therapy approach for this stage of disease (Stinchcombe, Fried, Morris, & Socinski, 2006). Keller et al. conducted a randomized trial to determine the role of thoracic radiotherapy alone versus combination chemotherapy plus thoracic radiotherapy in preventing local recurrence and prolonging survival in patients with completely resected stage II or IIIa NSCLC (2000). The 488 patients were randomly assigned to receive either four 28-day cycles of cisplatin and etoposide with concurrent radiotherapy versus radiotherapy alone. The combined modality patients had a treatment-associated mortality rate of 1.6% versus 1.2% in the radiotherapy alone group (Keller, et al., 2000). The median survival for the combined modality group was 38 months versus 39 months in the group that was given radiotherapy alone, and the researchers concluded that the addition of cisplatin and etoposide did not decrease the risk of intrathoracic recurrence or prolong survival in patients with completely resected stage II or IIIa NSCLC (Keller, et al., 2000). However, a phase III study that was performed to determine whether concurrent or sequential treatment with radiotherapy and chemotherapy improved survival in unresectable stage III NSCLC with 320 patients showed that a significantly superior median survival duration was achieved for the patients in the concurrent therapy group (16.5 months) versus sequential therapy (13.3 months). The chemotherapy was a combination of cisplatin, vindesine, and mitomycin (Furuse, et al., 1999).

In a prospective randomized trial, radiotherapy alone, sequential chemotherapy and radiotherapy, and comcomitant chemotherapy and radiation therapy in unresectable NSCLC were studied (Dasgupta, Dasgupta, Basu, & Majumdar, 2006). The 103 patients were randomized to receive radiotherapy alone; neoadjuvant therapy with cisplatin and etoposide for three cycles followed by radiotherapy and three more cycles of the same chemotherapy regimen; and radiotherapy with concurrent chemotherapy (cisplatin and etoposide), followed by two more cycles of chemotherapy with the same regimen (Dasgupta, et al., 2006). The toxicities were more significant in the combined modality groups; however, the researchers concluded that they were manageable. The chemotherapy groups had a decreased time to distant metastasis (65% for radiotherapy alone versus 48.6% for the neoadjuvant group and 44.4% for the concurrent group) (Dasgupta, et al., 2006). However, at the 2-year follow-up, the overall survival for the groups that received combined modality did not show any benefit, although response rates and disease-free survival DFS were positively affected.

There is interest in improving the response rates of combined modality treatments for locally advanced NSCLC, including using higher doses of thoracic radiation (Blackstock & Govindan, 2007). Although cisplatin and etoposide have been the focus of much of combined modality research, other agents have been used as well. It is accepted that concomitant therapies produce better results than sequential therapy; however, the most efficacious dose of radiation is still at question. Socinski et al. (2008) published the results of a randomized phase II trial of induction chemotherapy followed by concurrent chemotherapy and dose-escalated thoracic conformal radiotherapy (74 Gy) in stage III non-small cell lung cancer. Patients were randomized to receive induction chemotherapy with either carboplatin and paclitaxel or carboplatin with gemcitabine in combination with concurrent radiotherapy at 74 Gy (Socinski, et al., 2008). There was higher pulmonary toxicity in the carboplatin–gemcitabine group, which led to the closure of that arm of the study. The median survival time was 24.3 months, and this result will be compared to a standard dose of radiotherapy in a randomized phase III trial.

Platinum and Pemetrexed

Pemetrexed, a folate antagonist, was studied in combination with cisplatin (AC) versus gemcitabine plus cisplatin (GC) in 1725 patients with stage IIIb/IV NSCLC who had not received prior therapy before. The median survival was 10.3 months in the AC arm versus 10.3 months in the GC arm with median PFS of 4.8 and 5.1 months for AC and GC patients, respectively.

In September 2008, the cominbation of cisplatin with pemetrexed was approved for the initial treatment of patients with locally advanced or metastatic non-squamous NSCLC. It is not indicated for patients with squamous cell disease.

Second- and Third-Line Therapies for Non-Small Cell Lung Cancer

After the initial acceptance of the role of chemotherapy for NSCLC in the first-line setting, interest has grown in possible second- and third-line chemotherapy options for this disease. Currently, docetaxel, pemetrexed, and erlotinib are approved as second-line therapies for NSCLC. As noted previously, single agent docetaxel has activity against this tumor type and can produce longer survival in patients on this agent versus BSC (Shepherd, et al., 2000). Fossella and colleagues studied docetaxel monotherapy in 373 patients who were randomized to single docetaxel (in two different doses, 100 mg/m2 or 75 mg/m2) versus vinorelbine or ifosfamide (2000). The overall response rates were 10.8% for the higher docetaxel dose and 6.7% with the 75 mg/ m2 dose versus 0.8% response for the vinorelbine or ifosfamide patients. Overall survival was not significantly different between the three groups; however, the 1-year survival was greater with the 75 mg/m2 docetaxel patients than the control treatment. The researchers concluded that this randomized trial offered patients meaningful benefit when receiving docetaxel at the 75 mg/m2 dose (Fossella, et al., 2000). Additionally, docetaxel-associated toxicity was more significant at the higher dose in one phase II trial, particularly hematologic toxicity (Quoix, et al., 2004).

Pemetrexed is a novel agent that functions as a multitargeted antifolate agent (Onn, et al., 2006). Its activity in both recurrent and progressive NSCLC has been reported in several studies (de Marinis & Grossi, 2008). Smit and colleagues conducted a phase II trial that evaluated pemetrexed against NSCLC in a second-line setting (2003). A group of 81 patients was assigned to receive pemetrexed based on whether the first-line therapy that was given had included a platinum regimen, and the response rate for the platinum-pretreated group was 4.5% versus 14.1% in the nonplatinum-treated group. The median duration of response was 6.8 months, with a median survival time of 5.7 months. The researchers concluded that this new therapy was active in a second-line setting in nonplatinum-pretreated patients with NSCLC who progressed within 3 months of first-line therapy (Smit, et al., 2003).

Phase III studies were conducted with Hanna and colleagues (2004). The researchers examined pemetrexed versus docetaxel in patients who had previously been treated with one prior chemotherapy regimen for advanced NSCLC. The patients were randomized to either receive pemetrexed (with vitamin B12, folic acid, and dexamethasone or docetaxel [75 mg/m2]). A group of 571 patients was entered into the study, and the overall response rates were 9.1% and 8.8% (for pemetrexed and docetaxel, respectively). The median PFS was 2.9 months for both arms, with a 1-year survival rate of 29.7% for each arm. Although the researchers concluded that pemetrexed had a clinically equivalent efficacy outcome as compared to docetaxel, they felt that the novel therapy had much fewer side effects than docetaxel and should be considered a standard therapy in the second-line setting when available for therapy (Hanna, et al., 2004). Pemetrexed is the only therapy that has been directly compared to an active chemotherapy agent (docetaxel) in the second-line setting (de Marinis & Grossi, 2008).

Current guidelines now recognize pemetrexed in combination with platinum as a reasonable first-line therapy option for patients who have a performance status of 0-1 and nonsquamous histology (NCCN 2008a). Additionally, recently presented data at the American Society of Clinical Oncology (ASCO) 2008 meeting showed that maintenance therapy with pemetrexed administered after the induction of platinum-based chemotherapy doubled the time to progression for patients with advanced NSCLC (Ciuleanu, et al., 2008). The researchers studied 663 patients, and the patients who received the maintenance therapy had a significantly longer PFS than the placebo group (4.04 months versus 1.97 months, $p <$ 0.0001). The best responses to this agent are seen in patients who do not have squamous cell tumors (Ciuleanu, et al., 2008). As an antifolate agent, nurses must assure that patients receive folic acid and vitamin B12 to protect against

treatment-related hematologic and gastrointestinal toxicities; renal toxicity should be monitored as well.

Targeted Therapies

One of the most intriguing changes in the treatment of NSCLC in the second- or third-line setting has been the development of targeted therapies. These specific therapies are selective in their action and toxicities versus traditional chemotherapy with its more general toxicities. Two of the best-studied categories in the treatment of this cancer include the epidermal growth factor receptor (EGFR) inhibitor agents and the vascular endothelial growth factor (VEGF) receptor (see Figures 5–1, 5–2, and 5–3).

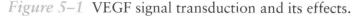

Figure 5–1 VEGF signal transduction and its effects.

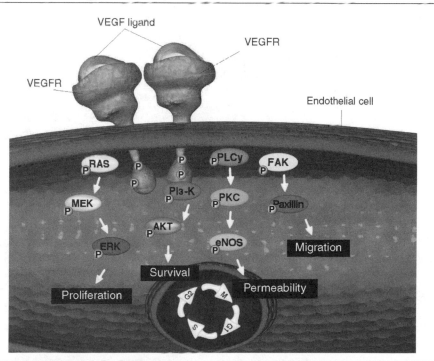

Source: Reprinted with permission from the Institute for Medical Education and Research.

Figure 5–2 Mechanisms of action of common targeted therapies used in solid tumors.

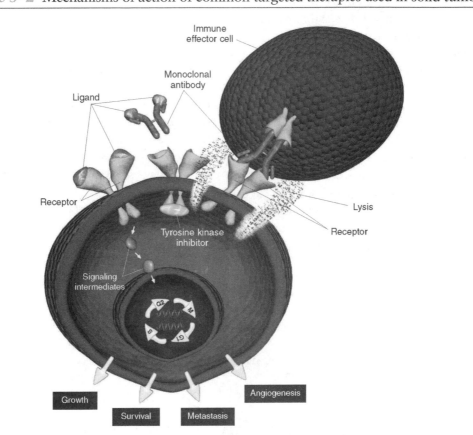

Source: Reprinted with permission from the Institute for Medical Education and Research.

The EGFR is overexpressed typically in 80–90% of patients with NSCLC (Kollmansberger, et al., 2006). The EGFR is part of the ERBB family of cell membrane receptors and is integral to cellular growth and survival (Gridelli, et al., 2007a). The receptor is made up of three segments: an extracellular domain that has the ability to bind to specific ligands (i.e., epidermal growth factor, epiregulin, transforming growth factor, among others), a transmembrane domain, and an intracellular domain in which the tyrosine kinase activity occurs (Gridelli, et al., 2007a). When the tyrosine kinase domain is activated, autophosphorylation occurs, which subsequently activates the EGFR-mediated signal transduction pathways leading to key components of cellular survival, inhibition of apoptosis, angiogenesis, and metastasis (Gridelli, et al., 2007a). The EGFR inhibitors have an important role in epithelial cancers due to the generally high expression levels of the ligands and receptors in this family (Gridelli, et al., 2007a). The oral

Figure 5–3 Receptor tyrosine kinases (RTKs).

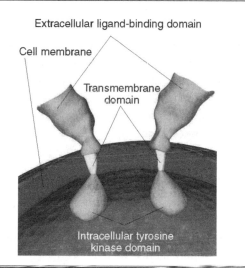

Extracellular ligand-binding domain

Cell membrane

Transmembrane domain

Intracellular tyrosine kinase domain

Source: Reprinted with permission from the Institute for Medical Education and Research.

EGFR inhibitors include gefitinib and erlotinib; the monoclonal antibodies for EGFR inhibition include panitumumab and cetuximab; however, these two agents are not approved in the treatment of lung cancer.

The vascular endothelial growth factor receptor (VEGFR) represents an intriguing target for cancer treatment. Although vasculogenesis is important physiologically for embryo development, wound healing, muscle and bone growth, and menstruation, normally the effects are short lived. However, angiogenesis is important in cancer as well, and it can promote the growth of tumors, facilitating metastasis (Franson & Lapka, 2005). The vasculature is disorganized and highly permeable in tumor tissue compared to the organized appearance of vasculature in normal tissue, and this abnormality can contribute to migration and accumulation of en-

dothelial cells (Ferrara, 2004). Interstitial fluid pressure can increase, and when combined with the inefficient blood flow inside tumors, chemotherapy efficacy can be negatively affected. Therefore, the inhibition of angiogenesis in cancer treatment is of increasing importance. The monoclonal antibody (moAb) bevacizumab was originally approved for the treatment of metastatic colorectal cancer in 2004, and as such, it directly inhibits the binding of VEGF to the cell receptor. The indications for this agent have now been expanded to include other tumor types, such as lung (approved in 2006) and most recently breast (Viale, 2007). Jain reports that anti-angiogenic agents can help to inhibit the development of new blood vessels and inhibit tumor growth; additionally higher VEGF levels can cause a disorganized and "leaky" vasculature within the tumor itself, which could inhibit delivery of chemotherapy to the tumor (2001).

Although there are both monoclonal antibodies (large molecules that must be given intravenously) and small-molecule tyrosine kinase inhibitor (TKI) agents (which are given orally) in the EGFR family, the TKI agents are currently approved in the treatment of advanced NSCLC. These two agents are gefitinib and erlotinib. The monoclonal antibody cetuximab has also been under study in the treatment of lung cancer, but it is not approved in this setting as of this writing.

Gefitinib

Gefitinib was originally granted accelerated approval in the United States for the treatment of NSCLC based on data from two research trials (de Marinis & Grossi, 2008). Kris et al. reported on a double-blind phase II trial with 216 patients randomized to receive either gefitinib at 500 mg/day or 250 mg/day (2003). The drug was well tolerated, and the researchers reported improved symptoms of disease in 43% of patients, with partial radiographic responses in 12% of the 250 mg arm versus 9% at the 500 mg/day dose (Kris, et al., 2003). The overall survival at 1 year for both groups was 25%. Fukuoka and colleagues studied the efficacy and tolerability of the two doses of gefitinib as well in a multi-institutional randomized phase II trial of previously treated patients with advanced NSCLC (2003). A group of 210 patients was entered on trial, and the results showed improvement in symptoms of 40.4%, with median PFS times of 2.7 and 2.8 months and median overall survival times of 7.6 and 8.0 months. However, drug toxicities were more frequently noted in the patients who received the higher dose (Fukuoka, et al., 2003). Common toxicities included diarrhea, rash, and elevations in liver enzymes (ALT), but grade 3 or 4 adverse events were noted in only 1.5% of the patients who received the 250 mg/d dose versus 4.7% of the patients who received 500 mg/d.

Although the preceding data led to the approval of the agent in the United States, the indication was changed in 2005 based on data from the confirmatory trials, which did not meet its primary objective (de Marinis & Grossi, 2008). Thatcher et al. conducted a phase III trial in which gefitinib plus BSC was given as a second-line or third-line treatment for patients with locally advanced or metastatic NSCLC (2005). This large trial had 1692 patients randomized to gefitinib at 250 mg/day with BSC versus placebo and BSC. The primary end point was survival, and at a median follow-up of 7.2 months, the median survival was significantly different between the two groups (5.6 months for gefitinib and 5.1 months for placebo). These data precipitated the change in drug indication

to use in patients who were already receiving and benefiting from it, or use in clinical trials (Thatcher, et al., 2005). However, in analyses of the subgroup populations, significantly longer survival for gefitinib was noted in patients of Asian origin, with median survival of 9.5 months versus 5.5 months. Subsequently, further study has shown that the clinical predictors of Asian origin, female gender, patients with adenocarcinoma, and patients who have never smoked, may be linked with responsiveness to gefitinib (Han, et al., 2006). The epidermal growth factor receptor mutation has also been linked to responsiveness to this agent (Han, et al., 2006). More recently, Costa, Kobayashi, Tenen, and Huberman reported in an analysis of 101 patients from published trials on EGFR-mutant patients and gefitinib and concluded that monotherapy with this agent leads to objective response in most patients who have the EGFR mutations (2007).

Erlotinib

Erlotinib is currently approved for the treatment of patients with locally advanced or metastatic non-small cell lung cancer after failure of at least one prior chemotherapy regimen; it is not recommended in combination with platinum-based chemotherapy (Tarceva prescribing information). Several key trials support its use in NSCLC. A trial led by Shepherd and colleagues examined the use of erlotinib in NSCLC after the failure of first- or second-line chemotherapy (2005). A group of 731 patients was randomized in a placebo-controlled, double-blind trial (49% had received two prior chemotherapy regimens, and 93% had received platinum-based chemotherapy). Response rates for the erlotinib patients was 8.9% versus less than 1% in the placebo group, with a median duration of response of 7.9 months for the treated patients versus 3.7 months for the placebo group. Overall survival was 6.7 months for the erlotinib patients and 4.7 months for placebo ($p < 0.001$) (Shepherd, et al., 2005). Tsao et al. studied patients in a clinical trial of erlotinib versus placebo, examining the tumor-biopsy samples from the participants to determine if drug response was related to the expression by the tumor of EGFR and EGFR gene amplification and mutations (2005). Although the patients in whom an EGFR mutation was present seemed to increase the responsiveness to the agent, it was not indicative of a survival benefit, and in multivariate analysis, neither EGFR expression nor the number of EGFR copies was associated with patient survival.

When its effectiveness as monotherapy was established, interest in the combination of a targeted therapy with conventional chemotherapy was heightened. Erlotinib was studied in combination with chemotherapy agents to determine the efficacy and safety of this therapy. Gatzemeirer and colleagues (2007) reported on a phase III study of erlotinib in combination with cisplatin and gemcitabine in advanced NSCLC. This was a large trial of 1,172 patients; however, the combination of erlotinib with cisplatin and gemcitabine showed no survival benefit (Gatzemeirer, et al., 2007). In a small subset of patients who had never smoked, overall survival (OS) and PFS were increased for those patients who received the erlotinib combination. The TRIBUTE trial studied erlotinib in combination with carboplatin and paclitaxel chemotherapy in advanced NSCLC. Herbst et al. examined 1,059 patients in a phase III trial that randomized erlotinib in combination with carboplatin and paclitaxel against placebo with chemotherapy (2005). There was no survival advantage for those patients who received the combination of erlotinib with standard chemotherapy and no difference in median survival or median time to progression (TTP). The subgroup of nonsmokers did have improved OS in the erlotinib arm (Herbst, et al., 2005). Therefore, the current indication remains as monotherapy.

Interest in the response of patients to erlotinib after failing gefitinib has sparked research in this area. Cho et al. reported on a phase II study of erlotinib in this setting with stage IIIB/IV or metastatic NSCLC who had received two or three prior chemotherapy regimens and with progressive disease within 4 months of gefitinib therapy (2007). There were 21 patients entered into the study (five of those patients had EGFR mutations). The disease control rates and response rates for all patients were 28.6% and 9.5%, and the mediation duration of disease control was 125 days. The patients who had stable disease while on gefitinib had a much higher disease control rate: 75% versus 17.6% in nonstable disease patients, leading the researchers to conclude that erlotinib may be a potential therapeutic option for the treatment of advanced NSCLC patients with wild-type EGFR (lacking EGFR mutations) who had stable disease on gefitinib (Cho, et al., 2007).

In general, gefitinib and erlotinib as monotherapy agents have a 10–20% response rate and a 30–50% symptom improvement rate in patients with advanced NSCLC who have been previously treated and are refractory to chemotherapy and represent a new direction in the treatment of this patient population (Cascone, Morelli, & Ciardiello, 2006). However, their effectiveness has been established against BSC versus pemetrexed as compared to active chemotherapy. Despite this, great interest remains in the TKI agents, and as further information is obtained from trials that examine the role of EGFR mutations (as in the current data on KRAS mutations and EGFR monoclonal antibodies), a more significant role for the TKI agents may yet be discovered.

Combination targeted therapies, such as dual inhibition, may represent the next area of clinical focus. Because cancer cells have redundant signaling pathways, blockage of one specific area of a pathway is often inadequate because signaling may occur via another cellular pathway, stimulating tumor growth and metastasis. Using the strategy of dual inhibition of the EGFR could help prevent this problem. Ramalingam and colleagues, who studied patients with advanced or metastatic NSCLC previously treated with platinum therapy (2008), recently reported the results of that phase I study. The patients received escalating doses of weekly cetuximab (100, 200, and 250 mg/m2) and fixed doses of gefitinib (250 mg/day orally) until disease progression or toxicity. The available tumor samples were examined for expression of EGFR, number of EGFR gene copies and mutations, and KRAS mutations, and the results showed that treatment was generally well tolerated at every dose level (Ramalingam, et al., 2008). Expected EGFR toxicities of skin rash and electrolyte changes were observed; three patients experienced infusion reactions with the monoclonal antibody treatment. Out of the 13 patients, four achieved stable disease (31%). The researchers determined that the combination is safe and may have modest activity in advanced or metastatic NSCLC. Further studies are needed to determine the overall benefit of dual inhibitor therapy; this trial did not show any responses to therapy (Ramalingam, et al., 2008).

The EGFR inhibitor monoclonal antibodies are continuing to be studied in NSCLC, and ce-

tuximab in combination with chemotherapy has shown promise in the treatment of this disease. A small phase I/II study of cetuximab with paclitaxel and carboplatin in stage IV patients showed that response rate, time to progression, and median survival were improved compared to chemotherapy alone (Thienelt, et al., 2005). Cetuximab in combination with gemcitabine and platinum was studied in 65 patients randomized to receive the novel combination (with cisplatin or carboplatin) showing that first-line therapy with cetuximab with chemotherapy was safe and well tolerated. Results suggested that improvements in response rate, time to progression, and median survival were noted, but larger studies are needed. The most recently presented data from ASCO in 2008 discussed the combination of cetuximab with cisplatin and vinorelbine, showing increased overall survival in advanced EGFR NSCLC compared with chemotherapy alone in a large trial (FLEX) that involved 1,125 patients. The OS was 11.3 months in the group with cetuximab versus 10.1 months in the control group; the 1-year survival was 47% in the cetuximab group versus 42% in the control group (Pirker, et al., 2008). The regimen significantly increases costs of therapy for NSCLC for the 1.4 month survival benefit; the main toxicity noted was the papular-pustular rash associated with EGFR inhibitor therapies.

Combining of other targeted therapy agents has also been studied with conventional chemotherapy agents in this disease. A phase I study of an EGFR monoclonal antibody (EMD 72000 or matuzumab) was studied in combination with paclitaxel in EGFR-positive advanced NSCLC in a study of 18 chemotherapy-naïve patients or pretreated patients. The combination appeared to be well tolerated and showed evidence of antitumor activity (Kollmansberger, et al., 2006).

Further studies of targeted therapy agents and chemotherapy drugs are needed to continue the evaluation of the role of these combinations.

Common toxicities associated with the EGFR inhibitor agents include rash, diarrhea, and changes in electrolytes. Less commonly or rarely seen is the side effect of interstitial lung disease. Hypersensitivity can occur with the intravenously administered agents.

Bevacizumab

The pivotal trial leading to the approval of bevacizumab in NSCLC studied 878 patients with recurrent or advanced NSCLC (stage IIIB or IV) and assigned them to receive either chemotherapy with paclitaxel and carboplatin alone or paclitaxel and carboplatin plus bevacizumab (Sandler, et al., 2006). The primary end point was overall survival. The median survival was 12.3 months in the group receiving chemotherapy plus bevacizumab versus 10.3 months in the chemotherapy alone group. The median PFS in the two groups was 6.2 and 4.5 months, respectively; however, the rates of clinically significant bleeding were 4.4% in the bevacizumab group compared to 0.7% in the chemotherapy alone group. There were also 15 treatment-related deaths in the bevacizumab combination group, five of those from pulmonary hemorrhage (Sandler, et al., 2006). The authors concluded that these increased toxicities must be considered against the perceived survival benefit with the addition of bevacizumab to standard chemotherapy in this tumor type (Sandler, et al., 2006).

Based on the trial results, there is interest in the combination of bevacizumab with other chemotherapy agents, and currently ongoing trials are examining the VEGF inhibitor agents with docetaxel and carboplatin, as well as acizumab, pemetrexed, and carboplatin in phase II trials (Gridelli, Maione, Rossi, & De Marinis, 2007c). A trial conducted by Davila et al. examined the combination of gemcitabine and oxaliplatin with the addition of bevacizumab in a phase II study (2006). The small trial of 26 patients showed no bleeding complications with a response rate of 31%. Patel, Hensing, and Villafor evaluated pemetrexed and carboplatin with bevacizumab and found that out of the 39 patients enrolled in the study, one complete response and 20 partial responses PRs were obtained with an overall response rate of 55% (2007). Currently, the FDA indication is for bevacizumab to be administered in combination with carboplatin and paclitaxel for the initial treatment of patients with unresectable, locally advanced, recurrent, or metastatic nonsquamous NSCLC (Cohen, Gootenberg, Keegan, & Pazdur, 2007).

Ongoing trials will continue to address the potential of targeted therapy in advanced non-small cell lung cancer. Sorafenib and sunitinib (multitargeted agents), as well as vandetanib, are in phase III trials for refractory NSCLC; other experimental compounds are under study. These evolving treatment strategies offer patients continued hope against a daunting disease entity.

Side effects frequently seen with bevacizumab are bleeding, wound healing complications, hypertension, and proteinuria. Less commonly seen or more rare side effects include reversible posterior leukoencephalopathy, nasal septum perforation, fistula formation, and bowel perforation. Hemorrhage can occur in some patients; pulmonary hemorrhage was seen in patients with lung cancer in the clinical trials. Patients with squamous cell histology had a higher incidence of pulmonary hemorrhage; the drug is not approved for patients with this disease.

Summary of National Comprehensive Cancer Center Practice Guidelines in Oncology v.1.2009 and ASCO Guidelines for Advanced or Unresectable NSCLC

There are national guidelines that help to direct the ordering clinician into optimal treatment choices. These guidelines are made up of panel groups of expert clinicians in the specific field who review the evidence and make suggestions for therapy based on that evidence. To that end, ASCO has published a guideline with recommendations for unresectable NSCLC, calling for chemotherapy in association with definitive thoracic irradiation in selected patients with unresectable locally advanced NSCLC and chemotherapy in selected patients with stage IV NSCLC, although the guidelines have not been updated since 2003, and major changes have occurred in the treatment of this cancer (Pfister, et al., 2004). The specific agents recommended in this guideline are a two-drug combination given for first-line treatment, with nonplatinum-containing regimens as an alternative to platinum-based therapy if needed, and single agents as appropriate for poorer PS patients as well as elderly patients. The duration of therapy for the ASCO guideline is four cycles of platinum-based therapy for unresectable stage III patients, and no more than six cycles for responding patients with stage IV disease (four cycles for patients who are not responding to therapy). Treatment for longer periods may cause chronic treatment-related toxicities that may outweigh the potential benefits of therapy (Onn, et al., 2006).

The most recent 2008 update by the National Comprehensive Cancer Network (NCCN) for NSCLC has comprehensive treatment information regarding the systemic therapies for advanced or metastatic disease. The NCCN does remark on the benefits of platinum-based chemotherapy for its ability to prolong survival and improve symptom control but states that no specific platinum-based cytotoxic combination is clearly superior in this setting (NCCN, 2008a). There are multiple options for first-line therapy, including bevacizumab plus chemotherapy or chemotherapy alone in patients with good PS with advanced or recurrent NSCLC. Patients with nonsquamous histology may benefit from a cisplatin/pemetrexed combination versus cisplatin/gemcitabine and cetuximab with vinorelbine/cisplatin. This is indicated in patients with PS of 0-2 who have advanced or recurrent NSCLC and meet the criteria for cetuximab treatment (NCCN, 2008a). Those criteria are specific and include patients with stage IIIB disease or IV, EGFR expression by innunohistochemistry, age over or equal to 18 years, PS of 0-2, no known brain metastases, and no prior chemotherapy or anti-EGFR therapy (NCCN, 2008a). The guidelines state that two drug regimens are preferred over three drug regimens (excepting bevacizumab), and that cisplatin-based combinations are superior to BSC, with cisplatin or carboplatin effective in combination with paclitaxel, docetaxel, gemcitabine, vinorelbine, irinotecan, etoposide, and vinblastine. Due to the available data on EGFR TKI inhibitors, if patients have known active EGFR mutation or gene amplification and have never smoked, erlotinib plus or minus chemotherapy could be considered (NCCN, 2008a). Options for the second-line setting include single agent docetaxel, pemetrexed, or erlotinib, which is superior to BSC in the third-line setting for survival (NCCN, 2008a).

Resectable Non-Small Cell Lung Cancer

Patients who present with early disease may be eligible for initial surgery, which is often followed by chemotherapy or radiation therapy to improve disease outcome. The following section discusses the role of combined modality therapy in both adjuvant and neoadjuvant settings.

Combined Modality Therapy: Adjuvant and Neoadjuvant Treatment of NSCLC

Although many patients present with advanced or unresectable NSCLC, there are some patients who are resectable and go on to receive further therapy. These patients typically undergo surgery plus or minus radiation therapy, and the role of chemotherapy is specific to the stage of the patient. Adjuvant chemotherapy was not considered a standard of care until recent data determined benefit in stage I–IIIA patients (Pisters, et al., 2007b). ASCO has published a recent guideline in conjunction with Cancer Care Ontario. These guidelines are similar to the most recent version of the NCCN in their recommendations for treatment with chemotherapy in this setting. Although stage IA patients are not recommended to receive chemotherapy, stages IB through IIIA have a role for chemotherapy; however, it is not recommended routinely for IB. In general, the use of adjuvant

chemotherapy regimens with alkylating agents is not recommended because it is not beneficial to survival (Pisters, et al., 2007b).

Stages IA and IB

The Cancer Care Ontario (CCO)/ASCO guidelines do not recommend chemotherapy in stage IA patients due to the lack of evidence for adjuvant cisplatin-based chemotherapy in this setting (Pisters, et al., 2007b). If patients are able to be completely resected in stage IB disease, is is recommended that they not use chemotherapy routinely. The data for this recommendation come from an abstract presented in 2005 at ASCO evaluating 12 reports with over 6000 patients in the adjuvant setting. The results showed that the benefit for early stage IA patients was not significant (Bria, et al., 2005).

Stages II–IIIA

Scagliotti and colleagues conducted a randomized study of adjuvant chemotherapy for completely resected stage I, II, or IIIA NSCLC patients (2003). This was a large study with 1209 patients randomly assigned to receive mitomycin, vindesine, and cisplatin or no treatment after complete surgical resection. Although there was no statistically significant difference between the two patient groups in OS or PFS, the researchers felt that poor compliance with this particular regimen should lead future studies to explore more effective treatment. They did find, however, that disease stage and gender were associated with survival (Scagliotti, et al., 2003). A pivotal trial conducted by the International Adjuvant Lung Cancer Trial (IALT) Collaborative Group randomly assigned patients to either receive three or four cycles of cisplatin-based chemotherapy or to observation, with OS as the primary end point (IALT, 2004). There were 1,867 patients in total, with 36.5% stage I disease, 24.2% stage II, and 39.3% stage III. The chemotherapy group received cisplatin, which was given in conjunction with etoposide, vinorelbine, vinblastine, or vindesine. The chemotherapy patients had a significantly higher survival rate versus those randomized to observation (44.5% versus 40.4%). The conclusion of the researchers was that cisplatin-based adjuvant chemotherapy does improve survival in patients who have completely resected NSCLC (IALT, 2004). Douillard and colleagues studied the role of adjuvant vinorelbine plus cisplatin versus observation in patients with completely resected stage IB–IIIA NSCLC in a randomized, controlled trial with 840 patients (2006). The patients in the chemotherapy group had a median survival of 65.7 months versus 43.7 months in the observation group, leading the researchers to conclude that the combination increased survival times for those patients in the study (Douillard, et al., 2006).

For stage IIIA patients, adjuvant cisplatin-based chemotherapy is recommended based on the data from the LACE meta-analysis, which found a benefit for cisplatin therapy in stage III patients in the pooled analysis. This corroborates the improvements seen in the IALT and ANITA trials for overall survival in this stage of disease (Pisters, et al., 2007b).

The recommendations from CCO/ASCO are that physicians should help patients in interpreting the direct benefit from adjuvant therapy in NSCLC, and they point out that the LACE data calculate the absolute benefit for increases in 5-year survival from 64% to 67% for stage IB NSCLC, from 39% to 49% for stage II disease, and from 26% to 39% in stage III NSCLC (Pisters, et al., 2007b). Additionally, chemo-

therapy in this setting versus observation carries a higher incidence of toxicities and side effects, which may affect the patients' QOL; therefore any discussion of potential treatment should consider the short- and long-term effects of these therapies for patients, including the possibility of treatment-related death (Pisters, et al., 2007b).

Based on the available data, while carboplatin has a clear role in the advanced or unresectable setting, the agent should not be administered routinely in the adjuvant setting, and the CCO/ASCO guidelines recommend as an initial choice the use of cisplatin with vinorelbine for the greatest survival benefit. However, if clinicians cannot adopt that regimen, the recommendation is that clinicians choose one cisplatin-based chemotherapy regimen and use it consistently to improve safety (Pisters, et al., 2007b).

Neoadjuvant Chemotherapy for NSCLC

In the interest of improving outcomes for this disease, researchers have explored the notion of neoadjuvant therapy prior to definitive resection. Gottfried and colleagues reported on the results of a phase III trial for patients with locally advanced stage IIB, IIIA, and IIIB NSCLC (2008). The primary endpoint of the study was 2-year survival, and data was obtained from 143 assessable patients. Because of the low inclusion rate, efficacy of a adjuvant chemotherapy could not be assessed; however, after three cycles of vinorelbine, ifosfamide, and cisplatin, 82 patients (57.3%) had an objective response, and after a median of 32 days postchemotherapy, 69% of the patients (107) went on to operation with complete resection in 74% of them (Gottfried, et al., 2008). Previous studies have shown that patients who receive cisplatin neoadjuvant therapy followed by radiation therapy (RT) over RT alone have shown a small benefit, but neoadjuvant therapy followed by chemoradiotherapy has not been proven superior (Glynne-Jones & Hoskin, 2007). Pisters et al. reported an abstract on the S9900 study (closed when chemotherapy became standard in the adjuvant treatment of NSCLC) and noted that PFS and OS showed a trend in favor of induction paclitaxel–carboplatin, supporting its use in operable NSCLC and recommended randomized trials comparing induction to adjuvant chemotherapy in the future (Pisters, et al., 2007a). Therefore, the role of neoadjuvant therapy is not yet established in this tumor type. However, randomized studies that compare sequential therapy versus concurrent treatment have been shown to be beneficial, at the cost of greater toxicity (Glynne-Jones & Hoskin, 2007).

Most patients with NSCLC will eventually relapse and die of their disease. Although surgery was historically the mainstay of therapy for this tumor type, combining radiation therapy and chemotherapy has improved the outcome of selected patients with NSCLC and is now considered to be the standard of care for stage III patients.

Treatment of the Elderly Patient with NSCLC

Nearly one-third of patients with NSCLC are aged 70 or older, and these patients are at higher risk for cormorbid conditions and decreased organ function (Onn, et al., 2006). However, this fact should not translate into denial of treatment for this patient population, and studies have shown that older age should not be the sole factor in whether or not to treat a patient with

cancer (Devlin & Langer, 2007). For some patients, single-agent chemotherapy versus combination chemotherapy may be more appropriate in the palliative setting, but there are trials showing efficacy in this population of patients (Devlin & Langer, 2007).

Cisplatin with gemcitabine or vinorelbine was evaluated in elderly patients in two phase I/II trials (Gridelli, et al., 2007b). There were 159 patients older than 70 years of age who had a PS of 0–1 enrolled in the trials, and they received cisplatin and gemcitabine or vinorelbine every 21 days (Gridelli, et al., 2007b). Cisplatin and gemcitabine were given without unacceptable toxicity with objective responses in 43.5% of the patients and a median PFS and OS of 25.3 and 43.6 weeks. The cisplatin and vinorelbine were tolerated well, with 82% reporting acceptable toxicity, and objective responses seen in 36.1% of patients with median PFS and OS of 21.1 and 33.1 weeks, respectively. This led the researchers to conclude that both combinations are feasible and active in this patient population (Gridelli, et al., 2007b). The results of an ECOG trial reported by Langer et al. looked at older patients in the context of cisplatin-based chemotherapy and compared outcomes of patients aged 70 years and older to younger patients (2002). This was a randomized phase III trial of cisplatin plus either etoposide or paclitaxel in chemotherapy-naïve patients with stages III or IV NSCLC. The results showed that response rate, toxicity, and survival in fit, elderly NSCLC patients who received platinum-based treatment was fairly similar to those results seen in the younger patient population. However, as might be expected, because of existing comorbidities in the older patients, more leukopenia and neuropsychiatric toxicity was noted, although the researchers cautioned that advanced age alone should not bar patients from the appropriate treatment for their lung cancer (Langer, et al., 2002).

Ramalingam et al. recently reported on the ECOG trial 4599 that examined elderly, advanced-stage NSCLC patients who were treated with bevacizumab in combination with carboplatin and paclitaxel in a subset analysis to determine outcome (2008). Twenty-six percent of the patients ($n = 224$) were elderly in this randomized trial; there was a trend toward higher response rate and PFS with carboplatin and paclitaxel with bevacizumab versus carboplatin and paclitaxel alone (Ramalingam, et al., 2008). Although the elderly patients had higher incidences of neutropenia, bleeding, and proteinuria with the triple drug combination compared to the younger patients, the researchers concluded that there was also no obvious improvement in survival and recommended prospective evaluation of this combination in elderly patients (Ramalingam, et al., 2008).

Two of the strategies recommended for elderly patients may be to consider substituting carboplatin for cisplatin in the adjuvant setting and increased use of neoadjuvant treatment to reduce perioperative comorbidities and possible problems with compliance (see Table 5–2; Langer, 2008).

Small Cell Lung Cancer

Small cell lung cancer (SCLC) behaves differently from the other types of lung cancer (Onn, et al., 2006). It is a more aggressive disease and is known for its early systemic spread of disease (Onn, et al., 2006). In fact, this aggressiveness is the key feature in this disease; therefore patients with SCLC usually have a short overall survival (Onn, et al., 2006). Before systemic treatment with chemotherapy became available, the median survival duration was 12 weeks for patients with limited-stage disease and 5 weeks for patients with extensive-stage disease, with most patients rarely surviving longer than 35 weeks

Table 5–2 Considerations for Elderly and Chemotherapy Options for Lung Cancer

Strategy	Rationale
Substitute carboplatin for cisplatin in adjuvant setting	Carboplatin is less myelosuppressive than cisplatin; decreased nausea and vomiting; decreased renal toxicity
Consider increased use of neoadjuvant treatment initially to reduce perioperative comorbidities	Initial therapy could reduce tumor burden and potentially reduce surgical risks and comorbidities
Strategize to increase compliance with therapies	Pill counts with oral therapies; frequent phone calls to assess for side effects of therapy and promote early intervention; patient diaries
Geriatric assessments	Can help to monitor and assess for frailty (assist in predicting ability to withstand more aggressive therapy), mental status, and emotional status

Source: Based on data from Langer, 2008; NCCN, 2008; Viale & Sommers, 2007.

(Onn, et al., 2006). When chemotherapy became accepted in the treatment of SCLC, these dismal statistics improved significantly. However, as a disease entity, SCLC remains formidable.

Staging of SCLC differs significantly from NSCLC. The system is much simpler for this tumor type; patients are staged as limited-stage disease or extensive-stage disease, reflecting the specific nature of this type of lung cancer. Small cell lung cancer is considered to be not only more aggressive than NSCLC, but it is also known for its propensity for early and widespread metastasis. It is also known for the frequency of paraneoplastic syndromes, and in a positive note, its sensitivity to treatment with chemotherapy (Lally, Urbanic, Blackstock, Miller, & Perry, 2007). Because of SCLC's chemoresponsiveness, this treatment plays a major role in the therapy for this disease. Radiation and occasionally surgery (in limited-stage disease) also play a role in the treatment of SCLC. Selected pivotal trials will be reviewed in the treatment of this tumor type.

Chemotherapy in Extensive-Stage Small Cell Lung Cancer and Summary of National Comprehensive Cancer Network Practice Guidelines in Oncology v.2.2008

Treatment with chemotherapy is the standard of care for SCLC; however, most patients will develop recurrence of disease and ultimately succumb to this tumor type. This section will review the role of chemotherapy and the current NCCN practice guidelines for treatment of SCLC.

Cisplatin and Etoposide Combination

Although SCLC is extremely chemosensitive, with impressive response rates of 70–85% and complete response rates of 20–30%, almost all patients relapse (Lally, et al., 2007). The NCCN treatment guidelines call for patients to receive combination chemotherapy, including supportive care regimens, if there is not brain metastases or localized symptomatic sites (NCCN, 2008b). If there are symptomatic sites, the recommendation is chemotherapy plus or minus symptomatic field radiation therapy, and for patients with extensive stage and positive brain metastases, chemotherapy may be administered first for asymptomatic patients prior to radiation therapy or after radiation if patients present as symptomatic (NCCN, 2008b).

Although the combination of cyclophosphamide, doxorubicin, and vincristine (CAV) has been a recommended chemotherapy regimen for this disease, the current standard of therapy for SCLC is the drug combination of cisplatin and etoposide. This has not changed significantly since the 1980s (Evans, et al., 1985). The combination of CAV was compared to etoposide and cisplatin in at least two studies. Fukuoka et al. reported that response rates for cisplatin and etoposide were 78% versus 55% for CAV, although complete response rates were similar (1991).

Evans et al. reported on the effectiveness of the combination of etoposide and cisplatin in 31 patients with SCLC who couldn't receive doxorubicin in most cases due to comorbidities (1985). Out of the 28 evaluable patients, 43% achieved a complete response, with partial responses in 43%. The median duration of response for the patients with limited disease ($n = 11$) was 39 weeks, and for those patients with extensive disease, it was 26 weeks (Evans, et al., 1985). Median survival time for the entire group of patients was 70 weeks (Evans, et al., 1985). The current NCCN recommendations are to offer cisplatin and etoposide, carboplatin and etoposide, cisplatin and irinotecan, carboplatin and irinotecan, or cyclophosphamide, doxorubicin, and vincristine as initial therapy for extensive-stage disease. The recommendation for the CAV regimen is not uniform consensus (NCCN, 2008b).

Carboplatin versus Cisplatin

Clinicians have been able to successfully replace cisplatin with carboplatin for patients who are unable to tolerate toxicities of cisplatin as well (Lally, et al., 2007). The results of the JCOG 9702 randomized phase III trial showed that carboplatin plus etoposide versus split doses of cisplatin with etoposide in elderly or poor-risk patients with extensive SCLC showed no significant difference between response rate (73% versus 73%) and overall survival (carboplatin combination had 10.6 months versus 9.9 months in the cisplatin group; Okamoto, et al., 2007). The researchers concluded that although cisplatin and etoposide are the standard of care, carboplatin could be substituted as an alternative if a risk–benefit ratio is being considered (Okamoto, et al., 2007).

Cisplatin Plus Irinotecan

Noda and colleagues studied the role of irinotecan hydrochloride, a topoisomerase I inhibitor approved in the treatment of metastatic colorectal cancer (mCRC), in combination with cisplatin for the treatment of SCLC (2002). The researchers sought to answer the question of superiority for the two treatment regimens and conducted a multicenter, randomized phase III trial with 154 evaluable patients. The median survival for the irinotecan with cisplatin group was 12.8 months

versus 9.4 months for the cisplatin with etoposide group, and the proportion of patients surviving at 2 years was 19.5% for the new regimen versus 5.2% in the etoposide with cisplatin group (Noda, et al., 2002). However, severe or life-threatening diarrhea occurred more frequently in the irinotecan with cisplatin group versus more frequent severe or life-threatening myelosuppression in the etoposide with cisplatin patients versus the new regimen (Noda, et al., 2002). The researchers concluded that irinotecan in combination with cisplatin represented an effective therapy for metastatic or extensive-stage SCLC. However, Hanna et al. also compared the two regimens in a group of patients with previously untreated extensive-stage disease SCLC in a randomized phase III trial (2006). Cisplatin and etoposide (EP) or irinotecan plus cisplatin (IP) was given to 241 patients who were randomly assigned in a 2:1 ratio (IP $n = 221$ and EP $n = 110$). In this trial the patients received treatment for at least four cycles until progressive disease or until intolerable toxicity was reached. There was no significant difference in response rates (48% versus 43.6%), median time to progression (4.1 months versus 4.6 months), or overall survival (9.3 months versus 10.2 months). These researchers concluded that there was no improvement in survival for IP versus EP, and the toxicities were specific to the individual agents given (Hanna, et al., 2006). Irinotecan is not approved in the treatment of SCLC.

Cisplatin, Etoposide, and Paclitaxel

The combination of the confirmed active agents cisplatin and etoposide was studied in a randomized phase III Intergroup trial with or without paclitaxel in patients with extensive-stage SCLC (Niell, et al., 2005). The trial enrolled 587 patients who were randomly assigned to the standard therapy of cisplatin and etoposide or cisplatin, paclitaxel, and etoposide followed by granulocyte colony-stimulating factor on days 4–18. The two regimens were given every 3 weeks for six cycles (Niell, et al., 2005). The median failure-free survival time was 5.9 months for the standard combination and 6 months for the triple regimen, with overall response rates of 68% of etoposide–cisplatin and 75% for the new combination, with median overall survival time of 9.9 months for etoposide–cisplatin and 10.6 months for cisplatin, etoposide, and paclitaxel (Niell, et al., 2005). The researchers concluded that the addition of paclitaxel did not improve time to progression or survival in patients with extensive-stage SCLC and had significant more toxicity, with 6.5% toxic deaths associated with the regimen versus 2.4% in etoposide and cisplatin patients. Although paclitaxel has an FDA indication in the treatment of patients with NSCLC, it does not presently have one for SCLC.

Two drug combinations are considerably more effective than single agent therapy. Although three-drug regimens have been studied as previously discussed, the addition of the third agent confers higher toxicity with increased response rates and does not improve median survival as compared to the cisplatin and etoposide combination (Lally, et al., 2007). Recently reported research on new combinations is available in abstract form. Syrigos et al. reported in abstract form on the results of a phase II trial that examined topotecan, carboplatin, and etoposide (2007). The study reported that 46 chemotherapy-naïve patients with extensive disease and PS 0–2 were enrolled in the trial; all of the patients were smokers. Carboplatin AUC 5 was given on day one, with irinotecan on day two, and three days of etoposide every 21 days in repeated cycles. The overall response rate was 52.2%, with a mean overall survival of 16.3 months, and a 1-year survival rate of 43.47% (Syrigos, et al., 2007). The regimen was well tolerated with one fatal thrombocytopenic death, and 19.5% of the patients had grade III/IV neutropenia. The researchers concluded that the triple regimen is effective and well tolerated for the patients in the poor prognosis group of extensive disease SCLC, and it is comparable to the standard of etoposide–cisplatin (Syrigos, et al., 2007).

Researchers have attempted other tactics to increase survival, including administration of additional cycles of chemotherapy; however, treatment over four to six cycles of any regimen with chemotherapy has not been seen as a successful strategy. Maintenance therapy has produced mixed results as well, and failure of second-line therapy may be related to the relatively rapid development of drug resistance (Lally, et al., 2007).

Second-Line Therapy for Extensive-Stage SCLC

When the disease has relapsed, patients who receive second therapy generally have a poor prognosis (Onn, et al., 2006). If the disease relapses within 3 months of the original first-line treatment, the disease is generally considered to be refractory (versus those who relapse more than 3 months after original treatment and are considered to be sensitive) (Onn, et al., 2006).

Topotecan

As of this writing, the only FDA-approved therapy in the second-line setting is topotecan, which can be administered either intravenously or orally. Topotecan was studied against cyclophosphamide, doxorubicin, and vincristine (CAV) in a randomized, multicenter study of patients with SCLC who had relapsed at least 60 days after completing their first-line therapy and who had an ECOG status of less than or equal to two (von Pawel, et al., 1999). The response rates achieved in patients who were treated with topotecan (24.3%) were at least as effective as those in the CAV group (18.3%), and the median survival was 25 weeks for topotecan versus 24.7 weeks for the CAV group. More patients experienced symptom improvement in the topotecan group as well, leaving the researchers to conclude that this is an active regimen in this setting (von Pawel, et al., 1999). Building on the data obtained from this study, other researchers have examined topotecan in combination with additional chemotherapy agents to see if increased efficacy could be achieved. Combinations with docetaxel, vinorelbine, and cisplatin have reported positive results in some patients (Morgensztern, Perry, & Govindan, 2007; Beldner, et al., 2007; Sorensen, et al., 2008).

Giving topotecan sequentially versus alternating administration of cisplatin–etoposide and topotecan in previously untreated extensive-stage SCLC patients was also studied; the researchers concluded that both regimens resulted in comparable efficacy and tolerability for patients with similar dose reductions for toxicity required in both arms (Ignatiadis, et al., 2005).

Additional Chemotherapy Strategies in the Second-Line Setting

The alternation of chemotherapy with maintenance therapy was hoped to combat the drug resistance that occurs frequently with SCLC, but positive data has not been consistent (Onn, et al., 2006). Additional strategies include dose intensity, a technique that has gained prominence in the treatment of patients with breast cancer (Onn, et al., 2006). New drug therapies and combinations in relapsed SCLC have been reported in abstract form. Pemetrexed, a therapy now approved in NSCLC, was studied in SCLC patients with relapsed disease. The phase II trial enrolled eligible patients with limited- or extensive-stage SCLC, PS 0–2, with only one prior chemotherapy regimen (Raju, et al., 2007). Pemetrexed was given every 21 days, with 121 patients enrolled in the study. The preliminary clinical benefit rates of 20% and 17.4% represented what was thought to be modest activity at a dose of 500 mg/m2, and although higher doses can be given without significantly more toxicity, the efficacy did not increase (Raju, et al., 2007). Irinotecan and paclitaxel was studied in patients with recurrent disease following one prior chemotherapy regimen in one trial (Owonikoko, et al., 2007). Although 55 patients were enrolled, this preliminary abstract reports data available for 32 patients showing the objective response rate after a maximum of six cycles was 37%, with median survival of 19.6 weeks and a 1-year survival of 15% (Owonikoko, et al., 2007). Ongoing trials of a novel microtubule inhibitor (vinflunine) are being tested in this setting, and early data on gemcitabine and irinotecan show that the combination is well tolerated and active as well (Nishio, et al., 2007).

Chemotherapy in Limited-Stage Small Cell Lung Cancer

Approximately 40% of SCLC patients are diagnosed with limited-stage disease using the two-tier system of staging for this tumor type (Socinski & Bogart, 2007). These patients have slightly better 5-year survival rates in the Surveillance Epidemiology and End Results database analysis (Govindan, et al., 2006). Because of the chemosensitivity and radiosensitivity of this disease, both treatments are standard in the therapy recommendations for limited-stage SCLC (Socinski & Bogart, 2007). Although the disease is very sensitive initially to chemotherapy alone, most patients relapse with recurrent disease. Therefore the role of thoracic radiation therapy has become integrated into standard therapy for SCLC, and this combined approach has improved 5-year survival rates, greater than 20% for some patients (Faivre-Finn, Lorigan, West, & Thatcher, 2005). The current NCCN guidelines call for chemotherapy as the primary therapy for limited stage SCLC and recommend a combination of cisplatin and etoposide or carboplatin and etoposide, although when given with radiation therapy the cisplatin and etoposide regimen is preferred (NCCN, 2008b).

For some patients, surgical resection can play a role in early disease as well. The chemotherapy options for treatment of these patients include the combinations of cisplatin and etoposide and CAV, which were previously reviewed in the discussion of extensive-stage disease (Lee, Morris, Fried, & Socinski, 2006). Sundstrom et al. studied the efficacy of cisplatin and etoposide as compared to CAV in a randomized phase III trial with a 5-year follow-up and determined that cisplatin and etoposide are superior to CAV in limited-stage patients with SCLC, but it is seemingly equivalent in patients with extensive-stage disease (2002). However, etoposide and cisplatin have become the preferred regimen because they are easily given in conjunction with thoracic radiotherapy for limited-stage SCLC.

A practice guideline for the role of combination chemotherapy in the initial management of limited-stage SCLC was published in 2004 and is based on a systematic review of 50 random-ized controlled trials (Laurie, Logan, Markman, Mackay, & Evans, 2004). The chemotherapy regimens reviewed in the trial were CAV and etoposide–cisplatin; the analysis could not conclusively show a true superiority for either regimen, although when treating for cure, one trial showed an improvement with the use of etoposide–cisplatin versus an anthracycline regimen (Laurie, et al., 2004). The guideline did not find evidence for the use of maintenance chemotherapy, and there was insufficient evidence to support dose-intensive regimens in standard practice. The conclusion of the guideline was to consider etoposide–cisplatin as the preferred chemotherapy regimen for patients with limited stage SCLC whenever concurrent thoracic radiotherapy is to be used and to consider CAV as an alternative (while avoiding the use of concurrent anthracycline with radiotherapy) (Laurie, et al., 2004).

Although improvements have been made in the survival of this tumor type, there are few long-term survivors, and research continues in the study of new drugs and new combinations of therapy.

The Role of Targeted Therapy in Small Cell Lung Cancer

Heightened interest in the use of targeted therapy in NSCLC has prompted researchers to explore its role in SCLC. Interestingly, most SCLC express the c-KIT oncoprotein (a member of the tyrosine kinase family), which provides a basis for studying the effects of tyrosine kinase inhibitors specific to this protein. Johnson et al. conducted a phase II study of imatinib in patients with small cell lung cancer ($n = 19$); however, there were no objective responses with a median time to progression of 0.8 months and 1.2 months in the previously untreated and sensitive-relapse groups (2003). Samples of tissue showed that 21% of the patients had the c-KIT receptor (Johnson, et al., 2003).

Another trial examined the role of imatinib in c-KIT expressing SCLC with 29 evaluable patients (Dy, et al., 2005). Patients with disease progression less than 3 months were enrolled in arm A, while arm B contained patients with disease progression greater than or equal to 3 months after previous treatment. Median survival was 3.9 and 5.3 months, with median times to progression of 1 and 1.1 months for both arms of the study. Because of the early disease progression and early deaths seen in arm A, enrollment was temporarily suspended. With no objective responses and no confirmed stable disease at greater than 6 weeks after starting therapy, the researchers concluded that imatinib therapy failed to show any clinical activity in spite of selecting patients for the c-KIT protein (Dy, et al., 2005). The benefit of thalidomide when given to patients after two courses of etoposide, cisplatin, cyclophosphamide, and 4'-epidoxorubicin (PCDE) was studied in a phase III double-blinded, placebo-controlled study of extensive-disease SCLC patients (Pujol, et al., 2007). The 119 patients were randomly assigned to receive four additional PCDE cycles plus thalidomide or placebo. However, although the patients who were treated with thalidomide had a longer survival compared to placebo, the difference was not statistically significant, and there was more neuropathy in those patients. There was some benefit noted in patients with a PS of 1 or 2, leading the researchers to conclude that more studies are needed to determine the role of anti-angiogenesis agents in the treatment of SCLC (Pujol, et al., 2007).

Although some of the results have proven to be disappointing, and targeted therapy agents have not yet gained a prominent place in the treatment of this disease, ongoing research in this area is continuing to evaluate angiogenesis and other novel targeted therapies in the treatment of this disease.

Treatment of the Elderly Patient with Small Cell Lung Cancer

The results of combination chemotherapy with irinotecan and cisplatin in elderly patients greater than or equal to 65 years of age were reported recently (Kim, et al., 2008). This phase II study enrolled 46 previously untreated elderly patients with extensive-stage disease who received irinotecan with cisplatin every 4 weeks until six cycles were reached. The median age of the patients was 70 years, and a complete and partial response was observed in 19.6% and 56.5%, respectively (Kim, et al., 2008). The overall response rate was 76.1%, and the overall median survival was 10.4 months. Although there were major toxicities noted, including neutropenia, leukopenia, infection, and diarrhea, the results indicated that combination chemotherapy with these two agents is an effective treatment for elderly patients who have a good ECOG PS (Kim, et al., 2008). Irinotecan was also studied in combination with carboplatin and granulocyte colony-stimulating factor (G-CSF) support in elderly patients with SCLC (Okamoto, et al., 2006). Three different AUC and irinotecan dose levels were used, and patients were stratified to doses using history of prior chemotherapy, PS level, or greater age (75 years or more). Eighteen patients were enrolled in the study, and the response rate was 89%, with two complete responses and 14 partial responses. The median survival time was 13.3 months, with a 1-year survival rate of 62%, leading the researchers to conclude that this regimen is an effective and nontoxic one for this patient population (Okamoto, et al., 2006).

Toxicities of Chemotherapies for Lung Cancer

Medical oncology nurses are well versed in the management of multiple toxicities associated with conventional chemotherapy treatments, either as single agent protocols or combination therapy regimens. Nurses who specialize in radiation oncology are becoming more familiar with the chemotherapy regimens utilized in the combined modality treatments of this cancer because many patients will receive both therapies during the course of their disease.

In most cases, combination chemotherapy protocols have more side effects associated with their administration. The adverse event profiles of most chemotherapy agents include myelosuppression, gastrointestinal side effects (diarrhea, nausea, and vomiting), alopecia with specific therapies, potential for hypersensitivity, and agent-specific neuropathies (see Table 5–3). Practicing oncology nurses are familiar with the strategies used to combat these common toxicities. The administration of growth factors is commonly done to combat neutropenia and anemia associated with treatment. Antiemetics are given for most, if not all, regimens given for the treatment of lung cancer. Typical regimens are depicted in Table 5–4. However, the newer targeted therapies carry a unique side effect profile that requires special awareness by oncology nurses with regard to assessment and early intervention (see Table 5–5).

Tyrosine Kinase Inhibitor Adverse Events

Erlotinib is a commonly given therapy for NSCLC and is currently approved for that indication. When blocked by the EGFR inhibitor therapy, interruption of the hair follicle growth and maintenance can produce a characteristic papular–pustular rash. The other most commonly seen side effect associated with erlotinib therapy is diarrhea, although other side effects occur in conjunction with this agent as well. The skin rash can be severe and dose limiting; however, there is an association between the appearance and severity of skin rash and survival for patients with epithelial malignancies, such as lung and head and neck cancer (Rudin, et al., 2008). At the present time, it is difficult to predict who will suffer more significant toxicity with EGFR inhibitor therapy; however, researchers are attempting to define predictive markers and determine if the polymorphisms in EGFR are associated with the toxicity and efficacy of therapy (Rudin, et al., 2008).

In the clinical trials, erlotinib produced any grade of rash in 75% of the patients, with grade 3 rash in 8% and grade 4 rash in less than 1% (Tarceva prescribing information). Diarrhea occurred in 54% of patients (any grade) with grade 3 or 4 diarrhea in 7% of the patients. Dose modification may be necessary in patients whose diarrhea is unable to be managed with loperamide, and special caution should be taken to avoid dehydration and subsequent complications with renal toxicity. If dose reduction is undertaken, the dose should be reduced in 50 mg increments. Oncology nurses should be aware that drug–drug and drug–food interactions can occur with erlotinib, and if patients develop an acute onset of new or progressive pulmonary

Table 5-3 Chemotherapy Toxicities

System	Cisplatin (Platinol)	Carboplatin (Paraplatin)	Vinorelbine (Navelbine)	Paclitaxel (Taxol)	Docetaxel (Taxotere)	Irinotecan (Camptosar)	Ifosfamide (Ifex)	Gemcitabine (Gemzar)	Pemetrexed (Alimta)
Bone marrow	Neutropenia	Neutropenia; thrombocytopenia	Myelosuppression	Neutropenia	Neutropenia	Neutropenia	Neutropenia; thrombocytopenia	Myelosuppression	Myelosuppression
Gastrointestinal	N/V (severe)	N/V (moderate)	N/V; severe constipation		Should not be given with bilirubin at upper limit of normal or elevated SGOT and/or SGPT	N/V; acute and delayed onset diarrhea	N/V; anorexia, diarrhea, constipation	N/V; mild to moderate hepatic toxicity rare	N/V
Neurologic	Peripheral neuropathies	Peripheral neuropathies, less severe than cisplatin	Severe peripheral neuropathy 1%	Cumulative; may require dosage adjustment for subsequent courses	Severe neurosensory symptoms, may require dose adjustment			Mild paresthesias	Sensory neuropathy
Cardiovascular			Chest pain 5%; rare MI	Severe conduction abnormalities in < 1% of patients; hypotension, bradycardia, and hypertension	Severe fluid retention; requires premedication; hypotension			Edema (general and peripheral) reported	Hypertension higher in patients older than 65 years of age vs. younger patients
Renal	Acute and chronic nephrotoxicity	Uncommon as compared to cisplatin				Rare cases identified in patients who became volume depleted from N/V or diarrhea	Hemorrhagic cystitis; requires uroprotective agent (mesna)	Mild proteinuria and hematuria commonly reported	Should not be given to patients with CrCl < 45 ml/min

Hypersensitivity	Acute reactions can occur; more common in later cycles	Reported in 2% of patients; more common in later cycles		Severe; requires premedication	Severe; requires premedication	Severe reactions observed			
Other			Vesicant; interstitial lung changes and ARDS reported	Requires non-PVC tubing and 0.22 micron filter for administration	Cutaneous side effects including rash and nail toxicities	Patients who are homozygous for UGT1A1*28 allele are at increased risk for neutropenia	CNS side effects seen in 12%, including hallucinations/confusion	Flulike symptoms reported; fever incidence in clinical trials 41%; rash reported in 30%; pulmonary toxicity	Need for folate and vitamin B12 supplementation to reduce treatment-related hematologic and gastrointestinal toxicity; dyspnea; skin rash is reduced in patients who receive premedication with steroids

Source: Data taken from prescribing information.

Table 5–4 Acute and Delayed Setting Antiemetic Recommendations for Patients Undergoing Chemotherapy

Acute Setting

Organization	Highly Emetogenic (HEC)	Moderately Emetogenic
ASCO	Aprepitant or fosaprepitant (3-day regimen) in combination with a serotonin antagonist and steroid; + or − lorazepam	Serotonin antagonist with steroid
ONS	Aprepitant or fosaprepitant (3-day regimen) in combination with a serotonin antagonist and steroid; + or − lorazepam	Aprepitant, serotonin antagonist with steroid
MASCC	Aprepitant or fosaprepitant (3-day regimen) in combination with a serotonin antagonist and steroid; + or − lorazepam	Serotonin antagonist with steroid
NCCN	Aprepitant or fosaprepitant (3-day regimen) in combination with a serotonin antagonist and steroid; + or − lorazepam	Serotonin antagonist with steroid; aprepitant or fosaprepitant (3-day regimen) for patients receiving specific chemotherapy agents[a]

Delayed Setting

Organization	Highly Emetogenic (HEC)	Moderately Emetogenic
ASCO	Steroid and aprepitant	For non AC patients, steroid or serotonin antagonist
ONS	Steroid and aprepitant	Aprepitant, or serotonin antagonist or steroid or metoclopramide + or − diphenhydramine
MASCC	Steroid and aprepitant	Steroid alone; if cannot be used then serotonin antagonist
NCCN	Steroid and aprepitant	If using aprepitant or fosaprepitant on day 1, then continue on days 2 and 3 in combination with serotonin antagonist and steroid

ASCO (American Society of Clinical Oncology) guidelines updated 2006
ONS (Oncology Nursing Society) "Putting Evidence into Practice" guidelines updated 2007
MASCC (Multinational Association of Supportive Care in Cancer) guidelines updated 2008
NCCN (National Comprehensive Cancer Network) guidelines updated 2008
[a]Consider aprepitant in anthracycline/cyclophosphamide (AC) combinations, carboplatin, cyclophosphamide, doxorubicin, epirubicin, ifosfamide, irinotecan, or methotrexate.

Table 5-5 Selected Toxicities of Biotherapy Agents

System	Bevacizumab (Avastin)	Cetuximab (Erbitux)	Gefitinib[a] (IRESSA)	Erlotinib (Tarceva)
Gastrointestinal	Perforation	Diarrhea	Diarrhea; hepatotoxicity; N/V	Diarrhea; hepatotoxicity; N/V
Dermatological		Papular–pustular rash; paronychia, hair and eyelash growth changes	Papular–pustular rash; dry skin; ocular symptoms	Papular–pustular rash; conjunctivitis
Pulmonary		ILD	ILD	ILD
Renal	Proteinuria; nephrotic syndrome			Renal failure
Alterations in electrolytes		Hypomagnesemia, hypokalemia, hypocalcemia		
Cardiovascular	Hypertension; arterial thrombotic events; CHF			
Other	RPLS; fistula development; nasal septum perforation; wound healing complications; hemorrhage; neutropenia	Infusion reactions; some geographic areas have increased reactions[b]	Potential for drug–drug interactions	Potential for drug–drug interactions

CHF: Congestive heart failure

ILD: Interstitial lung disease

RPLS: Reversible posterior leukoencephalopathy syndrome

[a]Gefitinib is indicated as monotherapy for the continued treatment of locally advanced or metastatic non-small cell lung cancer after failure of platinum-based and docetaxel chemotherapies in patients who are benefiting or have benefited from gefitinib.

[b]Cetuximab has been linked to significantly higher grade 3 and 4 infusion reactions in patients who reside in certain southeastern states, such as Tennessee and North Carolina.

Source: Data taken from prescribing information.

symptoms, it may reflect the development of interstitial lung disease, which necessitates interruption of therapy until it is completely evaluated with appropriate diagnostics (Tarceva prescribing information). Management of the EGFR-associated rash has proved to be challenging for clinicians; however, there are small evidenced-based trials that have been published to help guide appropriate treatments. Proposed treatment strategies are shown in Figure 5–4.

Cetuximab is associated with the potential for electrolyte changes, interstitial lung disease (ILD), and diarrhea. Although diarrhea and electrolyte changes can be monitored and managed with appropriate interventions, including antidiarrheal agents and repletion of needed electrolytes, interstitial lung disease can be fatal. Patients with suspected ILD should have prompt evaluation of symptoms and may require cessation of therapy.

Figure 5–4 **EGFR rash care strategies.**

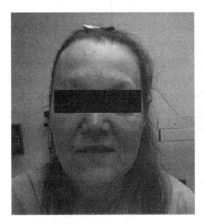 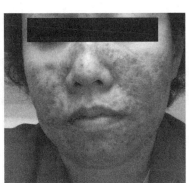 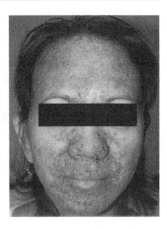

Figure A: Mild EGFR rash

Possible care strategies:
- Mild soaps
- Protective sun cream
- Emollients
- Clindamycin gel
- If necessary, steroid cream
- Colloidal oatmeal lotion

Figure B: Moderate EGFR rash

Possible care strategies:
- Mild soaps
- Protective sun cream
- Emollients
- Clindamycin gel
- If necessary, steroid cream
- Tetracycline analogs (doxycycline or minocycline)
- Colloidal oatmeal lotion

Figure C: Severe EGFR rash

Possible care strategies:
- Mild soaps
- Protective sun cream
- Emollients
- Clindamycin gel
- If necessary, steroid creams or consideration of short oral course of steroids
- Tetracycline analogs (doxycycline or minocycline)
- Colloidal oatmeal lotion

Source: Based on information from Lynch, et al., 2007; Alexandrescu, et al., 2007; Scope, et al., 2007. Pictures courtesy of Pamela Hallquist Viale, RN.

VEGFR Inhibitor Agent Adverse Effects

Administration of bevacizumab, a VEGF inhibitor monoclonal antibody, has a unique side effect profile as well. As an inhibitor of VEGF, this agent can delay wound healing and bleeding may occur. In the clinical trials with bevacizumab, increased incidences of arterial thrombosis, hypertension, bleeding, and bowel perforation occurred. Although older patients were at higher risk, oncology nurses should be aware of potential complications associated with bevacizumab therapy. Proteinuria can be increased, and it is recommended to monitor urinary protein regularly. Postmarketing side effects of reversible posterior leukoencephalopathy (RPLS) and nasal septum perforation have occurred, and subsequent label changes reflect those toxicities. If patients have signs and symptoms of RPLS (which can occur with conventional chemotherapy treatments as well), such as visual changes, headaches, and/or confusion while on therapy with bevacizumab, prompt evaluation and discontinuation of the agent should occur (Ozcan, Wong, & Hari, 2006). In most cases, nasal septum perforation represents a cosmetic challenge, but it is one that does not necessitate cessation of drug therapy. In the clinical trials of bevacizumab in lung cancer, some patients experienced hemoptysis, with several fatalities (Avastin prescribing information). If patients have recent hemoptysis (described as greater than or equal to one half teaspoon of red blood), they should not receive this targeted therapy agent (Avastin prescribing information). The most recent drug warning regarding this agent refers to the possibility of tracheoesophageal (TE) fistula, which occurred in a study of concurrent chemotherapy and radiation in conjunction with bevacizumab in patients with limited-stage small cell lung cancer (with three fatalities); this agent is not approved for use in SCLC.

Conclusion

Lung cancer remains a daunting disease. Although there are vastly more treatment options available for patients with this common cancer, ultimately many will eventually relapse and die of their disease. However, chemotherapy (often in conjunction with other treatment options, such as radiation therapy and surgery) plays a now prominent role in the treatment of both NSCLC and SCLC, offering prolonged survival and in some cases contributing to cure in a small number of patients. Ongoing and future research will continue to address optimal chemotherapy strategies for the treatment of both NSCLC and SCLC, while targeted therapy options represent a growing and exciting area of treatment for lung cancer. Identification of biomarkers (such as KRAS and a number of EGFR gene copies) may help clinicians determine appropriate candidates for specific targeted therapy agents. Additional targeted therapy agents are being studied, and although initial studies with bortezomib in SCLC were disappointing, ongoing studies of this proteasome inhibitor agent combined with chemotherapy are continuing to evaluate this therapy. Immunotherapy and lung cancer vaccines are also under study. Because lung cancer remains a leading cause of cancer-related death and many patients present with advanced disease at diagnosis, improvements in therapeutic strategies are being explored in ongoing studies. Oncology nurses should be aware of the many treatment options for this disease and their role in the management of toxicities associated with chemotherapy and targeted therapy treatments.

References

Albain, K. S., Crowley, J. J., LeBlanc, M., & Livingston, R. B. (1991). Survival determinants in extensive-stage non-small-cell lung cancer: The Southwest Oncology Group experience. *Journal of Clinical Oncology, 9*(9), 1618–1626.

Belani, C. P., Lee, J. S., Socinski, M. A., Robert, F., Waterhouse, D., Rowland, K., et al. (2005). Randomized phase III trial comparing cisplatin-etoposide to carboplatin-paclitaxel in advanced or metastatic non-small cell lung cancer. *Annals of Oncology, 16*(7), 1069–1075.

Beldner, M. A., Sherman, C. A., Green, M. R., Garrett-Mayer, E., Chaudhary, U., Meyer, M. L., et al. (2007). Phase I dose escalation study of vinorelbine and topotecan combination chemotherapy in patients with recurrent lung cancer. *BMC Cancer, 7*, 231.

Blackstock, A. W., & Govindan, R. (2007). Definitive chemoradiation for the treatment of locally advanced non-small cell lung cancer. *Journal of Clinical Oncology, 25*(26), 4146–4152.

Bonomi, P., Kim, K., Fairclough, D., Cella, D., Kugler, J., Rowinsky, E., et al. (2000). Comparison of survival and quality of life in advanced non-small cell lung cancer patients treated with two dose levels of paclitaxel combined with cisplatin versus etoposide with cisplatin: Results of an Eastern Cooperative Oncology Group trial. *Journal of Clinical Oncology, 18*(3), 623–631.

Bria, E., Gralla, J., Raftopoulos, H., Ferretti, G., Felici, G., Nistico, C., et al. (2005). Does adjuvant chemotherapy improve survival in non small cell lung cancer (NSCLC)? A pooled-analysis of 6494 patients in 12 studies, examining survival and magnitude of benefit. *2005 ASCO Annual Meeting Proceedings. Journal of Clinical Oncology, 23*(16S), Pt. I of II (June 1 Suppl.), 7140.

Bunn, P. A., Jr., & Thatcher, N. (2008). Introduction. *The Oncologist, 13*(Suppl. 1), 1–4.

Cardenal, F., Lopez-Cabrerizo, M. P., Anton, A., Alberola, V., Massuti, B., Carrato, A., et al. (1999). Randomized phase III study of gemcitabine-cisplatin versus etoposide-cisplatin in the treatment of locally advanced or metastatic non-small-cell lung cancer. *Journal of Clinical Oncology, 17*(1), 12–18.

Cascone, T., Morelli, M. P., & Ciardiello, F. (2006). Small molecule epidermal growth factor receptor (EGFR) tyrosine kinase inhibitors in non-small cell lung cancer. *Annals of Oncology, 17*(Suppl. 2), ii46–ii48.

Cho, B. C., Im, C. K., Park, M. S., Kim, S. K., Chang, J., Park, J. P., et al. (2007). Phase II study of erlotinib in advanced non-small-cell lung cancer after failure of gefitinib. *Journal of Clinical Oncology, 25*(18), 2528–2533.

Ciuleanu, T. E., Brodowicz, T., Belani, C. P., Kim, J., Krzakowski, M., Laack, R., et al. (2008). Maintenance pemetrexed plus best supportive care (BSC) versus placebo plus BSC: A phase III study [Abstract 8011]. *Journal of Clinical Oncology, 26*, Retrieved September 19, 2008 from http://www.asco.org/ASCO/Abstracts+%26+Virtual+Meeting/Abstracts?&vmview=abst_detail_view&confID=55&abstractID=31696.

Cohen, M. H., Gootenberg, J., Keegan, P., & Pazdur, R. (2007). FDA drug approval summary: Bevacizumab (Avastin) plus carboplatin and paclitaxel as first-line treatment of advanced/metastatic recurrent nonsquamous non small cell lung cancer. *The Oncologist, 12*(6), 713–718.

Costa, D. B., Kobayashi, S., Tenen, D. G., & Huberman, M. S. (2007). Pooled analysis of the prospective trials of gefitinib monotherapy for EGFR-mutant non-small cell lung cancers. *Lung Cancer, 58*(1), 95–103.

Crino, L., Scagliotti, G. V., Ricci, S., de Marinis, F., Rinaldi, M., Gridelli, C., et al. (1999). Gemcitabine and cisplatin versus mitomycin, ifosfamide, and cisplatin in advanced non-small-cell lung cancer: A randomized phase III study of the Italian Lung Cancer Project. *Journal of Clinical Oncology, 17*(11), 3522–3530.

Dasgupta, A., Dasgupta, C., Basu, S., & Majumdar, A. (2006). A prospective and randomized study of radiotherapy, sequential chemotherapy radiotherapy and comcomitant chemotherapy-radiotherapy in unresectable non small cell carcinoma of the lung. *Journal of Cancer Research and Therapeutics, 2*(2), 47–51.

Davila, E., Lilenbaum, R., Raez, L., Seigel, L., Tseng, J., & Graham, P. (2006). Phase II trial of oxaliplatin and gemcitabine with bevacizumab in first-line advanced non-small cell lung cancer (NSCLC). *Journal of Clinical Oncology, 24*(Suppl. 18), 673S.

De Marinis, F., & Grossi, F. (2008). Clinical evidence for second- and third-line treatment options in advanced non-small cell lung cancer. *The Oncologist, 13*(Suppl. 1), 14–20.

Devlin, J. G., & Langer, C. J. (2007). The 800-lb gorilla we all ignore: Treatment of NSCLC in elderly and PS 2 patients. *Clinical Advances in Hematology and Oncology, 5*(3), 216–233.

Douillard, J. Y., Rosell, R., De Lena, M., Carpagnano, F., Ramlau, R., Gonzales-Larriba, J. L., et al. (2006). Adjuvant vinorelbine plus cisplatin versus observation in patients with completely resected stage IB-IIIA non-small-cell lung cancer (Adjuvant Navelbine International Trialist Association [ANITA]): A randomised controlled trial. *Lancet Oncology, 7*(9), 719–727.

Dy, G. K., Miller, A. A., Mandrekar, S. J., Aubry, M. C., Langdon, R. M., Morton, R. F., et al. (2005). A phase II trial of imatinib (ST 1571) in patients with c-kit expressing relapsed small cell lung cancer: A CALGB and NCCTG study. *Annals of Oncology, 16,* 1811–1816.

Evans, W. K., Shepherd, F. A., Feld, R., Osoba, D., Dang, P., & Deboer, G. (1985). VP-16 and cisplatin as first-line therapy for small-cell lung cancer. *Journal of Clinical Oncology, 3*(11), 1471–1477.

Faivre-Finn, C., Lorigan, P., West, C., & Thatcher, N. (2005). Thoracic radiation therapy for limited-stage small cell lung cancer: Unanswered questions. *Clinical Lung Cancer, 7*(1), 23–29.

Ferrara, N. (2004). Vascular endothelial growth factor as a target for anticancer therapy. *The Oncologist, 9*(Suppl. 1), 2–10.

Fossella, F. V., DeVore, R., Kerr, R. N., Crawford, J., Natale, R. R., Dunphy, F., et al. (2000). Randomized phase III trial of docetaxel versus vinorelbine or ifosfamide in patients with advanced non-small cell lung cancer previously treated with platinum containing regimens. *Journal of Clinical Oncology, 18*(12), 2354–2362.

Fossella, F., Pereira, J. R., von Pawel, J., Pluzanska, A., Gorbounova, V., Kaukel, E., et al. (2003). Randomized, multinational, phase III study of docetaxel plus platinum combinations versus vinorelbine plus cisplatin for advanced non-small cell lung cancer: The TAX 326 study group. *Journal of Clinical Oncology, 21* (16), 3016–3024.

Franson, P. J., & Lapka, D. V. (2005). Antivascular endothelial growth factor monoclonal antibody therapy: A promising paradigm in colorectal cancer. *Clinical Journal of Oncology Nursing, 9*(1), 55–60.

Fukuda, M., Soda, H., Fukuda, M., Kinoshita, A., Nakamura, Y., Nagashima, S., et al. (2007). Irinotecan and cisplatin with concurrent split-course radiotherapy in locally advanced nonsmall-cell lung cancer: A multiinstitutional phase 2 study. *Cancer, 110*(3), 606–613.

Fukuoka, M., Furuse, K., Saijo, H., Nishiwaki, Y., Ikegami, H., Tamura, T., et al. (1991). Randomized trial of cyclophosphamide, doxorubicin, and vincristine versus cisplatin and etoposide versus alternation of these regimens in small-cell lung cancer. *Journal of the National Cancer Institute, 83*(12), 855–861.

Fukuoka, M., Yano, S., Giaccone, G., Tomura, T., Nakagawa, K., Douillard, J. Y., et al. (2003). Multiinstitutional randomized phase II trial of gefitinib for previously treated patients with advanced non-small cell lung cancer. *Journal of Clinical Oncology, 21*(12), 2237–2246.

Furuse, K., Kukuoka, M., Kawahara, M., Nishikawa, H., Takada, Y., Kudoh, S., et al. (1999). Phase III study of concurrent versus sequential thoracic radiotherapy in combination with mitomycin, vindesine, and cisplatin in unresectable stage III non-small cell lung cancer. *Journal of Clinical Oncology, 17*(9), 2692–2699.

Gatzemeirer, U., Pluzanska, A., Szczesna, A., Kaukel, E., Roubec, J., De Rosa, F., et al. (2007). Phase III study of erlotinib in combination with cisplatin and gemcitabine in advanced non-small cell lung cancer: The Tarceva Lung Cancer Investigation Trial. *Journal of Clinical Oncology, 25*(12), 1545–1552.

Glynne-Jones, R., & Hoskin, P. (2007). Neoadjuvant cisplatin chemotherapy before chemoradiation: A flawed paradigm? *Journal of Clinical Oncology, 25*(33), 5281–5286.

Gottfried, M., Ramlau, R., Krzakowski, M., Ziolo, G., Olechnowicz, H., Koubkova, L., et al. (2008). Cisplatin-based three drugs combination (NIP) as induction and adjuvant treatment in locally advanced non-small cell lung cancer: Final results. *Journal of Thoracic Oncology, 3*(2), 152–157.

Govindan, R., Page, N., Morgensztern, D., Read, W., Tierney, R., Vlahiotis, A., et al. (2006). Changing epidemiology of small-cell lung cancer in the United States over the last 30 years: Analysis of the surveillance, epidemiologic, and end results database. *Journal of Clinical Oncology, 24*(28), 4539–4544.

Gridelli, C., Bareschino, M. A., Schettino, C., Rossi, A., Maione, P., & Ciardiello, F. (2007a). Erlotinib in non-small cell lung cancer treatment: Current status and future development. *The Oncologist, 12*(7), 840–849.

Gridelli, C., Maione, P., Illiano, A., Piantedosi, F. V., Favoretto, A., Bearz, A., et al. (2007b). Cisplatin plus gemcitabine or vinorelbine for elderly patients with advanced non-small cell lung cancer: The MILES-2P studies. *Journal of Clinical Oncology, 25*(29), 4663–4669.

Gridelli, C., Maione, P., Rossi, A., & De Marinis, F. (2007c). The role of bevacizumab in the treatment of non-small cell lung cancer: Current indications and future developments. *The Oncologist, 12*(10), 1183–1193.

Han, S. W., Kim, T. Y., Lee, K. H., Hwang, P. G., Jeon, Y. K., Oh, D. Y., et al. (2006). Clinical predictors versus epidermal growth factor receptor mutation in gefitinib-treated non-small cell lung cancer patients. *Lung Cancer, 54*(2), 201–207.

Hanna, N., Bunn, P.A. Jr., Langer, C., Einhorn, L., Guthrie, T. Jr., Beck, T., et al. (2006). Randomized phase III trial comparing irinotecan/cisplatin with etoposide/cisplatin in patients with previously untreated extensive-stage disease small-cell lung cancer. *Journal of Clinical Oncology, 24*(13), 2038–2043.

Hanna, N., Shepherd, F. A., Fossella, F. V., Pereira, J. R., de Marinis, F., von Pawel, J., et al. (2004). Randomized phase III trial of pemetrexed versus docetaxel in patients with non-small cell lung cancer previously treated with chemotherapy. *Journal of Clinical Oncology, 22*(9), 1589–1597.

Herbst, R. S., Prager, D., Hermann, R., Fehrenbacher, L., Johnson, B. E., Sandler, A., et al. (2005). TRIBUTE: A phase III trial of erlotinib hydrochloride (OSI-774) combined with carboplatin and paclitaxel chemotherapy in advanced non-small cell lung cancer. *Journal of Clinical Oncology, 23*(25), 5892–5899.

Hotta, K., Fujiwara, Y., Matsuo, K., Suzuki, T., Kiura, K., Tabata, M., et al. (2007). Recent improvement in the survival of patients with advanced nonsmall cell lung cancer enrolled in phase III trials of first-line, systemic chemotherapy. *Cancer, 109*(5), 939–948.

Ignatiadis, M., Mavroudis, D., Veslemes, M., Boukovinas, J., Syrigos, K., Agelidou, M., et al. (2005). Sequential versus alternating administration of cisplatin/etoposide and topotecan as first-line treatment in extensive-stage small-cell lung cancer: Preliminary results of a phase III trial of the Hellenic Oncology Research Group. *Clinical Lung Cancer, 7*(3), 183–189.

International Adjuvant Lung Cancer Trial (IALT) Collaborative Group. (2004). Cisplatin-based adjuvant chemotherapy in patients with completely resected non-small cell lung cancer. *The New England Journal of Medicine, 350*(4), 351–360.

Jain, R. K. (2001). Normalizing tumor vasculature with anti-angiogenic therapy: A new paradigm for combination therapy. *Nature Medicine, 7,* 978–989.

Johnson, B. E., Fischer, T., Fischer, B., Dunlop, D., Rischin, B., Silberman, S., et al. (2003). Phase II study of imatinib in patients with small cell lung cancer. *Clinical Cancer Research, 9*(16 Pt 1), 5880–5887.

Keller, S. M., Adak, S., Wagner, H., Herskovic, A., Komaki, R., Brooks, B. J., et al. (2000). A randomized trial of postoperative adjuvant therapy in patients with completely resected stage II or IIIA non-small-cell lung cancer. Eastern Cooperative Oncology Group. *The New England Journal of Medicine, 343*(17), 1217–1222.

Kelly, K., Crowley, J., Bunn, P. A., Presant, C. A., Grevstad, P. K., Moinpour, C. M., et al. (2001). Randomized phase III trial of paclitaxel plus carboplatin versus vinorelbine plus cisplatin in the treatment of patients with advanced non-small cell lung cancer: A Southwest Oncology Group Trial. *Journal of Clinical Oncology, 19*(13), 3210–3218.

Kim, H. G., Lee, G. W., Kang, J. H., Kang, M. H., Hwang, I. G., Kim, S. H., et al. (2008). Combination chemotherapy with irinotecan and cisplatin in elderly patients (>/= 65 years) with extensive-disease small-cell lung cancer. *Lung Cancer, 61*(2), 220–226.

Kollmansberger, C., Schittenhelm, M., Honecker, F., Tillner, J., Weber, D., Oeschsle, K., et al. (2006). A phase I study of the humanized monoclonal anti-epidermal growth factor receptor (EGFR) antibody EMD 72000 (matuzumab) in combination with paclitaxel in patients with EGFR-positive advanced non-small-cell lung cancer (NSCLC). *Annals of Oncology, 17*(6), 1007–1013.

Kris, M. G., Natale, R. B., Herbst, R. S., Lynch, T. J., Prager, D., Belani, C. P., et al. (2003). Efficacy of gefitinib, an inhibitor of the epidermal growth factor receptor tyrosine kinase, in symptomatic patients with non-small cell lung cancer: A randomized trial. *Journal of the American Medical Association, 290*(16), 2149–2158.

Lally, B. E., Urbanic, J., Blackstock, A. W., Miller, A. A., & Perry, M. C. (2007). Small cell lung cancer: Have we made any progress over the last 25 years? *The Oncologist, 12*(9), 1096–1104.

Langer, C. J. (2008). Resectable non-small cell lung cancer in the elderly: Is there a role for adjuvant treatment? *Drugs & Aging, 25*(3), 209–218.

Langer, C. J., Manola, J., Bernardo, P., Kugler, J. W., Bonomi, P., Cella, D., et al. (2002). Cisplatin-based therapy for elderly patients with advanced non-small cell lung cancer: Implications of Eastern Cooperative Oncology Group 5592, a randomized trial. *Journal of the National Cancer Institute, 94*(3), 173–181.

Laurie, S. A., Logan, D., Markman, B. R., Mackay, J. A., & Evans, W. K. (2004). Practice guideline for the role of combination chemotherapy in the initial management of limited stage small cell lung cancer. *Lung Cancer, 43*(2), 223–240.

Lee, C. B., Morris, D. E., Fried, D. B., & Socinski, M. A. (2006). Current and evolving treatment options for limited stage small cell lung cancer. *Current Opinion in Oncology, 18*(2), 162–172.

Mok, T. S., Ho, S., Chan, G., Ho, W. M., Wong, H., Chan, A. T., et al. (2007). Sequential chemotherapy with combination irinotecan and cisplatin followed by docetaxel for treatment-naïve patients with advanced non-small cell lung cancer. *Journal of Thoracic Oncology, 2*(9), 838–844.

Molina, J. R., Adjei, A. A., & Jett, J. R. (2006). Advances in chemotherapy of non-small cell lung cancer. *Chest, 130*(4), 1211–1219.

Morgensztern, D., Perry, M. C., & Govindan, R. (2007). A phase II study of topotecan and docetaxel in patients with sensitive relapse small cell lung cancer. *Acta Oncologica, 10*, 1–2.

National Comprehensive Cancer Network (NCCN) (2007). NCCN clinical practice guidelines in oncology: Senior Adult Oncology, V.2.2007. Retrieved September 20, 2008 from http://www.nccn.org/professionals/physician_gls/PDF/senior.pdf.

National Comprehensive Cancer Network (NCCN). (2008a). *NCCN clinical practice guidelines in oncology: Non-small cell lung cancer. V.1.2009.* Retrieved September 20, 2008, from http://www.nccn.org/professionals/physician_gls/PDF/nscl.pdf.

National Comprehensive Cancer Network (NCCN). (2008b). *NCCN clinical practice guidelines in oncology: Small cell lung cancer. V.1.209.* Retrieved September 20, 2008, from http://www.nccn.org/professionals/physician_gls/PDF/sclc.pdf.

Niell, H. B., Herndon, J. E., Miller, A. A., Watson, D. M., Sandler, A. B., Kelly, K., et al. (2005). Randomized phase III Intergroup trial of etoposide and cisplatin with or without paclitaxel and granulocyte colony-stimulating factor in patients with extensive stage small-cell lung cancer: Cancer and Leukemia Group B Trial 9732. *Journal of Clinical Oncology, 23*(16), 3752–3759.

Nishio, M., Ohyanagi, F., Horikike, A., Okano, Y., Satoh, Y., Sakae, O., et al. (2007). Phase II trial of gemcitabine and irinotecan in previously treated patients with small-cell lung cancer. *2007 ASCO Annual Meeting Proceedings. Journal of Clinical Oncology, 25*(18S), Pt. I. (June 20 Suppl.), 7718.

Noda, K., Nishwaki, Y., Kawahara, M., Negoro, S., Sugiura, T., Yokoyama, A., et al. (2002). Irinotecan plus cisplatin compared with etoposide plus cisplatin for extensive small-cell lung cancer. *The New England Journal of Medicine, 346*(2), 85–91.

Non-Small Cell Lung Cancer Collaborative Group. (1995). Chemotherapy in non-small cell lung cancer: A meta-analysis using updated data on individual patients from 52 randomised clinical trials. *British Medical Journal, 311*(7010), 899–909.

Okamoto, H., Naoki, K., Narita, Y., Hida, N., Kunikane, H., & Watanabe, K. (2006). A combination chemotherapy of carboplatin and irinotecan with granulocyte colony-stimulating factor (G-CSF) support in elderly patients with small cell lung cancer. *Lung Cancer, 53*(2), 197–203.

Okamoto, H., Watanabe, K., Kunikane, H., Yokoyama, A., Kudoh, S., Asakawa, T., et al. (2007). Randomised phase III trial of carboplatin plus etoposide vs split doses of cisplatin plus etoposide in elderly or poor-risk patients with extensive disease small-cell lung cancer: JCOG 9702. *British Journal of Cancer, 97*, 162–169.

Onn, A., Vaporciyan, A. A., Chang, J. Y., Komaki, R., Roth, J. A., & Herbst, R. S. (2006). Cancer of the lung. In D. W. Kufe, R. C. Bast Jr., W. N. Hait, W. K. Hong, R. E. Pollack, R. R. Weichselbaum, et al. (Eds.), *Cancer Medicine 7* (pp. 1179–1224). Hamilton, Ontario: BC Decker.

Owonikoko, T. K., Ramalingam, S., Forster, J., Shuai, Y., Evans, T., Gooding, W. E., et al. (2007). Phase II study of irinotecan and paclitaxel for patients with recurrent small cell lung cancer (SCLC). *2007 ASCO Annual Meeting Proceedings. Journal of Clinical Oncology, 25*(18S), Pt. I (June 20 Suppl.), 18011.

Ozcan, C., Wong, S. J., & Hari, P. (2006). Reversible posterior leukoencephalopathy syndrome and bevacizumab. *The New England Journal of Medicine, 354*(9), 980–982.

Patel, J. D., Hensing, T. A., & Villafor, V. (2007). Pemetrexed and carboplatin plus bevacizumab for advanced non-squamous non-small cell lung cancer (NSCLC): Preliminary results. *Journal of Clinical Oncology, 25*(Suppl. 18), 409S.

Pfister, D. G., Johnson, D. H., Azzoli, C. G., Sause, W., Smith, T. J., Baker, S., et al. (2004). American Society of Clinical Oncology treatment of unresectable non-small-cell lung cancer guideline: Update 2003. *Journal of Clinical Oncology, 22*(2), 330–353.

Pirker, R., Szczesna, A., von Pawel, J., Krzakowski, M., Ramlau, R., Park, K., et al. (2008). FLEX: A randomized, multicenter, phase III study of cetuximab in combination with cisplatin/vinorelbine (CV) versus CV alone in the first-line treatment of patients with advanced non-small cell lung cancer (NSCLC). [Abstract 3]. *Journal of Clinical Oncology, 26*(May 20 Suppl.). Retrieved September 19, 2008, from http://www.asco.org/ASCO/Abstracts+%26+Virtual+Meeting/Abstracts?&vmview=abst_detail_view&confID=55&abstractID=30338.

Pisters, K., Vallieres, E., Bunn, P. A., Jr., Crowley, J., Chansky, K., Ginsberg, R., et al. (2007a). S9900: Surgery alone or surgery plus induction (ind) paclitaxel/carboplatin (PC) chemotherapy in early stage non-small cell lung cancer (NSCLC): Follow-up on a phase III trial. *2007 ASCO Annual Meeting Proceedings. Journal of Clinical Oncology, 25*(18S; June 20 Suppl.; Post-Meeting Edition), 7520.

Pisters, K. M. W., Evans, W. K., Azzoli, C. G., Kris, M. G., Smith, C. A., Desch, C. E., et al. (2007b). Cancer Care Ontario and American Society of Clinical Oncology adjuvant chemotherapy and adjuvant radiation therapy for stages I-IIIA resectable non-small-cell lung cancer guidelines. *Journal of Clinical Oncology, 25*(34), 5506–5518.

Planchard, D., Bourgeois, H., Adoun, M., Paitel, J. F., Blanc, P., Genet, D., et al. (2006). Gemcitabine, ifosfamide, and cisplatin combination (GIP) in treatment of patients with locally advanced or metastatic non-small cell lung cancer: Results of a phase II study. *American Journal of Clinical Oncology, 29*(4), 345–351.

Pujol, J. L., Breton, J. L., Gervais, R., Tanguy, M. L., Quoix, E., David, P., et al. (2007). Phase III double-blind, placebo-controlled study of thalidomide in extensive-disease small-cell lung cancer after response to chemotherapy: An Intergroup Study FNCLCC cleo04–IFCT 00-01. *Journal of Clinical Oncology, 25*(25), 3945–3951.

Quoix, E., Lebeau, B., Depierre, A., Ducolone, A., Moro-Sibilot, D., Milleron, B., et al. (2004). Randomised, multicentre phase II study assessing two doses of docetaxel (75 or 100 mg/m2) as second-line monotherapy for non-small cell lung cancer. *Annals of Oncology, 15*(1), 38–44.

Raju, R. N., Neubauer, M. A., Smith, D. A., Richards, D. A., Asmar, L., Cunneen, J. L., et al. (2007). Pemetrexed (P) in relapsed small cell lung cancer (SCLC): Preliminary results of a phase II trial. *2007 ASCO Annual Meeting Proceedings. Journal of Clinical Oncology, 25*(18S), Pt. I (June 20 Suppl.), 7716.

Ramalingam, S., & Belani, C. (2008). Systemic chemotherapy for advanced non-small cell lung cancer: Recent advances and future directions. *The Oncologist, 12* (Suppl. 1), 5–13.

Ramalingam, S. S., Dahlberg, S. E., Langer, C. J., Gray, R., Belani, C. P., Brahmer, J. R., et al. (2008). Outcomes for elderly, advanced-stage non-small cell lung cancer patients treated with bevacizumab in combination with carboplatin and paclitaxel: Analysis of Eastern Cooperative Oncology Group Trial 4599. *Journal of Clinical Oncology, 26*(1), 60–65.

Rapp, E., Pater, J. L., Willan, A., Cormier, Y., Murray, N., Evans, W. K., et al. (1988). Chemotherapy can prolong survival in patients with advanced non-small-cell lung cancer: Report of a Canadian multicenter randomized trial. *Journal of Clinical Oncology, 6*(4), 633–641.

Rosell, R., Gatzemeier, U., Betticher, D. C., Keppler, U., Macha, H. N., Pirker, R., et al. (2002). Phase III randomized trial comparing paclitaxel/carboplatin with paclitaxel/cisplatin in patients with advanced non-small-cell lung cancer: A cooperative multinational trial. *Annals of Oncology, 13*(10), 1539–1549.

Rudin, C. M., Liu, W., Desai, A., Karrison, T., Jiang, X., Janisch, L., et al. (2008). Pharmacogenomic and pharmacokinetic determinants of erlotinib toxicity. *Journal of Clinical Oncology, 26*(7), 1119–1127.

Sandler, A., Gray, R., Perry, M. C., Brahmer, J., Schiller, J. H., Dowlati, A., et al. (2006). Paclitaxel-carboplatin alone or with bevacizumab for non-small cell lung cancer. *The New England Journal of Medicine, 355*(24), 2542–2550.

Sandler, A. B., Nemunaitis, J., Denham, C., von Pawel, J., Cormier, Y., Gatzemeier, U., et al. (2000). Phase III trial of gemcitabine plus cisplatin versus cisplatin alone in patients with locally advanced or metastatic non-small cell lung cancer. *Journal of Clinical Oncology, 18*(1), 122–130.

Scagliotti, G. V., Fossati, R., Torri, V., Crino, L., Giaccone, G., Silvano, G., et al. (2003). Randomized study of adjuvant chemotherapy for completely resected stage I, II, or IIIA non-small cell lung cancer. *Journal of the National Cancer Institute, 95*(19), 1453–1461.

Schiller, J. H., Harrington, D., Belani, C., Langer, C., Sandler, A., Krook, J., et al. (2002). Comparison of four chemotherapy regimens for advanced non-small cell lung cancer. *The New England Journal of Medicine, 346*(2), 92–98.

Shepherd, F. A., Dancey, J., Ramlau, R., Mattson, K., Gralla, R., O'Rourke, M., et al. (2000). Prospective randomized trial of docetaxel versus best supportive care in patients with non-small cell lung cancer previously treated with platinum-based chemotherapy. *Journal of Clinical Oncology, 18*(10), 2095–2103.

Shepherd, F. A., Pereira, J. R., Ciuleanu, T., Tan, E. H., Hirsh, V., Thongprasert, S., et al. (2005). Erlotinib in previously treated non-small cell lung cancer. *The New England Journal of Medicine, 353*(2), 123–132.

Smit, E. F., Mattson, K., von Pawel, J., Manegold, C., Clarke, S., & Postmus, P. E. (2003). ALIMTA (pemetrexed disodium) as second-line treatment of non-small-cell lung cancer: A phase II study. *Annals of Oncology, 14*(3), 455–460.

Socinski, M. A., Blackstock, A. W., Bogart, J. A., Wang, X., Munley, M., Rosenman, J., et al. (2008). Randomized phase II trial of induction chemotherapy followed by concurrent chemotherapy and dose-escalated thoracic conformal radiotherapy (74 Gy) in stage III non-small cell lung cancer: CALGB 30105. *Journal of Clinical Oncology, 26*(15), 2457–2463.

Socinski, M. A., & Bogart, J. A. (2007). Limited stage small cell lung cancer: The current status of combined-modality therapy. *Journal of Clinical Oncology, 25*(26), 4137–4145.

Sorensen, M., Lassen, U., Palshof, T., Jensen, B. B., Johansen, J., Jensen, P. B., et al. (2008). Topotecan and cisplatin in combination with concurrent twice-daily chemoradiation in limited disease small cell lung cancer: A Danish Oncological Lung Cancer Group (DOLG) phase II trial. *Lung Cancer, 60*(2), 252–258.

Stinchcombe, T. E., Fried, D., Morris, D. E., & Socinski, M.A. (2006). Combined modality therapy for stage III non-small cell lung cancer. *The Oncologist, 11*(7), 809–823.

Sundstrom, S., Bremnes, R. M., Kaasa, S., Aasebo, U., Hatlevoll, R., Dahle, R., et al (2002). Cisplatin and etoposide regimen is superior to cyclophosphamide, epirubicin, and vincristine regimen in small cell lung cancer: Results from a randomized phase III trial with 5 years' follow up. *Journal of Clinical Oncology, 20*(24), 4665–4672.

Syrigos, K., Katirtzoglou, N., Charpidou, A., Botsis, T., Karapanagiotou, E., Dilana, K., et al. (2007). Irinotecan, carboplatin and etoposide regimen in extensive disease small cell lung cancer: Phase II trial. *2007 ASCO Annual Meeting Proceedings. Journal of Clinical Oncology, 25*(18S), Pt. I (June 20 Suppl.), 18153.

Thatcher, N., Chang, A., Parikh, P., Rodrigues, P. J., Ciuleanu, T., von Pawel, J., et al. (2005). Gefitinib plus best supportive care in previously treated patients with refractory advanced non-small cell lung cancer: Results from a randomised, placebo-controlled, multicentre study (Iressa Survival Evaluation in Lung Cancer). *Lancet, 366*(9496), 1527–1537.

Thienelt, C. D., Bunn, P. A., Hanna, N., Rosenberg, A., Needle, M. N., Long, M. E., et al. (2005). Multicenter phase I/II study of cetuximab with paclitaxel and carboplatin in untreated patients with stage IV non-small cell lung cancer. *Journal of Clinical Oncology, 23*(34), 8786–8793.

Tsao, M. S., Sakurada, A., Cutz, J. C., Zhu, C. Q., Karnel-Reid, S., Squire, J., et al. (2005). Erlotinib in lung cancer: Molecular and clinical predictors of outcome. *The New England Journal of Medicine, 353*(2), 133–144.

United States Food and Drug Administration. (2008). *ALIMTA (pemetrexed disodium): Injection, powder, lyophilized, for solution for intravenous use.* Retrieved November 11, 2008, from http://www.fda.gov/cder/foi/label/2008/021462s0151b1.pdf

Viale, P. H. (2007). The biology of angiogenesis. *Oncology: Nurse Edition, 21*(14), 5–11.

Viale, P. H., & Sommers, R. (2007). Nursing care of patients receiving chemotherapy for metastatic colorectal cancer. *Seminars in Oncology Nursing, 23*, 22–35.

von Pawel, J., Schiller, J. H., Shepherd, F. A., Fields, S. Z., Kielsbauer, J. P., Chrysson, N. G., et al. (1999). Topotecan versus cyclophosphamide, doxorubicin, and vincristine for the treatment of recurrent small cell lung cancer. *Journal of Clinical Oncology, 17*(2), 658–667.

Wozniak, A. J., Crowley, J. J., Balcerzak, S. P., Weiss, G. R., Spiridonidis, C. H., Baker, L. H., et al. (1998). Randomized trial comparing cisplatin with cisplatin plus vinorelbine in the treatment of advanced non-small-cell lung cancer: A Southwest Oncology Group Study. *Journal of Clinical Oncology, 16*(7), 2459–2465.

New Advances in Radiotherapy for Lung Cancer

Giselle J.
Moore-Higgs

Kenneth R. Olivier

Introduction

Historically, radiotherapy has been an integral component of treatment for lung cancer. However, despite the advances in understanding lung cancer pathogenesis, the use of combined modality treatment approaches, and improved radiotherapy techniques, the long-term survival rate remains dismal. The majority of patients, particularly those with advanced disease, die from persistent thoracic disease after treatment and/or from the development of distant metastases. In view of the poor local control rate following conventional radiotherapy, there is a clear need for methods to improve efficacy. The three main reasons for local failure after radiotherapy are: (1) geographic misses due to inadequacy of imaging tools for staging and radiotherapy planning; (2) geographic misses due to respiratory tumor motion during radiation delivery; and (3) inadequate radiation dose because of the potential for significant toxicity (Chang, et al., 2008).

The successful outcome of radiotherapy depends on a clear definition of target volume, the optimal radiation dose and fractionation schedules, and proper radiation portal arrangement to secure the optimal dose distribution within the target volume (Choi, 2000). Unfortunately, "standard" radiotherapy techniques have several problems that have hindered the ability to improve outcomes. A number of innovative treatment approaches using radiotherapy are under investigation in an attempt to enhance local disease control with less normal tissue toxicity. These approaches include radiation dose escalation, altered fractionation schedules, improvements in radiation dose distribution, brachytherapy procedures using radioactive seeds, use of radioprotectors (i.e., amifostine), and chemoradiation schemes. In addition, measures to overcome hypoxic tumor cells are under investigation. These include the use of high linear energy transfer (LET) beams, radiotherapy under hyperbaric conditions, the use of hypoxic cell sensitizers, and hyperthermia (Choi, 2000).

This chapter will provide a brief overview of the standard radiotherapy procedures for lung cancer as well as address several new radiation technologies and clinical trials aimed at addressing the current limitations of normal tissue damage and improvements in dose distribution.

Standard Therapy: Non-Small Cell Lung Cancer

Radiotherapy has been an important component of treatment of non-small cell lung cancer (NSCLC). It has been used extensively in the definitive and postoperative setting and more recently in trials evaluating preoperative treatment. Patients with NSCLC who are appropriate candidates for radiotherapy fall into one of the following categories:

- Medically inoperable stage I and II NSCLC: Commonly seen in patients with extensive tobacco histories. Most have other smoking-related diseases, such as coronary artery disease, chronic obstructive pulmonary disease, and peripheral vascular disease, which render them inoperable even though definitive resection might be indicated.
- Unresectable stage III NSCLC: Advanced local disease in the thoracic cavity.
- Postoperative therapy in stages II and III NSCLC: For positive or close surgical margins or lymph node involvement.
- Superior pulmonary sulcus tumor: Presenting in the apex of the lung and that is unresectable secondary to its invasion into a number of critical structures.
- Metastatic spread of disease: Outside the thoracic cavity (i.e., brain, bone, adrenal gland); usually treated with palliative therapy.
- Recurrent disease: Includes endobronchial lesions that obstruct the bronchi.

The NCCN (2008) guidelines for the treatment of NSCLC recommend that modern three-dimensional conformal radiation therapy techniques with computed tomography (CT), or CT/positron emission tomography (PET)-based treatment planning should be used on all patients who receive radiation therapy for lung cancer. In addition, whenever feasible, respiratory management techniques should be incorporated in the radiation setup and delivery to individualize respiratory motion and/or decrease dose to the normal tissues, respectively (NCCN, 2008).

Primary Radiation Therapy

Medically inoperable patients with early stage disease (stage I and II) are usually offered radiotherapy with or without chemotherapy. Although the results are not as good as those for patients selected for surgery, definitive radiation offers patients a chance of cure. Treatment is usually tailored to the individual, taking into consideration tumor volume as well as overall health. The treatment usually includes radiation to the primary lesion as well as the regional lymphatics to a dose of 50–65 Gy over a 5- to 6-week period. A new alternative approach in these patients is the use of stereotactic body radiotherapy (SBRT), which uses high doses (48–60 Gy) given in few fractions. SBRT has achieved local control rates comparable to surgery, with few side effects if carefully delivered (McGarry, Papiez, Williams, Whitford, & Timmerman, 2005; Nagata, et al., 2005).

Until recently, patients with stage IIIA or IIIB NSCLC also received radiotherapy to doses of 50–65 Gy using daily fractionation over a 5- to 6-week period of time. Randomized trials have compared standard daily radiotherapy (60 Gy) with twice-daily treatment of a higher dose (69.6 Gy) and with an accelerated regimen that delivered 54 Gy over 2.5 weeks. Both altered fractionation schedules resulted in improved survival (Khuri, Keller, & Wagner, 1999).

The combination of chemotherapy and radiotherapy is the standard treatment approach for locally advanced NSCLC in patients with a good performance status. A number of randomized trials have evaluated combined chemotherapy and radiotherapy as a method to improve outcomes in stage III disease. Current approaches include induction chemotherapy for several cycles followed by radiotherapy or concurrent chemoradiation. Cisplatin, vinblastine, carboplatin, and paclitaxel have all been used in these trials. Radiotherapy is usually given to a dose of 60 to 70 Gy over 5 to 7 weeks. An analysis of five RTOG trials studying chemoradiotherapy for NSCLC (88-04, 88-08 [chemo-RT arm], 90-15, 91-06, and 92-04) was undertaken to determine if patients with NSCLC and positive supraclavicular nodes (SN+) have a similar outcome to other patients with stage IIIB NSCLC negative supraclavicular nodes (SN2) when treated with modern chemoradiotherapy. In this series, the outcome for patients with supraclavicular metastases who were treated with modern chemoradiotherapy appeared to be similar to that of other stage IIIB patients. This supports the rationale for continuing to enroll SN+ patients in aggressive chemoradiotherapy clinical trials for locally advanced NSCLC (Machtay, et al., 1999).

In advanced disease (stage IV), patient care is individualized and usually palliative. The goal of treatment is to relieve symptoms, including shortness of breath, airway obstruction, pain, or neurologic symptoms. The primary site is treated with radiotherapy consisting of 30 Gy over a 2-week period. Bone, brain, and adrenal metastasis may also be treated with short courses of palliative radiotherapy (8–30 Gy).

Preoperative Radiation Therapy

Preoperative radiation therapy with or without chemotherapy has been used for patients with stage III disease. Advantages of preoperative therapy include delivery of therapy to better-oxygenated tumors and better-vascularized tissue. Preoperative chemoradiation should be avoided if pneumonectomy is required to avoid postoperative pulmonary toxicity (NCCN, 2008). Surgery in a field that has received 60 Gy can be difficult, because important landmarks may disappear and increase the risk of a surgical complication. The NCCN guidelines (2008) recommend a total dose of 45–50 Gy in 1.8–2 Gy fractions to treat all volumes of gross disease in the preoperative chemoradiation setting.

Research from the Cleveland Clinic shows promising results in terms of tumor response, disease control, survival, and toxicity after short-course induction chemoradiotherapy and surgical resection in patients with stage III disease. Patients received 12-day induction therapy of a 96-hour continuous infusion of cisplatin (20 mg/m2 per day), 24-hour infusion of paclitaxel (175 mg/m2), and concurrent accelerated fractionation radiotherapy (1.5 Gy twice daily) to a dose of 30 Gy, followed by surgical resection 4 weeks later and a second postoperative identical course of chemotherapy and concurrent radiotherapy (30–33 Gy). This regimen resulted in good tumor response and downstaging, with 71% of those who underwent thoracotomy able to be resected for cure. Thirty-one patients were downstaged to mediastinal node negative (stage

0, I, or II) status. The median survival was modestly improved compared with historical controls. Induction toxicity resulted in hospitalization of 18 patients (40%) for neutropenic fever (Rice, et al., 1998).

Postoperative Radiation Therapy

The role of radiotherapy in stage I and II disease has been primarily as postoperative adjuvant therapy in patients with close or positive margins or N1 or N2 disease. However, the appropriate role of postoperative radiotherapy remains ill defined despite a number of randomized trials. The trials have been hindered by a lack of uniformity of patient selection and the use of non-CT guided treatment planning approaches. In a meta-analysis of nine randomized trials that assessed postoperative radiotherapy in NSCLC, there was no significant improvement in disease-free or overall survival, and there was a 21% increase in mortality (PORT MTG, 1998). This meta-analysis used outdated radiotherapy methods and has been criticized as irrelevant with current radiotherapy techniques. Enthusiasm for carefully selected patients with positive mediastinal nodes remains and is commonly used in clinical practice. A recent European trial using chemotherapy and adjuvant therapy (Douillard, et al., 2006) showed a trend toward improved survival in patients with positive mediastinal nodes treated with radiotherapy. They also showed a potentially harmful effect of radiotherapy given to patients with no evidence of mediastinal node involvement.

Endobronchial Brachytherapy

Endobronchial occlusion is a common and potentially life-threatening complication. Endobronchial irradiation has also been used to palliate symptoms arising from partial airway obstruction (Khuri, et al., 1999). In palliative care, 50–100% of patients have reported symptomatic relief. Studies also report that two-thirds to three-fourths of the remainder of the patient's life is symptom improved or symptom free (Mehta, 1996).

Standard Treatment: Small Cell Lung Cancer

The routine use of thoracic radiotherapy in small cell lung cancer (SCLC) is limited to those patients with cancer restricted to the thorax. In these patients radiotherapy is used in combination with chemotherapy to improve survival. Doses range from 45 Gy given in 1.5 Gy fractions twice daily to 70 Gy given in 2 Gy daily fractions. The techniques used to treat SCLC are essentially the same as those used in NSCLC. The pattern of failure in SCLC is slightly different than NSCLC, which has prompted a notable difference in management from a radiotherapy perspective.

SCLC has a strong propensity to spread to the brain (up to 50% of patients develop brain metastases during the course of treatment). Given the high incidence of brain metastases, radiotherapy has an established role in preventing that pattern of spread through the use of prophylactic cranial irradiation (PCI). This has a proven survival benefit (Auperin, et al., 1999).

New Technologies

There have been two major advances in technology that have significantly impacted the planning and delivery of radiation and have resulted in increased selectivity of irradiation to the tumor and a decrease in the dose to the normal tissues and critical structures. The first is the availability of new techniques in medical imaging, which have greatly improved the three-dimensional delineation of tumors and critical tissue structures. This includes computed tomography (CT), magnetic resonance imaging (MRI), and positron emission tomography (PET). The other advancement is the development of high-precision technologies for beam delivery that allow better dose distribution within the target and spare a larger portion of normal tissue than conventional radiotherapy.

Image Guided Treatment Planning

The use of diagnostic and planning CT and MRI has greatly improved the accuracy of tumor localization in treatment planning. Both of these imaging studies have undergone significant advances that have improved both the clarity of the image and the accuracy of recognizing benign versus malignant densities. Another imaging study that has had a significant impact on the identification of local and metastatic disease is the PET scan. The PET scan is an imaging technique that relies on metabolic properties of the tumors. Glycolysis is increased in tumor tissue, and PET detects increased uptake of fluorodeoxyglucose (FDG), a glucose analog radiopharmaceutical, in malignant tissue. For tumor volume delineation and characterization, PET has brought an additional dimension to the management of lung cancer patients by allowing the incorporation of crucial functional and molecular images in radiotherapy treatment planning (i.e, direct evaluation of tumor metabolism, cell proliferation, apoptosis, hypoxia, and angiogenesis) (Lecchi, Fossati, Elisei, Orecchia, & Lucignani, 2008).

In lung cancer PET imaging is useful in evaluating both parenchymal lung nodules and mediastinal nodes as well as detecting distant metastasis that may not otherwise be detected. PET/CT has been shown to improve targeting accuracy in 25% to 50% of cases (Chang, et al., 2008). The increased use of FDG–PET has been associated with a stage migration in patients with NSCLC, which may partially account for improvements in survival as compared with historical controls (Morgensztern, Goodgame, Baggstrom, Gao, & Govindan, 2008).

A major obstacle to radiotherapy target delineation has been respiration-induced target motion (also known as intrafractional tumor motion), which can add considerable geometrical uncertainty to the radiation treatment (Chang, et al., 2008). Such motion requires enlargement of the treatment field portals to cover the movement of the tumor during treatment. The development of four-dimensional CT with multislice detectors and faster imaging reconstruction has facilitated the ability to obtain images while patients breathe and to assess organ motion (Nehmeh & Erdi, 2008). Four-dimensional CT involves acquiring oversampled CT information and correlating these data with information about the respiratory cycle. The four-dimensional techniques can be classified into three groups: respiratory control, gating, and tracking (van Meerbeeck, Meersschout, De Pauw, Madani, & De Neve, 2008). Respiratory control techniques involve assisted or voluntary pausing of respiration in a selected phase of the respiratory cycle. Irradiation is performed during the respiratory pauses and is turned off when the respiratory motion resumes. Gating means enabling irradiation when the motion amplitude coincides with a preselected sector of the respiratory cycle and halting the beam when the respiratory motion travels outside this sector.

Tracking involves intentionally moving the irradiating beam so that it follows the movement of the tumor. Each of these techniques has its benefits and requires some degree of assessment of the patient's ability to participate in the procedure.

Another technique that is gaining a lot of attention is "dose painting." This concept is an attempt to address the issue of dose inhomogeneity that has plagued traditional treatment planning techniques. Using the newer imaging modalities mostly based on PET, functional MRI, and magnetic resonance spectroscopy, radiobiological information about the tumor can be integrated into intensity-modulated radiation therapy (IMRT) planning (van Meerbeeck, et al., 2008). Tumor regions of higher radiation resistance may, in the future, be painted with an escalated dose while radiation-sensitive regions receive conventional or even lower dose levels (van Meerbeeck, et al., 2008).

Intensity-Modulated Radiation Therapy

Recently, an advanced form of three-dimensional conformal radiation therapy (CRT), called intensity-modulated radiation therapy (IMRT), has been introduced. IMRT is a new technology that delivers radiation more precisely to the tumor while relatively sparing the surrounding normal tissues. Its aim is to overcome previous limitations by adding modulation of beam intensity to beam shaping (Tubiana & Eschwège, 2000). IMRT has wide application in most aspects of radiation oncology because of its ability to create multiple targets and multiple avoidance structures, to treat different targets simultaneously to different doses, as well as to weight targets and avoidance structures according to their importance. By delivering radiation with greater precision, IMRT has been shown to minimize acute treatment-related morbidity while making dose escalation feasible, which may ultimately improve local tumor control.

IMRT has also introduced a new accelerated fractionation scheme known as simultaneous modulated accelerated radiation therapy (SMART) boost. By shortening the overall treatment time, SMART boost has the potential of improving tumor control in addition to offering patient convenience and cost savings.

In lung cancer, very little has been published on the role of IMRT. Graham (2001) speculated that this may be due to concern about the respiratory movement during treatment. The resultant intensity-modulated calculations may not be reproducibly produced during treatment, and heterogeneity factors may not be reproducibly accounted for in some IMRT systems. To overcome these concerns, it will take time and continued improvement in the treatment planning technology.

Particle Beam Radiation Therapy

Proton beam therapy, as the name implies, uses protons to fight cancer. Protons are stable, positively charged subatomic particles with a mass 1800 times that of an electron. These characteristics allow the proton's dose of radiation to be released at an exact shape and depth within the body (Optivus Technology, 2008). Proton beam radiation is unlike megavoltage X-rays in that it has weight and mass and usually an electric charge. Massive cyclotrons and synchrotrons use enormous amounts of energy to accelerate protons for therapeutic use. Proton beams have been used for treatment since the mid-1950s, but for most of that time only in physics laboratories. Proton therapy provides the radiation oncologist with a highly precise method of placing radiation within a patient when compared with conventional radiotherapy using megavoltage X-rays (photons) or electrons.

Both conventional megavoltage X-ray therapy and proton beam therapy work in the same way. They produce cellular changes that damage DNA and kill the cell. Megavoltage X-ray therapy delivers this damage via a wave of energy that has neither a charge nor mass and relies on the probability of interaction between the wave and the cellular contents. Because of the large number of waves and reliable probabilities of interaction, the dose of radiotherapy is both consistent and predictable. A dose of radiotherapy is also given to surrounding structures because of this probability of interaction. This pattern of energy placement results in damage to healthy tissues and prevents the radiation oncologist from prescribing a sufficient dose of radiation to control the disease.

Protons, on the other hand, are charged particles with a known mass. Because you can control the energy of the proton, you can better determine the dose delivery to tissues. These energies determine how deeply in the body protons will deposit their maximum energy. As the protons move through the body, they slow down, causing increased interaction with orbiting electrons.

Maximum interaction with electrons occurs as the protons approach their targeted stopping point. Thus, maximum energy is released within the designated tumor volume. The surrounding healthy cells receive significantly less injury than the cells in the designated volume. As a result of protons' dose-distribution characteristics, the radiation oncologist can increase the dose to the tumor while reducing the dose to surrounding normal tissues. This allows the

dose to be increased beyond that which less-conformal radiation will allow. This has the potential for fewer harmful side effects, more direct impact on the tumor, and increased tumor control. Currently this treatment is very expensive and available at only a few institutions in North America.

Several publications address the role of proton beam radiotherapy in lung cancer. The majority of them address methods and tools for beam design. Bush and colleagues (1999a) published the results of a prospective study to evaluate the efficacy and toxicity of conformal proton beam radiotherapy for early-stage, medically inoperable NSCLC. Preliminary results indicated that proton beam radiotherapy can be used safely in this group of patients. Disease-free survival and local control appear to be good and compare favorably with previously reported conventional photon irradiation. In another recent publication, Bush and colleagues (1999b) reported on a study that was undertaken to determine the frequency and severity of pulmonary injury revealed by CT in patients who had undergone conformal proton (to a limited volume) radiotherapy. They compared the findings with those from a group of patients who had undergone a combination of photon and conformal proton (to a larger volume) radiotherapy. They concluded that proton radiotherapy was associated with a lower frequency of pulmonary injury than the combined regimen. Injury correlated well with the volume of normal lung that was irradiated.

Clinical Trials

Currently, the National Cancer Institute (NCI) has approximately 100 clinical trials registered for the treatment of lung cancer with radiotherapy either alone or in combination with a systemic or surgical modality. Of these, the majority are for NSCLC. Most of the trials are being conducted by the NCI or one of the cooperative groups, including the Radiation Therapy Oncology Group (RTOG) or the European Organisation for Research and Treatment of Cancer (EORTC). Other trials are being conducted by either single or multi-institutional groups. The focus of the trials appears to be on the following:

- What is the value of altered-fractionation and image guided radiotherapy in the treatment of NSCLC?
- What is the optimal sequencing of radiotherapy with various chemotherapy agents?
- What is the role of treatments such as photodynamic therapy in combination with endobronchial brachytherapy?
- What is the role of other systemic therapies such as biologicals and complementary therapies?
- What is the efficacy of agents that can reduce the toxicity of radiotherapy, thus allowing dose escalation?

It has been established that novel radiotherapy administration schedules and techniques as well as chemotherapy regimens for combined modality therapy are essential for improving the management of lung cancer. A number of phase I and phase II randomized trials of new chemoradiation regimens are currently enrolling patients.

Role of Nursing

With the continued evolution of radiotherapy, the role of nursing becomes more important in this field. In a disease such as lung cancer that has a large number of patients and an overall dismal outcome, it is important that radiation oncology nurses take an active role in the enrollment of patients in clinical trials that may offer a superior result. In addition, nurses should be proactive in the accurate assessment of the patient at the time of diagnosis and throughout treatment to provide quality care to the individual and also to provide accurate data for the clinical trial evaluation. Finally, nurses should be actively involved in the development of clinical trials to ensure that the outcomes evaluation includes quality of life evaluations and not just tumor response and localized tissue reactions.

Nurses also must remain proactive in their own education and participate in opportunities to learn more about the new technologies and their impact on patients. As the primary providers of patient and family education, it is important to provide accurate information at a level that the patient and family can understand. This requires deciphering complicated technology into simplistic terms. Patient education materials should be updated on a regular basis to reflect the ongoing changes in the planning and execution of the treatment protocol.

Conclusion

The role of radiotherapy in lung cancer continues to evolve as technology allows radiation oncologists to find new approaches to treatment in an attempt to improve the current dismal outcome of this disease. Although many patients with advanced disease may not benefit from the new technology, patients with inoperable early-stage disease may. It is important that healthcare providers remain current on the new approaches to treating this disease that are available through cooperative group trials and at numerous institutions and be open to enrolling patients in these trials.

References

Auperin, A., Arriagada, R., Pignon J., LePechoux, C., Gregor, A., Stephens, R. J., et al. (1999). Prophylactic cranial irradiation for patients with small cell lung cancer in complete remission. Prophylactic Cranial Irradiation Overview Collaborative Group. *New England Journal of Medicine, 341*(7), 476–484.

Bush, D. A., Dunbar, R. D., Bonnet, R., Slater, J. D., Cheek, G. A., & Slater, J. M. (1999a). Pulmonary injury from proton and conventional radiotherapy as revealed by CT. *AJR—American Journal of Roentgenology, 172*(3), 735–739.

Bush, D. A., Slater, J. D., Bonnet, R., Cheek, G. A., Dunbar, R. D., Moyers, M., et al. (1999b). Proton-beam radiotherapy for early-stage lung cancer. *Chest, 116*(5), 1313–1319.

Chang, J. Y., Dong, L., Liu, H., Starkschall, G., Balter, P., Mohan, R., et al. (2008). Image-guided radiation therapy for non-small cell lung cancer. *Journal of Thoracic Oncology, 3*(2), 177–186.

Choi, N. C. (2000). Cancer of the intrathorax. In C. C. Wang (Ed.), *Clinical radiation oncology: Indications, techniques, and results* (2nd ed., pp. 295–333). New York: Wiley-Liss.

Douillard, J., Rosell, R., De Lena, M., Carpagnano, F. L., Ramlau, R., Gonzales-Larriba, J. L., et al. (2006). Adjuvant vinorelbine plus cisplatin versus observation in patients with completely resected stage IB-IIIA non-small cell lung cancer (Adjuvant Navelbine International Trialist Association [ANITA]: A randomized controlled trial). *Lancet Oncology, 7*(9), 719–727.

Graham, M. V. (2001). NSCLC: Value of three-dimensional conformal radiotherapy: Pro. In B. Movsas, C. J. Langer, & M. Goldberg (Eds.), *Controversies in lung cancer: A multidisciplinary approach* (pp. 279–298). New York: Marcel Dekker.

Khuri, F. R., Keller, S. M., & Wagner, H., Jr. (1999). Non-small cell lung cancer and mesothelioma. In R. Pazdur & W. J. Hoskins (Eds.), *Cancer management: A multidisciplinary approach* (3rd ed.). Melville, NY: Research and Representation.

Lecchi, M., Fossati, P., Elisei, F., Orecchia, R., & Lucignani, G. (2008). Current concepts on imaging in radiotherapy. *European Journal of Nuclear Medicine and Molecular Imaging, 35*(4), 821–837.

Machtay, M., Seiferheld, W., Komaki, R., Cox, J. D., Sause, W. T., & Byhardt, R. W. (1999). Is prolonged survival possible for patients with supraclavicular node metastases in non-small cell lung cancer treated with chemoradiotherapy? Analysis of the Radiation Therapy Oncology Group experience. *International Journal of Radiation Oncology, Biology, Physics, 44*(4), 847–853.

Mehta, M. (1996). Endobronchial radiotherapy for lung cancer. In H. Pass, J. Mitchell, A. Johnson, & A. Turrisi (Eds.), *Lung cancer: Principles and practice* (pp. 741–751). Philadelphia: Lippincott-Raven.

McGarry, R., Papiez, L., Williams, M., Whitford, T., & Timmerman, R. D. (2005). Stereotactic body radiotherapy of early stage lung cancer. *International Journal of Radiation Oncology, Biology, Physics, 63*(4), 1010–1015.

Morgensztern, D., Goodgame, B., Baggstrom, M. Q., Gao, F., & Govindan, R. (2008). The effect of FDG-PET on the stage distribution of non-small cell lung cancer. *Journal of Thoracic Oncology, 3*(2), 135–139.

Nagata, Y., Takayama, K., Matsuo, Y., Norihisa, Y., Mizowki, T., Sakamoto, T., et al. (2005) Clinical outcomes of a phase I/II study of 48 Gy of stereotactic body radiotherapy in 4 fractions for primary lung cancer using a stereotactic body frame. *International Journal of Radiation Oncology, Biology, Physics, 63*(5), 1427–1431.

National Comprehensive Cancer Network (NCCN). (2008). *NCCN clinical practice guidelines in oncology: Non-small cell lung cancer. V.2.2008.* Fort Washington, PA: Author.

Nehmeh, S. A. & Erdi, Y. E. (2008). Respiratory motion in positron emission tomography/computed tomography: A review. *Seminars in Nuclear Medicine, 38*(3), 167–176.

Optivus Technology, Inc. (2008). *What is proton beam therapy?* Retrieved September 27, 2008, from www.optivus.com

PORT Meta-Analysis Trialists Group. (1998). Postoperative radiotherapy in non-small cell lung cancer: Systematic review and meta-analysis of individual patient data from nine randomized controlled trials. *Lancet, 352*(9124), 257–263.

Rice, T. W., Adelstein, D. J., Ciezki, J. P., Becker, M. E., Rybicki, L. A., Farver, C. F., et al. (1998). Short-course induction chemoradiotherapy with paclitaxel for stage III non-small cell lung cancer. *The Annals of Thoracic Surgery, 66*(6), 1909–1914.

Tubiana, M. & Eschwège, F. (2000). Conformal radiotherapy and intensity-modulated radiotherapy. Clinical data. *Acta Oncologica, 39*(5), 555–567.

van Meerbeeck, J. P., Meersschout, S., De Pauw, R., Madani, I., & De Neve, W. (2008). Modern radiotherapy as part of combined modality treatment in locally advanced non-small cell lung cancer: Present status and future prospects. *Oncologist, 13*(6), 700–708.

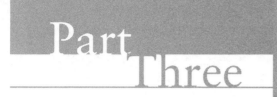

Part Three

Special Issues Facing Individuals with Lung Cancer

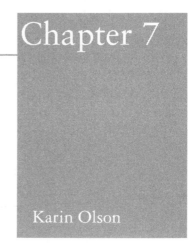

Chapter 7

Surviving Fatigue

Karin Olson

Studies over the past 2 decades have shown that fatigue is one of the most common and distressing symptoms experienced by individuals with cancer, and this is no less the case in the patient with lung cancer regardless of the stage of disease. The purpose of this chapter is to briefly review mechanisms of fatigue, to discuss related symptoms, and to outline strategies for managing fatigue.

Defining Fatigue

Many definitions of cancer-related fatigue can be found in the literature. For the purposes of this chapter, the current National Comprehensive Cancer Network (NCCN) definition of cancer-related fatigue is used. It states that cancer-related fatigue is "a distressing persistent, subjective sense of physical, emotional and/or tiredness or exhaustion related to cancer or cancer treatment that is not proportional to recent activity and interferes with usual functioning" (NCCN, 2008, p. FT-1). It would probably be unusual for patients to use the term "fatigue" when describing how they feel. The words "sluggish," "slow," "heavy," "worn out," "weary," "tired," or "exhausted" would be more commonly heard. The classic phrase "bone tired" typifies the experience of fatigue as described in Betty Ferrell's 1996 article. Indeed, one of the difficulties related to the study of fatigue is the conceptual distance between its various definitions in the scientific literature and the way fatigue is represented in everyday conversation.

The use of different definitions of fatigue in the literature makes it difficult to compare research findings. This discrepancy also hinders development of our theoretical understanding of fatigue as a clinical phenomenon. A lack of definition also results in poor communication between members of the healthcare team and between researchers and practitioners. Moreover, it creates difficulty for clinical decision making (for example, knowing what is a deviation from the usual fatigue associated with daily life or what is an expected level of fatigue at a particular stage in the cancer trajectory) (Glaus, Crow, & Hammond, 1996).

Piper (1993) stated that "in contrast to tiredness, subjective fatigue is perceived as unusual, abnormal or excessive whole-body tiredness, disproportionate to, or unrelated to activity or exertion" (p. 280). In a study of individuals with cancer in active treatment and palliative settings, Olson (2007a) defined the weariness of daily life as tiredness and found that fatigue could be distinguished from tiredness by an increase in anxiety; difficulty concentrating; loss of stamina earlier than expected; increased sensitivity to light, noise, taste, or touch; and a desire to withdraw from usual social interactions. These definitions begin to paint a picture for us that is noticeably different from the sensations we might experience following completion of a mentally challenging task that is relieved by rest or a good night's sleep.

Causes of Fatigue

The earliest reference to fatigue, appearing in the late 1700s, made reference to the existence of electric potentials in nerves and muscles of frog legs (Edwards, Toescu, & Gibson, 1995). By the late 1800s, Beard had written about the role of the chemical changes in the central nervous system that prevented the body from excreting the by-products of overused muscles (1869). Bartley and Chute (1947) provided the first paper on fatigue as a concept based on published studies in psychology, exercise, and physiology, and they described fatigue as feelings of lassitude and reduced energy due to an accumulating oxygen debt in muscles.

These studies provided a foundation for the work of Grandjean (1968), who described fatigue as a marker of central nervous system activity and said that it ranged from sleepy and tired to fresh and alert. Grandjean's work has given rise to the work of five nursing research groups with an interest in fatigue, including Ryden (1977), Piper (1986), Nail and Winningham (1993), Irvine, Vincent, Graydon, Bubela, and Thompson (1994), and Aaronson et al. (1999).

A second perspective on fatigue mechanisms grew from the work of Bartlett (1953), whose work was based on a stress theory as developed by Selye (1952, 1956, 1971). He argued that fatigue was a function of energy demand and that the sensations associated with fatigue were a result of excess energy demand. Bartlett's work provided a foundation for five additional research groups with an interest in fatigue: Cameron (1973), Rhoten (1982), Aistars (1987), Glaus (1993), and Olson (2007b).

A third possible fatigue mechanism features proinflammatory cytokines. This is particularly relevant to cancer-related fatigue, because these cytokines are sometimes given as part of treatment and are released in response to both tumor and cancer treatments. This approach links the cytokine network to the central nervous system and changes in behavioral processes; declines in activity, social and sexual behavior, food and water intake, and sleep; and increases in pain reactivity and cognitive alterations (Dantzer, 2001). Bower (2007) recently reported the results of a number of studies showing that inflammatory processes may be involved in both fatigue during treatment and fatigue that occurs long after treatment is finished. The inflammatory process has been included as one of the main drivers of decreased muscle endurance, a key component of fatigue in the recently proposed Edmonton Fatigue Framework (Olson, et al., 2008). Clearly a validated etiological model of fatigue has not yet been established, but the comments of Miaskowski and Portenoy (1998) regarding the likelihood that fatigue is the result of interactions between many factors are truer than ever before.

Cancer Treatment and Fatigue

Although fatigue is frequently one symptom in a cluster that might lead to diagnosis (Porock,

1999), clearly cancer treatment is a major event that causes and worsens fatigue. Cancer treatment-related fatigue can have such a negative impact that it almost eludes articulation. Fatigue research that has focused on the impact of treatment specifically on lung cancer confirms that fatigue is reported as a highly intense and severe symptom (Degner & Sloan, 1995; Ekfors & Petersson, 2004; Hollen, Gralla, Kris, & Potanovich, 1993; Kukull, et al., 1986; Lobchuk, Kristjanson, Degner, Blood, & Sloan, 1997; Okuyama, et al., 2001; Schag, Ganz, Wing, Sim, & Lee, 1994; Tishelman, Degner, & Mueller, 2000). Interestingly, Tishelman and colleagues found that, at least at the commencement of treatment, patients rate the importance of fatigue quite low even though it is often also rated as severe. There is insufficient information on how this perception may change over time, and it certainly points to the need for further investigation of symptom occurrence and distress in lung cancer.

A patient with lung cancer is quite likely to experience some combination of surgery, chemotherapy, and radiation therapy during the course of the illness. Because there is limited information on treatment-specific fatigue in lung cancer, much of the following information is general for all cancer types and therefore provides only a general guideline.

Each of these three major anticancer treatment modalities causes fatigue independently; thus, fatigue is cumulative with multiple modality treatment. Surgery presents a major trauma to the body, and additional resources for healing tissue are required. In addition, the effects of anesthesia, sedation, enforced bed rest, dehydration, missed meals, and indeed the psychological stress of surgery all add to the fatigue and weakness experienced after surgery (Oberle, Allen, & Lynkowski, 1994).

The incidence of fatigue in radiation therapy patients has been reported as 65–100%, depending on the cancer type and/or location of the tumor (Nail & Jones, 1995). In general, patients report that fatigue increases as treatment progresses, and it is worse at the end of each day (Love, Leventhal, Easterling, & Nerenz, 1989) and the end of each week and lasts for several months following treatment (Irvine, Vincent, Thompson, Bubela, & Graydon, 1991; Irvine, et al., 1994; Nail & Jones, 1995).

Interestingly, in a study of patients undergoing treatment for lung cancer, Beach, Siebeneck, Buderer and Ferner (2001) reported that that fatigue did not increase over the course of treatment; they attributed this finding to the fatigue assessment measure used and to the high level of fatigue among participants at the beginning of treatment. A study of quality of life during palliative radiation for non-small cell lung cancer (Langendijk, et al., 2001) showed a gradual increase in fatigue ratings over the course of the treatment. In this study, palliative radiation showed excellent improvement in hemoptysis and good pain control (particularly arm and shoulder pain) but poor palliation of cough and dyspnea. Throughout the course of the treatment there was also a decline in the physical and social functioning aspects of the quality of life measure, as well as a decline in the total score for quality of life. An unexpected finding was that emotional function remained comparatively high during palliative radiation, something the authors attributed to the maintenance of hope. Unfortunately, emotional function declined following completion of radiation. In their discussion, Langendijk and colleagues made it clear that tumor response is not a good surrogate for quality of life.

The same gradual decline in function and quality of life and increase in symptom distress—

in particular, fatigue—has been found in chemotherapy regimes for lung cancer (Muers & Round, 1993). For all cancer types, the impact of chemotherapy is well known, and overall it is estimated that 80% of patients report moderate to severe fatigue during treatment (Richardson & Ream, 1996).

Other Influencing Factors

Fatigue does not occur in isolation in the lung cancer patient. Many disease and treatment-related symptoms are concurrent, as are psychological and social sequelae of a cancer diagnosis, including anemia, effects and side effects of medications, psychological distress, cachexia/anorexia, metabolic disturbances, sleep disturbances, pulmonary impairment, pain, neuromuscular dysfunction, infection, sedentary lifestyle, smoking, excessive alcohol consumption, and comorbid conditions (Blesch, Paice, & Wickham, 1991; Groopman, 1998; Hickok, Morrow, & McDonald, 1996; Von Hoff, 1998).

As with fatigue itself, a nurse preparing to assess influencing factors must consider the validity of assessment instruments. It is not uncommon to use pencil-and-paper assessment approaches without determining first whether the approach has been validated against an acceptable gold standard. Many assessment tools for depression, for example, have only been validated against other similar instruments, rather than against a structured clinical interview, the accepted approach for the diagnosis of depression.

Three symptoms of particular importance in relation to fatigue in lung cancer are dyspnea, depression, and dietary intake. One of the most distinct symptoms with fatigue in lung cancer is dyspnea. Prevalence rates as high as 90% have been reported in individuals with lung cancer (Dudgeon, Lertzman, & Askew, 2001;

Kuo & Ma, 2002). Clearly, dyspnea and the accompanying problems of hypoxemia and anxiety are likely to affect physical and emotional function and exacerbate fatigue (Langendijk, et al., 2001; Luce & Luce, 2001; Tishelman, et al., 2000). Chan, Richardson, and Richardson (2005) showed that dyspnea, fatigue, and anxiety tend to occur together in patients with lung cancer and that the correlations between these symptoms remain high during treatment.

Many researchers report that depression is commonly associated with fatigue and with cancer in general. Estimates indicate that 15–25% of cancer patients experience depression (Henriksson, Isometsa, & Hietanen, 1995). Hopworth and Stephens (2000) reported that both fatigue and depression are strong predictors of quality of life in lung cancer patients, and that depression in patients is more likely than fatigue to cause emotional distress in family caregivers. Thus, it is important to manage depression not only for the comfort of the patient, but also to reduce distress in the family.

Judging from weight loss patterns in cancer patients, one could infer that dietary intake is frequently compromised. Indeed, there is some question about the number of kilocalories required per day by cancer patients, given issues related to the hypermetabolic state associated with tumor growth and symptoms such as infection, fever, and dyspnea (Watanabe and Bruera, 1996). Inadequate food intake may be compounded by symptoms such as anorexia, nausea and vomiting, diarrhea, bowel obstruction, and esophagitis. Reported mean dietary intakes of cancer patients are similar to the basal metabolic rates of the same or similar patient populations (Barber, Ross, Voss, Tisdale, & Fearon, 1999; Bosaeus, Daneryd, Svanberg, & Lundholm, 2001; Fearon, et al., 2003; Lindholm, Daneryd, Bosaeus, Korner, & Lindholm, 2004). Inadequate food intake in the presence of stress, immuno-suppressive chemotherapies, and fatigue is a serious problem, because it activates the innate immune response (inflammation) (Woods, Nail, Gilster, Winters, & Elsea, 2006) and suppresses T cell function, and it is associated with an increase in the risk of infection and a decrease in survival (Molle, Steffensen, Thiel, & Peterslund, 2006; Persson & Glimelius, 2002).

Posttreatment Fatigue

There is good evidence that fatigue continues to be a problem for many people posttreatment, including those who go on to become cancer survivors. Studies report moderate to severe fatigue in 33–75% of patients posttreatment in a variety of disease groups (Armer & Porock, 2001; Berglund, Boland, & Fornander, 1991; Bush, Hanerman, & Donaldson, 1995; Ferrell, et al., 1996; Schwartz, 1998; Whedon, Stearns, & Mills, 1995). In a study of lung cancer survivors, Fox and Lyon (2006) recently reported a symptom cluster comprised of depression and fatigue, both of which were correlated with quality of life.

Assessment and Management of Fatigue

With regard to daily and ongoing assessment, the NCCN guidelines recommend the use of a numeric rating scale where 0 equals no fatigue and 10 equals the worst possible fatigue, and where mild fatigue corresponds to a score of 1–3, moderate fatigue corresponds to a score of 4–6, and severe fatigue corresponds to a score of 7–10 (NCCN, 2008). Numerous other fatigue assessment tools have been developed, and while they may be reliable and valid, they are often too long to incorporate into busy clinical settings for screening purposes.

Fatigue is a multidimensional phenomenon with multiple potential causative factors that may work alone or together to produce overwhelming fatigue that affects all aspects of an individual patient's life. Given this complexity it is unlikely that a single intervention (e.g., treatment of anemia) is going to be the sole solution necessary to manage this symptom. It is clear that symptoms interrelate and compound one another (Lenz, et al., 1997). The management of fatigue can only be facilitated when all symptoms are assessed and managed effectively (Winningham, et al., 1994; Ream & Richardson, 1999). Despite the prevalence of fatigue in cancer patients and the extent to which it can interfere with daily activities, intervention research designed to prevent or ameliorate fatigue has only begun to emerge. Rest is still the most frequently recommended intervention in practice (Nail, et al., 1991; Ream & Richardson, 1999); however, it is now accepted in the research community that rest alone is generally not effective in returning cancer patients with fatigue to their previous level of functioning (Winningham, 1991). Unnecessary bed rest and prolonged sedentary periods can contribute significantly to the development of fatigue and weakness, which may result in rapid and potentially irreversible losses in energy and functioning.

Suggested interventions for the management of fatigue have been drawn from the NCCN practice guidelines for cancer-related fatigue. These guidelines are updated yearly, based on current evidence and consensus opinion of NCCN fatigue panel members. The patient's score on the fatigue numerical rating scale determines intervention recommendations. A summary of this approach is provided in Table 7–1, and the elements of a fatigue history are listed in Table 7–2. The reader is referred to www.nccn.org for the specific details of recommended interventions.

Table 7–1 Summary of Interventions for the Management of Cancer-Related Fatigue

Fatigue screen of 3 or less
- Educate the patient and family about the nature of fatigue and strategies for its management

Fatigue screen greater than 3
- Develop a focused history that includes disease status and treatment, review of systems, and fatigue history (see Table 7–2)
- Assess treatable contributing factors, including pain, emotional distress, anemia, sleep disturbance, nutrition, evaluation of medical interventions, activity level, and comorbidities

Table 7–2 Elements of a Fatigue History

Assessment	Criteria
Fatigue pattern	Onset, duration, and intensity Aggravating and alleviating factors
Disease pattern	Disease type Stage Infection/fever
Symptom pattern	Anemia Dyspnea Muscle wasting
Treatment pattern	Treatment history Treatment-related symptoms and side effects Current medication effects and side effects
Rest/activity pattern	Sleep, nap patterns, and sleep rituals Relaxation habits Activities of daily living Needed activities (e.g., attending treatment appointments)
Social pattern	Pastimes or preferred activities Support needs/resources Forthcoming family/social events
Work pattern	Employment Other care responsibilities (children, spouse, parents, etc.) Financial responsibilities/resources
Nutrition pattern	Intake Appetite Nausea/vomiting Diarrhea/constipation/obstruction

Until now, nursing research has focused on three core interventions: effective management of associated symptoms, maintenance/enhancement of activity (including exercise) balanced with rest, and management of emotional stress (including educational and psychosocial techniques). Furthermore, studies have shown benefit in patients using relaxation techniques or distraction. For example, simple measures such as listening to music or watching beautiful scenery can reduce cognitive fatigue (Cimprich, 1993; Lee, et al., 1994).

Research has shown some success in using a pharmacological approach for fatigue management with the use of low doses of psychostimulant drugs commonly associated in the treatment of attention-deficit/hyperactivity disorder (ADHD) (Feighner & Boyer, 1991; Fernandez, Adams, & Holmes, 1989). Clinical experience, principally in the palliative care population, suggests that in cancer patients these drugs improve the patient's sense of well-being, increase appetite, decrease fatigue, and are less sedating than antidepressants. Research continues with these drugs; however, in children with ADHD the appetite is suppressed, and it is not clear how the mechanism would be different in cancer patients. The side effects include insomnia, anxiety, and cardiac anomalies, particularly palpitations. In higher doses, some patients experience nightmares and have paranoid feelings. These drugs have not been specifically tested in the lung cancer population and should be used with extreme caution, particularly if the dyspnea associated with the lung cancer is already causing anxiety.

The correction of comorbidities, such as anemia or other metabolic imbalances, is an important step in the comprehensive approach to cancer-related fatigue. Anemia is prevalent with patients who have lung cancer, and transfusions are more likely to be needed by this patient pop-

ulation (Moliterno & Spivak, 1996). Epoetin alpha may also be used to treat symptomatic anemia in patients with cancer. Treatment efficacy of epoetin alpha varies among different neoplasms, with lung cancer patients having the highest response rate (Ludwig & Fritz, 1998).

Attention to nutrition has been minimal, but a good starting point is the current recommendations for each food group. It must be remembered that patients with lung cancer have not been the focus of interventional research in the nutrition area; thus, efforts to maintain dietary intake must be undertaken with good clinical judgment about the condition and ability of the patient.

The management of dyspnea is an essential component of fatigue management in patients with lung cancer. Dyspnea is an equally complex symptom as fatigue, and it is one that patients rate as both distressing and important (Tishelman, et al., 2000). Medications are an integral component of dyspnea management, and relevant drugs are listed in Table 7–3. Patients with chronic lung disease have increased minute ventilation at rest and during exercise, resulting in an increased production of carbon dioxide, lactic acidosis, and a heightened drive to breathe (American Thoracic Society, 1999a). Because dyspnea increases in proportion to the need to breathe, reducing the demand may diminish the sensation of breathlessness. Exercise increases aerobic capacity, decreases minute ventilation, and relieves dyspnea in COPD patients. This may have a similar effect in patients with lung cancer, but clinical trials are needed in this area (Casaburi, et al., 1991; O'Donnell, McGuire, Samis, & Webb, 1995). Dyspnea programs that have included education, respiratory care instruction, and psychosocial support have been reported to be beneficial for chronic lung disease and lung cancer patients (American Thoracic Society, 1999b; Ries, Kaplan, Limberg, & Prewitt, 1995).

Table 7–3 Management of Dyspnea

Intervention	Effects/Adverse Effects
Corticosteroids	Slows the rate of decline Improves mood Long-term use may cause muscle weakness and immune suppression
Anticholinergics	Decreases secretions
Oxygen therapy	Reduces pulmonary vascular resistance and survival in hypoxemic patients[a]
Opioids	Increases exercise tolerance and alleviates dyspnea[b]
Benzodiazepines	Decreases dyspnea by blunting the ventilatory drive[c] May cause drowsiness
Antidepressants	Decreased dyspnea found in one study requires further testing[d]
Improve nutrition	Increased body weight, increased respiratory and muscle strength, and thus decreased dyspnea[e]
Drain malignant pleural effusions	Drugs that stimulate appetite may enhance the sensation of breathlessness by increasing the drive to breathe

[a] Nocturnal Oxygen Therapy Trial Group, 1980.
[b] Light, et al., 1989.
[c] Man, Hsu, & Sproule, 1986.
[d] Smoller, Pollack, & Systrom, 1998.
[e] Efthimiou, Fleming, Gomes, & Spiro, 1988.

Fatigue at the End of Life

Extreme fatigue is a sign that death is imminent, as is an increasing disinterest in eating and increasing periods of sleep. A decision must be made at some time to stop active encouragement of interventions that are being used to ameliorate fatigue, for example, exercise or blood transfusions, and to focus the care purely on comfort. In the patient with lung cancer, dyspnea is most likely going to be the symptom that signals a patient's ability to continue. Hopefully, time will have been spent discussing patient preferences and wishes well before this happens. In any case, a reasonable time to suggest candid discussion about end-of-life decisions is when the patient remains dyspneic even at rest.

Conclusion

Fatigue is a complex, subjective symptom that is very prevalent at all stages of the cancer trajectory. For many years fatigue was a hidden and ignored symptom of cancer. Currently, its treatment, recent focus, and research effort in oncology nursing are providing a scientific basis for understanding fatigue, its impact, and management; this provides a foundation that is acknowledged and used by all the health professions. Despite an incomplete understanding of the mechanisms of fatigue, several research-based interventions have been tested with encouraging results. For the patient with lung cancer, education, time and sleep management, nutrition advice, and dyspnea management are all good interventions. Exercise should also be encouraged, as should quitting smoking. The use of psychostimulants has not been tested in the lung cancer patient and should be used with caution and under the care of a specialist. However, careful assessment and treatment of depression and weight loss should be pursued. Management of medications and evaluation of possible interactions of polypharmacy should be a priority.

Extreme fatigue is associated with serious illness, and it is also a sign of impending death; thus, fatigue has been feared as an indication that the end of life is inevitable and near. It is important that the nurse recognizes the signs of impending death and makes appropriate suggestions for how to approach fatigue as a part of dying, helping the patient and family to accept death as a natural part of life.

Fatigue is one of a constellation of symptoms that can adversely affect the patient with lung cancer and his or her family. It is not an easy symptom to treat, and its complexity requires the listening, empathic ear of the nurse to ensure that whatever the outcome, the patient and family feel they have had the best of care possible.

References

Aaronson, L., Teel, C., Cassmeyer, B., Neuberger, G., Pallikkathayil, L., Pierce, J., et al. (1999). Defining and measuring fatigue (state of the science). *Image—The Journal of Nursing Scholarship, 31*(1), 45–50.

Aistars, J. (1987). Fatigue in the cancer patient: A conceptual approach to a clinical problem. *Oncology Nursing Forum, 14*(6), 25–30.

American Thoracic Society. (1999a). Dyspnea: Mechanisms, assessment, and management: A consensus statement. *American Journal of Respiratory Critical Care Medicine, 159*(1), 321–340.

American Thoracic Society. (1999b). Pulmonary rehabilitation. *American Journal of Respiratory Critical Care Medicine, 159*(5 Pt 1), 1666–1682.

Armer, J., & Porock, D. (2001, July/September). Self-reported fatigue among women with post-breast cancer lymphedema. *Lymph Link (National Lymphedema Network Newsletter)*, 1–2, 4.

Barber, M., Ross, J., Voss, A., Tisdale, M., & Fearon, K. (1999). The effect of an oral nutritional supplement enriched with fish oil on weight loss in patients with pancreatic cancer. *British Journal of Cancer, 81*(1), 80–86.

Bartlett, F. (1953). Psychological criteria of fatigue. In W. Floyd & A. Welford (Eds.), *Symposium on fatigue* (pp. 1–5). London: H. K. Lewis.

Bartley, S., & Chute, E. (1947). *Fatigue and impairments in man.* New York: McGraw Hill.

Beach, P., Siebeneck, B., Buderer, N., & Ferner, T. (2001). Relationship between fatigue and nutritional status in patients receiving radiation therapy to treat lung cancer. *Oncology Nursing Forum, 28*(6), 1027–1031.

Beard, G. (1869). Neurasthenia, or nervous exhaustion? *Boston Medical and Surgical Journal, 3*(13), 217–221.

Berglund, G., Boland, C., & Fornander, T. (1991). Late effects of adjuvant chemotherapy and postoperative radiotherapy on quality of life among breast cancer patients. *European Journal of Cancer, 27*(9), 1075–1081.

Blesch, K. S., Paice, J. A., Wickham, R., Harte, N., Schnoor, D. K., Purl, S., et al. (1991). Correlates of fatigue in people with breast or lung cancer. *Oncology Nursing Forum, 18*(1), 81–87.

Bosaeus, I., Daneryd, P., Svanberg, E., & Lundholm, K. (2001). Dietary intake and resting energy expenditure in relation to weight loss in unselected cancer patients. *International Journal of Cancer, 93*(3), 380–383.

Bower, J. (2007). Cancer-related fatigue: Links with inflammation in cancer patients and survivors. *Brain, Behaviour, and Immunity, 21*(7), 863–871.

Bush, N. E., Hanerman, M., & Donaldson, G. (1995). Quality of life of 125 adults surviving 6–18 years after bone marrow transplantation. *Social Science and Medicine, 40*(4), 479–490.

Cameron, C. (1973). A theory of fatigue. *Ergonomics, 16*(5), 633–648.

Casaburi, R., Patessio, A., Ioli, F., Zanaboni, S., Donner, C. F., & Wasserman, K. (1991). Reductions in exercise lactic acidosis and ventilation as a result of exercise training in patients with obstructive lung disease. *American Review Respiratory Disease, 143*(1), 9–18.

Chan, C., Richardson, A., & Richardson, J. (2005). A study to assess the existence of the symptom cluster of breathlessness, fatigue, and anxiety in patients with advanced lung cancer. *European Journal of Oncology Nursing, 9*(4), 325–333.

Cimprich, B. (1993, April 16). Development of an intervention to restore attention in cancer patients. *Cancer Nursing, 16*(2), 83–92.

Dantzer, R. (2001). Cytokine-induced sickness behavior: Mechanisms and implications. *Annals of the New York Academy of Science, 933*, 222–234.

Degner, L. F., & Sloan, J. A. (1995). Symptom distress in newly diagnosed ambulatory cancer patients and as a predictor of survival in lung cancer. *Journal of Pain and Symptom Management, 10*(6), 423–431.

Dudgeon, D., Lertzman, M., & Askew, G. (2001). Physiological chances and clinical correlations of dyspnea in cancer outpatients. *Journal of Pain and Symptom Management, 21*(5), 373–379.

Edwards, R., Toescu, V., & Gibson, H. (1995). Historical perspective: A framework for interpreting pathobiological ideas on human muscle fatigue. In S. Gandevia, R. Enoka, A. McComas, D. Stuart, & C. Thomas (Eds.), *Fatigue* (pp. 481–494). New York: Plenum Press.

Efthimiou, J., Fleming, J., Gomes, C., & Spiro, S. G. (1988). The effect of supplementary oral nutrition in poorly nourished patients with chronic obstructive pulmonary disease. *American Review Respiratory Disease, 137*(5), 1075–1082.

Ekfors, H., & Petersson, K. (2004). A qualitative study of the experiences during radiotherapy of Swedish patients suffering from lung cancer. *Oncology Nursing Forum 31*(2), 329–334.

Fearon, K., von Meyenfeldt, M., Moses, A., van Geenen, R., Gouma, D., Giacosa, A., et al. (2003). Effect of a protein and energy dense n-3 fatty acid enriched oral supplement on loss of weight and lean tissue in cancer cachexia: A randomised double blind trial. *Gut 52*(10), 1479–1486.

Feighner, J. P., & Boyer, W. F. (1991). Selective serotonin re-uptake inhibitors: The clinical use of citalopram, fluoxetine, fluvoxamine, paroxetine and sertraline. *Perspectives in psychiatry* (Vol. 1). New York: John Wiley.

Fernandez, F., Adams, F., Holmes, V. F., Levy, J. K., & Neidhart, M. (1989). Methylphenidate for depressive disorders in cancer patients: An alternative to standard antidepressants. *Psychosomatics, 28*(9), 455–461.

Ferrell, B. R., Grant, M., Dean, G. E., Funk, B., & Ly, J. (1996). 'Bone tired': The experience of fatigue and its impact on quality of life. *Oncology Nursing Forum, 23*(10), 1539–1547.

Fox, S., & Lyon, D. (2006). Symptom clusters and quality of life in survivors of lung cancer. *Oncology Nursing Forum, 33*(50), 931–936.

Glaus, A. (1993). Assessment of fatigue in cancer and noncancer patients and in health individuals. *Supportive Care in Cancer, 1*, 305–315.

Glaus, A., Crow, R., & Hammond, S. (1996). A qualitative study to explore the concept of fatigue/tiredness in cancer patients and in healthy individuals. *European Journal of Cancer Care, 5*(Suppl. 2), 8–23.

Grandjean, E. (1968). Fatigue: Its physiological and psychological significance. *Ergonomics, 11*(5), 427–436.

Groopman, J. E. (1998). Fatigue in cancer and HIV/AIDS. *Oncology, 12*(3), 335–346, 351.

Henriksson, M. M., Isometsa, E. T., Hietanen, P. S., Aro, H. M., & Lonnqvist, J. K. (1995). Mental disorders in cancer suicides. *Journal of Affective Disorders, 36*(1–2), 11–20.

Hickok, J. T., Morrow, G. R., McDonald, S., & Bellg, A. J. (1996). Frequency and correlates of fatigue in lung cancer patients receiving radiation therapy: Implications for management. *Journal of Pain and Symptom Management, 11*(6), 370–377.

Hollen, P. J., Gralla, R. J., Kris, M. G., & Potanovich, L. M. (1993). Quality of life assessment in individuals with lung cancer: Testing the lung cancer symptom scale (LCSS). *European Journal of Cancer, 29A*(Suppl. 1), 551–555.

Hopwood, P., & Stephens, R. J. (2000). Depression in patients with lung cancer: Prevalence and risk factors derived from quality of life data. *Journal of Clinical Oncology, 18*(4), 893–903.

Irvine, D., Vincent, L., Graydon, J. E., Bubela, N., & Thompson, L. (1994). The prevalence and correlates of fatigue in patients receiving treatment with chemotherapy and radiotherapy. *Cancer Nursing, 17*(5), 367–378.

Irvine, D., Vincent, L., Thompson, L., Bubela, N., & Graydon, J. E. (1991). A critical appraisal of the research literature investigating fatigue in the individual with cancer. *Cancer Nursing, 14*(4), 188–199.

Kukull, W., McCorkle, R., & Driever, M. (1986). Symptom distress, psychosocial variables, and survival from lung cancer. *Journal of Psychosocial Oncology, 4*(1/2), 91–94.

Kuo, T., & Ma, F. (2002). Symptom distresses and coping strategies in patients with non-small cell lung cancer. *Cancer Nursing, 25*(4), 309–317.

Langendijk, J. A., Aaronson, N. K., de Jong, J. M. A., ten Vele, G. P. M., Muller, M. J., Lamers, R. J., et al. (2001). Prospective study on quality of life before and after radical radiotherapy in non-small cell lung cancer. *Journal of Clinical Oncology, 19*(8), 2123–2133.

Lee, K. A., Lentz, M. J., Taylor, D. L., Mitchell, E. S., & Woods, N. F. (1994). Fatigue as a response to environmental demands in women's lives. *Image, 26*(2), 149–154.

Lenz, E. R., Pugh, L. C., Milligan, R. A., Gift, A., & Suppe, F. (1997). The middle-range theory of unpleasant symptoms: An update. *Advances in Nursing Science, 19*(3), 14–27.

Light, R. W., Muro, J. R., Sato, R. I., Stansbury, D. W., Fischer, C. E., & Brown, S. E. (1989). Effects of oral morphine on breathlessness and exercise tolerance in patients with chronic obstructive pulmonary disease. *American Review of Respiratory Disease, 139*(1), 126–133.

Lobchuk, M. M., Kristjanson, L. J., Degner, L. F., Blood, P., & Sloan, J. A. (1997). Perceptions of symptom distress in lung cancer patients: I. Congruence between patients and primary family caregivers. *Journal of Pain and Symptom Management, 14*(3), 136–146.

Love, R. R., Leventhal, H., Easterling, D. V., & Nerenz, D. R. (1989). Side effects and emotional distress during cancer chemotherapy. *Cancer, 63*(3), 604–612.

Luce, J. M., & Luce, J. A. (2001). Management of dyspnea in patients with far-advanced lung disease: "Once I lose it, it's kind of hard to catch it...". *Journal of the American Medical Association, 285*(10), 1331–1337.

Ludwig, H., & Fritz, E. (1998). Anemia of cancer patients: Patient selection and patient stratification for epoetin treatment. *Seminars in Oncology, 25*(3, Suppl. 7), 35–38.

Lundholm, K., Daneryd, P., Bosaeus, I., Korner, U., & Lindholm, E. (2004). Palliative nutritional intervention in addition to cyclooxygenase and erythropoietin treatment for patients with malignant disease: Effects on survival, metabolism, and function—A randomized prospective study. *Cancer 100*(9), 1967–1977.

Man, G. C. W., Hsu, K., & Sproule, B. J. (1986). Effect of alprazolam on exercise and dyspnea in patients with chronic obstructive pulmonary disease. *Chest, 90*(6), 832–836.

Miaskowski, C., & Portenoy, R. K. (1998). Update on the assessment and management of cancer-related fatigue. *Principles and Practice of Supportive Oncology Updates, 1*(2), 1–10.

Moliterno, A., & Spivak, J. (1996). Anemia of cancer. *Hematology/Oncology Clinics of North America, 10*(2), 345–363.

Molle, I., Steffensen, R., Thiel, S., & Peterslund, N. (2006). Chemotherapy-related infections in patients with multiple myeloma: Associations with mannan-binding lectin genotypes. *European Journal of Haematology, 77*(1), 19–26.

Muers, M. F., & Round, C. E. (1993). Palliation of symptoms in non-small cell lung cancer: A study by the Yorkshire Regional Cancer Organisation Thoracic Group. *Thorax, 48*(4), 339–343.

Nail, L., & Jones, L. S. (1995). Fatigue side effects and treatment and quality of life. *Quality of Life Research, 4*(1), 8–16.

Nail, L., & Winningham, M. (1993). Fatigue. In M. Groenwald, M. Grogge, M. Goodman, & C. Yarbro (Eds.), *Cancer nursing: Principles and practice* (3rd ed., pp. 608–619). Sudbury, MA: Jones and Bartlett.

Nail, L. M., Jones, L. S., Greene, D., Schipper, D. L., & Jensen, R. (1991). Use and perceived efficacy of self-care in patients receiving chemotherapy. *Oncology Nursing Forum, 18*(5), 883–887.

National Comprehensive Cancer Network (NCCN). (2008). *Cancer-related fatigue.* Retrieved August 4, 2008, from www.nccn.org

Nocturnal Oxygen Therapy Trial Group. (1980). Continuous or nocturnal oxygen therapy in hypoxemic chronic obstructive lung disease: A clinical trial. *Annals of Internal Medicine, 93*(3), 391–398.

Oberle, K., Allen, M., & Lynkowski, P. (1994). Follow-up of same day surgery patients. *American Operating Room Nurses Journal, 59*(5), 1016–1025.

O'Donnell, D. E., McGuire, M., Samis, L., & Webb, K. A. (1995). The impact of exercise reconditioning on breathlessness in severe chronic airflow limitation. *American Journal of Respiratory Critical Care Medicine, 152*(6, Part 1), 2005–2013.

Okuyama, T., Tanaka, K., Akechi, T., Kugaya, A., Okamura, H., Nishiwaki, Y., et al. (2001). Fatigue in ambulatory patients with advanced lung cancer: Prevalence, correlated factors, and screening. *Journal of Pain and Symptom Management, 22*(1), 554–564.

Olson, K. (2007a). Fatigue in individuals with advanced cancer in active treatment and palliative settings. *Cancer Nursing, 30*(4), E1–E10.

Olson, K. (2007b). A new way of thinking about fatigue. *Oncology Nursing Forum, 34*(1), 93–99.

Olson, K., Turner, A. R., Courneya, K., Field, C., Man, G., Cree, M., et al. (2008). Possible links between behavioral and physiological indices of tiredness, fatigue, and exhaustion in advanced cancer. *Supportive Care in Cancer, 16*(3), 241–249.

Persson, C., & Glimelius, B. (2002). The relevance of weight loss for survival and quality of life in patients with advanced gastrointestinal cancer treated with palliative chemotherapy. *Anticancer Research, 22*(6B), 3661–3668.

Piper, B. (1993). Fatigue. In V. Carrieri-Kohlman, A. Lindsey, & C. West (Eds.), *Pathophysiological phenomena in nursing: Human responses to illness* (2nd ed., pp. 279–302). Philadelphia: Saunders.

Porock, D. (1999). Fatigue. In S. Aranda & M. O'Connor (Eds.), *Palliative care nursing: A guide to practice.* Melbourne, Australia: AUSMED Publications.

Ream, E., & Richardson, A. (1999). From theory to practice: Designing interventions to reduce fatigue in patients with cancer. *Oncology Nursing Forum, 26*(8), 1295–1303.

Rhoten, D. (1982). Fatigue and the postsurgical patient. In C. M. Norris (Ed.), *Concept clarification in nursing* (pp. 277–300). Rockville, MD: Aspen Publications.

Richardson, A., & Ream, E. (1996). The experience of fatigue and other symptoms in patients receiving chemotherapy. *European Journal of Cancer Care, 5* (Suppl. 2), 24–30.

Ries, A. L., Kaplan, R. M., Limberg, T. M., & Prewitt, L. M. (1995). Effects of pulmonary rehabilitation on physiologic and psychosocial outcomes in patients with chronic obstructive pulmonary disease. *Annals of Internal Medicine, 122*(11), 823–832.

Ryden, M. (1977). Energy: A crucial consideration in the nursing process. *Nursing Forum, 16*(1), 71–82.

Schag, C. A. C., Ganz, P. A., Wing, D. S., Sim, M. S., & Lee, J. J. (1994). Quality of life in adult survivors of lung, colon, and prostate cancer. *Quality of Life Research, 3*(2), 127–141.

Schwartz, A. (1998). Patterns of exercise and fatigue in physically active cancer survivors. *Oncology Nursing Forum, 25*(3), 485–491.

Selye, H. (1952). *The story of the adaptation syndrome.* Montreal, Canada: Acta.

Selye, H. (1956). *The stress of life.* New York: McGraw Hill.

Selye, H. (1971). *Hormones and resistance, Part 1.* New York, Springer.

Smoller, J. W., Pollack, M. H., Systrom, D., & Kradin, R. L. (1998). Sertraline effects on dyspnea in patients with obstructive airways disease. *Psychosomatics, 39*(1), 24–29.

Tishelman, C., Degner, L. F., & Mueller, B. (2000). Measuring symptom distress in patients with lung cancer: A pilot study of experienced intensity and importance of symptoms. *Cancer Nursing, 23*(2), 82–90.

Von Hoff, D. (1998). Asthenia: Incidence, etiology, pathophysiology, and treatment. *Cancer Therapeutics, 1,* 184–197.

Watanabe, S., & Bruera, E. (1996). Anorexia and cachexia, asthenia, and lethargy. *Hematology Oncology Clinics of North America, 10*(1), 189–206.

Whedon, M., Stearns, D., & Mills, L. E. (1995). Quality of life of long-term adult survivors of autologous bone marrow transplantation. *Oncology Nursing Forum, 22*(10), 1527–1535.

Winningham, M., Nail, L. M., Burke, M. B., Brophy, L., Cimprich, B., Jones, L. S., et al. (1994). Fatigue and the cancer experience: The state of the knowledge. *Oncology Nursing Forum, 21*(1), 23–36.

Winningham, M. L. (1991). Walking program for people with cancer. *Cancer Nursing, 14*(5), 270–276.

Woods, L., Nail, L., Gilster, A., Winters, K., & Elsea, C. (2006). Cancer chemotherapy-related symptoms: Evidence to suggest a role for proinflammatory cytokines. *Oncology Nursing Forum, 33*(3), 535–542.

Chapter 8

End-of-Life Care

Deborah Lowe
Volker

Doris Dickerson
Coward

Compassionate end-of-life care requires skillful attention to both the physical and psychological care needs of patients and their families. Fortunately, there has been substantial progress in understanding and managing care needs of the terminally ill. Provision of expert palliative care is now a professional mandate for all who work with persons facing the end of life. The term "palliative care" is defined as "the active total care of patients whose disease is not responsive to curative treatment. Control of pain, other symptoms, and of psychological, social, and spiritual problems, is paramount" (World Health Organization, 1990, p. 11). Traditionally, palliative care strategies are offered when the terminal phase of a disease is evident. However, there is growing recognition that palliative care should be integrated into care at the time of diagnosis of a life-threatening illness in which a cure is not expected. This chapter focuses on symptom management and ethical issues that are particularly germane to end-of-life care for persons with lung cancer. For a more comprehensive overview of palliative care as a specialty, the reader is referred to the many excellent resources available to guide practice (Berger, Shuster, & Von Roenn, 2006; Chochinov & Breitbart, 2000; Doyle, Hanks, Cherny, & Calman, 2004; Ferrell & Coyle, 2006; Hospice and Palliative Nurses Association, 2007; Matzo & Sherman, 2006; National Consensus Project for Quality Palliative Care, 2004; Zerwekh, 2006).

Symptom Management at End of Life

People with lung cancer typically present with advanced disease and symptoms on diagnosis (Cooley, 2000). Empirical studies show that there is some consistency in the types of symptoms most often seen. Specifically, problems associated with dyspnea, cough, anorexia, severe pain, fatigue, depression, anxiety, disruptions in outlook, and difficulty sleeping are often reported as problematic in advanced lung cancer (Claessens, et al., 2000; Krech, Davis, Walsh, & Curtis, 1992; Kurtz, Kurtz, Stommel, Given, & Given, 2000; McCarthy, Phillips, Zhong, Drews, & Lynn, 2000; Sarna, 1998; Sarna & Brecht, 1997; Vainio & Auvinen, 1996). With the exception of dyspnea, symptoms reported by patients with advanced lung cancer are common not only in end stage disease, but they are experienced by many newly diagnosed patients as well (Gift, Stommel, Jablonski, & Given, 2003; Kurtz, et al., 2000; Temel, Pirl, & Lynch, 2006).

For persons who are newly diagnosed with lung cancer, good communication among healthcare providers, patients, and family early in the care continuum is of prime importance. At the time of diagnosis, patients' concerns, preferences, life and treatment goals should be explored along with frank discussion of treatment options that promote both immediate and long-term goals (Griffin, et al., 2003; Lanken, et al., 2008). As patients approach the end of life, symptoms may increase in number and severity due to combined effects of treatment sequelae and progressive disease (Cooley, Short, & Moriarty, 2003). Soon after diagnosis, initiating a long-range plan of care (with the awareness that the plan is subject to change based on treatment effects and personal preferences) would be expected to enhance treatment decision making and emotional comfort at the end of life.

This section presents management of dyspnea, cough, pain, anxiety, and delirium. An overview of complementary and alternative measures used for symptom management in advanced cancer is included. Fatigue and anorexia are covered in Chapter 7, Surviving Fatigue, and Chapter 9, Nutritional Issues Facing Lung Cancer Individuals.

A systematic, ongoing approach to assessment of symptom distress in advanced lung cancer may be a first and important step in improving interventions to relieve patient discomfort (Griffin, Koch, Nelson, & Cooley, 2007). Comprehensive assessment includes intensity and quality, frequency, duration, and things that relieve or exacerbate symptoms (Matzo & Sherman, 2006). Anticipated or reported symptom distress can be captured by a variety of tools, such as the Symptom Distress Scale (SDS) (McCorkle & Young, 1978), the Edmonton Symptom Assessment System (ESAS) (Bruera, Kuehn, Miller, Selmser, & Macmillan, 1991), Memorial Symptom Assessment Scale (MSAS) (Portnoy, et al., 1994), and the M. D. Anderson Symptom Inventory (MDASI) (Cleeland, et al., 2000). Of these tools, the ESAS is especially useful for clinical (as opposed to research) palliative care settings to guide practice. The ESAS tool (see Figure 8–1) consists of nine numerical scales (0–10) that measure the patient's level of pain, tiredness, nausea, depression, anxiety, drowsiness, appetite, well-being, and shortness of breath. A 10th scale, labeled "other problem," can be used for an additional symptom as needed. Although the patient is the ideal person to complete the ESAS, family members, nurses, and other caregivers can complete the tool if the patient cannot do so. The ESAS tool can be used for assessments in both home and inpatient settings to determine the level of symptom control and need for change in interventions.

Clusters of symptoms in persons with lung cancer have been studied by nurse researchers recently (Gift, et al., 2003; Gift, Jablonski, Stommel, & Given 2004; Hoffman, Given, von Eye, Gift, & Given, 2007). Not surprisingly, certain symptoms—such as pain, fatigue, and insomnia—tend to occur together and are associated with limitations in functioning. The findings from this type of research reinforce the importance of systematic and comprehensive assessment of reported or anticipated symptoms. Early recognition of distress and the relationship among symptoms would be expected to lead to better relief of patients' symptom distress.

Figure 8–1 Edmonton Symptom Assessment System (ESAS numerical scale).

Please circle the number that best describes:

No pain	0	1	2	3	4	5	6	7	8	9	10	Worst possible pain
Not tired	0	1	2	3	4	5	6	7	8	9	10	Worst possible tiredness
Not nauseated	0	1	2	3	4	5	6	7	8	9	10	Worst possible nausea
Not depressed	0	1	2	3	4	5	6	7	8	9	10	Worst possible depression
Not anxious	0	1	2	3	4	5	6	7	8	9	10	Worst possible anxiety
Not drowsy	0	1	2	3	4	5	6	7	8	9	10	Worst possible drowsiness
Best appetite	0	1	2	3	4	5	6	7	8	9	10	Worst possible appetite
Best feeling of well-being	0	1	2	3	4	5	6	7	8	9	10	Worst possible feeling of well-being
No shortness of breath	0	1	2	3	4	5	6	7	8	9	10	Worst possible shortness of breath
Other problem	0	1	2	3	4	5	6	7	8	9	10	

Patient's Name: _____

Date: _____

Time: _____

Assessed By: _____

Source: Alberta Palliative Network.

Dyspnea

Dyspnea is a subjective symptom with both physiologic and affective components. Dyspnea, a prominent symptom in advanced lung cancer, may be both distressing and debilitating. Dyspnea is often present at the time lung cancer is diagnosed and nearly universal prior to the time of death (Kvale, Selecky, & Prakash, 2007). However, patients with advanced-stage lung cancer do not necessarily have the most severe symptoms of dyspnea (Smith, et al., 2001). Poor control of dyspnea may be especially frightening to patients and families due to fears that the patient will suffocate. Indeed, dyspnea in cancer patients may peak immediately before death (Mercadante, Casuccio, & Fulfaro, 2000).

The etiologic basis of dyspnea in people with lung cancer is often multidimensional. Dyspnea may arise due to direct tumor involvement, metastatic disease, treatment effects, debilitation associated with end-stage disease, and other concomitant syndromes such as COPD. Table 8–1 summarizes the common causative factors associated with lung cancer.

Assessment

Because dyspnea is a subjective response, self-report is the most reliable means of diagnosis. The focus of assessment is on ascertaining the

Table 8–1 Sources of Dyspnea in Lung Cancer

Airway obstruction by tumor, lymph nodes

Anemia

Atelectasis

Chronic obstructive pulmonary disease (COPD)

Deconditioning

Lymphangitis carcinomatosa

Pleural effusion

Pericardial effusion

Pneumonia

Radiation pneumonitis

Respiratory muscle weakness

Superior vena cava syndrome

Source: Ripamonti, 1999; Silvestri, 2000.

presence and severity of dyspnea, precipitating factors, relieving events or activities, and the effect of treatments. The use of a simple self-report scale, such as the ESAS tool, at each patient encounter is helpful for assessing dyspnea (and any anxiety, fear, or pain that is frequently associated with dyspnea) and for evaluating ongoing symptom management. It is difficult to determine the role anxiety may play in the sensation of dyspnea, because anxiety may contribute to dyspnea but may also be caused by dyspnea (Bruera, Schmitz, Pither, Neumann, & Hanson, 2000). Dyspnea-specific measurement tools are summarized within the Oncology Nursing Society (ONS) Putting Evidence into Practice evidence table for dyspnea interventions (http://www.ons.org/outcomes/volume2/dyspnea/EvidenceTable_dyspnea.shtml). Invasive or burdensome measures, such as arterial blood gas evaluation and pulmonary function tests, may not be appropriate in the context of end-of-life care. However, should the patient's anticipated life span and personal preference dictate as such, other diagnostic tests may be warranted to identify conditions that can be treated for symptomatic relief. For example, use of a chest X-ray to determine a pleural effusion may prompt a discussion of whether a thoracentesis would improve a patient's symptoms.

Treatment

Nonpharmacologic strategies are used in conjunction with pharmacologic interventions to decrease the impact of dyspnea. Additionally, some patients may benefit from more invasive treatments targeted to treat specific etiologic factors.

Nonpharmacologic strategies include the use of oxygen, increasing the circulation of cool air, positioning, modification of activity to conserve energy, and relaxation techniques (Matzo & Sherman, 2006). The aim of oxygen therapy is to reduce the respiratory drive and sensation of dyspnea by increasing alveolar oxygen tension (Zeppetella, 1998). However, there is insufficient evidence to recommend oxygen for dyspneic patients who are not hypoxic (Bruera, et al., 2003; DiSalvo, Joyce, Tyson, Culkin, & MacKay, 2008). In some patients with advanced cancer, air relieves dyspnea as effectively as does oxygen (Booth, Kelly, Cox, Adams, & Guz, 1996). This finding suggests that use of a fan, opening a window, or using an air conditioner to move air in the patient's room may relieve dyspnea.

Patient positioning and activity modification also are useful for relieving discomfort due to dyspnea. Most patients find that an upright position is more comfortable because it maximizes lung volume and vital capacity (Campbell,

1998); patients with an obstructed lung may prefer lying on the obstructed side for relief (Kemp, 1999). In the presence of concurrent COPD, patients may improve dyspnea by leaning forward on an overbed table or other support (Dudgeon, 2006). This position may improve inspiratory muscle strength and diaphragm expansion, reduce neck and upper costal neck muscle use, and decrease abdominal paradoxical breathing. Pursed lip breathing may be suggested if a patient is not familiar with using that strategy. Use of activity modification also reduces dyspnea by conserving oxygen consumption. Patients may also benefit from the use of assistive devices and strategies, such as a wheelchair, portable oxygen, or assistance with meals and other household maintenance activities. As a patient approaches death, simple activities, such as eating, bathing, and changing linens, may need to be paced in short segments so as not to worsen discomfort associated with severe dyspnea.

Behavioral interventions, such as relaxation techniques, can be an important adjunct to managing dyspnea. Gallo-Silver and Pollack (2000) suggest exercises designed to promote diaphragmatic breathing, alter breathing rate and rhythms, and enhance exhalation for lung cancer-related breathlessness. Research using behavioral interventions is discussed in the Complementary and Alternative Methods for Symptom Management section of this chapter.

Potential pharmacologic strategies to manage dyspnea include the use opioids, sedatives, and tranquilizers. Although systemic opioid therapy is clearly beneficial, the optimal drug, dose, and route have not been established (Bruera & Neumann, 1998). Oral and parenteral morphine has been used successfully to decrease anxiety, muscle tension, and restlessness, thereby reducing oxygen consumption and increasing respiratory comfort (Campbell, 1998; Jennings, Davies, Higgins, Gibbs, & Broadley, 2002). The usefulness of nebulized opioids remains uncertain. The goal of such therapy is to deliver the drug directly to opioid-sensitive airway receptors, thereby lowering the dosage required for effect and decreasing systemic side effects (Dudgeon, 2006). Two reports of evidence synthesis concluded that nebulized opioids were no more effective than nebulized saline in treating dyspnea in advanced disease (Jennings, et al., 2002; Joyce, McSweeney, Carrieri-Kohlman, & Hawkins, 2004). Because insufficient evidence exists to support the use of nebulized opioids to relieve dyspnea, ONS does not endorse use of the modality at this time (DiSalvo, et al., 2008).

Sedatives and tranquilizers are used for management of dyspnea and anxiety despite a lack of controlled clinical trials to support such practice (National Comprehensive Cancer Network [NCCN], 2008; Ripamonti & Fusco, 2002). Chlorpromazine, promethazine, diazepam, alprazolam, and prochlorperazine have all been used with varying degrees of success as either single agents or in combination with morphine (Dudgeon, 2006). Due to lack of conclusive evidence regarding usefulness of these drugs in managing terminal dyspnea, some practitioners recommend limiting their use to patients with coexisting anxiety or panic disorders (Bruera & Neumann, 1998; LeGrand & Walsh, 1999; Ripamonti, 1999). Steroids also are used to manage dyspnea, but efficacy has not been evaluated in controlled studies (Chan, Shan, Tse, & Thorsen, 2004).

The patient who experiences dyspnea due to excessive bronchial and oral secretions may benefit from anticholinergic drugs, such as hyoscyamine or scopolamine (Kazanowski, 2006; NCCN, 2008). Discontinuation of fluid support and use of a low-dose diuretic may be helpful if fluid overload contributes to symptoms associated with dyspnea (DiSalvo, et al., 2008). However, limiting fluid intake to reduce secretions at the end of life is a highly individualized patient decision and is based on weighing the benefits and burdens of other discomfort and symptoms caused by dehydration.

Cough

Cough can be a debilitating and distressing symptom for people with lung cancer. Although cough is often a presenting symptom with a new diagnosis of lung cancer, cough is also prevalent in end-stage disease (Cooley, 2000; Dudgeon, 2006). The physiologic mechanism of cough in lung cancer is multifaceted; cough can be triggered by a variety of sources, including tumor obstruction, radiation effects, infection, inflammation of the airways, increased sputum production, pneumothorax, bronchiectasis, and other concomitant diseases (Dudgeon, 2006). Regardless of the cause, unrelieved cough can interfere with breathing and sleep, leads to fatigue, and may cause exacerbation of pain, pathological rib fracture, hemoptysis, vomiting, syncope, stress incontinence, and fear that the cancer is progressing (Chan, et al., 2004; Dudgeon, 2006).

Assessment

Successful management of cough begins with assessment of the potential etiologies that may be treatable conditions. For example, cough caused by an angiotensin-converting enzyme (ACE) inhibitor drug could prompt a simple change to a different medication. Note whether the cough is productive or not, characteristics of sputum, factors that precipitate or relieve cough, and other associated symptoms (Dudgeon, 2006). As with assessment of dyspnea, diagnostic tests, such as a chest X-ray, spirometry, or other procedures, may or may not be warranted, depending on the patient's prognosis and personal preferences.

Treatment

Treatment of cough depends on the underlying cause, patient and family preferences for simply suppressing cough versus more aggressive treatment, and whether or not the cough is productive (Dudgeon, 2006; Kvale, Simoff, & Prakash, 2003). A variety of pharmacologic interventions may be useful for symptom management. Table 8–2 provides examples of oral agents and suggested dose ranges. Opioids are the most effective suppressants, while codeine is the most widely used (Kvale, et al., 2003; Temel, et al., 2006). Should cough be triggered by an infec-

---

Table 8–2 **Therapies for Cough**

Guaifenesin 2–4 tsp (200–400 mg) orally every 4 hours
  (maximum dose 2400 mg per day)

Guaifenesin with codeine 2 tsp orally every 12 hours
  (2 tsp contains 40 mg of codeine)

Benzonatate 100 mg orally every 4 hours as necessary
  (maximum dose 600 mg per day)

Codeine 10–20 mg orally every 4 hours as necessary

Oxycodone 5 mg orally every 4 hours
  (consider long-acting oxycodone when more than 3–4 doses are needed per day)

Source: Temel, Pirl, & Lynch, 2006, p. 243.

tion, a trial of oral antibiotics may produce symptom relief. Nebulized local anesthetics, such as lidocaine or bupivacaine, are also useful and easily administered. Patients must be cautioned not to eat or drink after treatments because the gag reflex will be suppressed for 1 hour or longer (Chan, et al., 2004). Patients with a history of COPD or smoking may also benefit from bronchodilator treatment (Bruera & Neumann, 1998); corticosteroids may be helpful to patients with postradiation lung damage and endobronchial tumors (Chan, et al., 2004).

Other supportive measures for a patient with cough include keeping the head of the bed elevated; provision of warm humidified air; avoidance of irritants, such as cigarette smoke or pungent chemicals; and provision of oral fluids to thin secretions (Dudgeon, 2006). Patients and families may worry that cough will cause massive bleeding and death due to exsanguination. Although some patients may be reassured by the knowledge that death due to massive hemoptysis is a very rare event, discussion of potential care measures, such as palliative sedation, may be warranted for this type of event. The concept of palliative sedation is presented in the Ethical Issues at the End of Life section of this chapter.

Pain Syndromes

From the moment of diagnosis through the end-of-life stage of illness, all people with lung cancer must receive expert pain management. For core concepts of pain management in cancer patients, the reader is referred to many excellent resources available to guide practice (American Pain Society, 2005; Ashburn & Rice, 1998; McGuire, Yarbro, & Ferrell, 1995; Paice & Fine, 2006). Unfortunately, many terminally ill patients still die painful deaths. In a study of 1,021 patients with advanced non-small cell

lung cancer, researchers found that 74% of participants experienced pain, and 50% reported that the pain affected their daily life activities (DiMaio, et al., 2004). In short, patients dying of lung cancer often experience severe, unrelieved pain (Kvale, et al., 2007).

Pain syndromes specific to lung cancer can vary depending on the type of location of the tumor and sites of metastatic disease. Patients with advanced local disease may experience pain in the chest wall, vertebrae, and brachial plexus (Silvestri, 2000). Typically, cancer pain at the end of life can be well controlled with oral, transdermal, rectal, or parenteral opioid and nonopioid analgesics (Paice & Fine, 2006).

Severe intractable neuropathic thoracic pain from locally advanced lung cancer may not respond to conventional approaches. A variety of other approaches have been tried with varying success. For example, interpleural analgesia can be accomplished by placement of a permanent, interpleural catheter for periodic instillation of an anesthetic agent, such as bupivacaine (Irick & Hostetter, 2000). Potential complications include pneumothorax, pleural effusion, catheter displacement or rupture, systemic reaction to the anesthetic agent, and Horner syndrome secondary to nerve blockage. However, Swarm, Karanikolas, and Cousins (2004) suggest that interpleural analgesia may be no more effective than spinal analgesia. Percutaneous cervical cordotomy has also been used with success (Bekar, Kocaeli, Abas, & Bozkurt, 2007). Both of these approaches reflect a high-technology approach to pain relief that may not be compatible with a particular patient's preferences for interventions at the end of life.

Pain secondary to bone metastases is a second type of pain syndrome experienced by people with end-stage lung cancer. Bone metastasis occurs in 50% of patients with lung cancer (Strohl

& Hawkins, 2006) and can represent a challenging clinical management problem. Radiation therapy is highly effective in treating local metastatic bone pain; approximately 80% of patients will achieve some pain relief (Hoskin, 2004). In most instances, external beam therapy is used; however, strontium 89 and samarium 153 are also useful approaches to target osteoblastic bone lesions in lung cancer (Lin & Ray, 2006). Because these agents can cause myelosuppression, they may not be suitable for patients with low blood counts. Additionally, because there is a delay in onset and timing of peak effect of strontium 89, its use is appropriate only for patients with at least a 3-month projected life span (Paice & Fine, 2006).

In addition to radiation, patients with bone metastasis may require pain management via narcotics and nonsteroidal anti-inflammatory drugs (NSAIDs) (Strohl & Hawkins, 2006). Metastatic bone pain also may be treated with other adjuvant drugs, such as bisphosphonates and corticosteroids. Bisphosphonates act by inhibiting bone resorption, thus decreasing bone breakdown, calcium release, and pain. In particular, pamidronate disodium induces analgesic effects within 2 to 4 weeks of starting treatment; either 60 mg every 2 to 4 weeks or 90 mg every 4 weeks can produce pain relief (Paice & Fine, 2006).

Anxiety

People with end-stage lung cancer may experience a variety of neurocognitive disorders related to metastatic disease to the brain, side effects of drugs, progressive decline in pulmonary function, and existential issues associated with facing the end of one's life. Disorders may include depression, anxiety, and delirium. Depression is a common, persistent problem in persons with

lung cancer; prevalence may be as high as 33% (Hopwood & Stephens, 2000). The reader is referred to Part IV, Psychosocial Issues of Individuals with Lung Cancer, for a complete discussion of depression and lung cancer. Anxiety and delirium management for end-stage lung cancer patients are reviewed in this chapter.

Anxiety refers to feelings of deep unease without an identifiable cause (Kazanowski, 2006). In the context of palliative care, anxiety can occur in response to poorly controlled symptoms, such as pain and dyspnea, abnormal metabolic states, hormone-producing tumors, and medication side effects (Payne & Massie, 2000). Anxiety may also increase as the patient becomes increasingly aware that death is approaching. Of note, most studies that have evaluated the presence of psychiatric symptoms in cancer patients have documented a higher prevalence of a mixture of anxiety and depression as opposed to anxiety alone (Payne & Massie, 2000).

Assessment

Assessment of an anxious patient must include a careful history and physical as well as a psychological evaluation. Detection of potential treatable factors that contribute to anxiety is critical to treatment decisions. For example, untreated pain and hypoxia can precipitate both anxiety and panic. Other sources of treatable anxiety include adverse reactions to medications or drug interaction effects (Kazanowski, 2006). Patients who have been taking high doses of opioids or benzodiazepines may experience anxiety and an acute withdrawal state should those drugs be withdrawn abruptly. Both kinds of drugs should be slowly tapered if given in high doses over a long period of time (Breitbart, Chochinov, & Passik, 2004). Patients may describe their anxiety with a variety of terms, such as restless, anxious, agitated, irritable, apprehensive, or fearful. Physiologic manifestations of anxiety can include tachycardia, shortness of breath, trembling, nausea, and insomnia.

Treatment

Treatment of anxiety includes both nonpharmacologic and pharmacologic strategies. Empathetic listening, discussion, and acknowledgment of the patient's anxiety is key. A variety of psychological approaches may be useful, including psychoeducational interventions to explain the predictable emotional phases people experience at the end of life, behavioral techniques to promote relaxation, individual psychotherapy, and participation in support groups (Payne & Massie, 2000).

Table 8–3 summarizes current pharmacologic approaches to management of anxiety in

Table 8–3 Pharmacotherapy of Anxiety in Terminal Illness

Generic Name	Approximate Daily Dosage Range (mg)	Route[a]
Benzodiazepines		
Very short acting		
midazolam	10–60 per 24 h	IV, SC
Short acting		
alprazolam	0.25–2.0 t.i.d.–q.i.d.	PO, SL
oxazepam	10–15 t.i.d.–q.i.d.	PO
lorazepam	0.5–2.0 t.i.d.–q.i.d.	PO, SL, IV, IM
Intermediate acting		
chlordiazepoxide	10–50 t.i.d.–q.i.d.	PO, IM
Long acting		
diazepam	5–10 b.i.d.–q.i.d.	PO, IM, IV, PR
clorazepate	7.5–15 b.i.d.–q.i.d.	PO
clonazepam	0.5–2 b.i.d.–q.i.d.	PO
Non-benzodiazepines		
buspirone	5–20 t.i.d.	PO
Neuroleptics		
haloperidol	0.5–5 q2–12 h	PO, IV, SC, IM
methotrimeprazine	10–20 q4–8 h	IV, SC, PO
thioridazine	10–75 t.i.d.–q.i.d.	PO
chlorpromazine	12.5–50 q4–12 h	PO, IM, IV
Antihistamine		
hydroxyzine	25–50 q4–6 h	PO, IV, SC
Tricyclic antidepressants		
clomipramine	25–100 q.i.d.	PO

[a]PO, per oral; IM, intramuscular; PR, per rectum; IV, intravenous; SC, subcutaneous; SL, sublingual; b.i.d., two times a day; t.i.d., three times a day; q.i.d., four times a day. Parenteral doses are generally twice as potent as oral doses; intravenous bolus injections or infusions should be administered slowly.
Source: Breitbart, Chochinov, & Passik, 2004.

terminal illness. Benzodiazepine drugs form the mainstay of treatment. The selection of drug and dose is highly individualized based on the underlying physiologic condition and age. Because the onset, distribution, and excretion of benzodiazepines are influenced by liver disease and decreased absorption in the GI tract, caution must be used in patients with advanced cancer (Stiefel, Berney, & Mazzocato, 1999). Long-acting drugs may cause prolonged sedation, daytime drowsiness, hangover, and dizziness. Intermediate- and short-acting drugs may be more tolerable and safer to use.

Delirium

The essential defining characteristics of delirium are disordered cognition and arousal (with disturbances in level of consciousness and attention) (Breitbart, et al., 2004). Delirium is characterized as a "disturbance of consciousness that is accompanied by a change in cognition that cannot be better accounted for by a pre-existing or evolving dementia" (Breitbart & Cohen, 2000, p. 77). The incidence of delirium in terminally ill cancer patients is variable, ranging from 44% to 85%, with elderly patients being more susceptible (Breitbart & Cohen, 2000). Typically, delirium evolves over a short time frame of hours to days and fluctuates in severity within each day over time. Other clinical features of delirium may include both hyperactive and hypoactive symptoms, such as nighttime agitation, daytime sleepiness, hallucinations, delusions, daytime agitation, disorientation, anxiety, fear, depression, confusion, sedation, irritability, anger, euphoria, apathy, and rapidly shifting emotions (Kuebler, Heidrich, Vena, & English, 2006). With the exception of the last day or two of life, delirium may

be reversible (Breitbart & Cohen, 2000). In the context of the last few days or hours of life, the onset of delirium may be described as terminal restlessness.

Assessment

Assessment of the patient experiencing delirium includes focus on potential sources of delirium as well as symptom evaluation. In the great majority of cases, the causes of delirium are multifactorial. Sources of delirium include both direct effects of cancer (such as brain metastasis) on the central nervous system and indirect effects, including metabolic encephalopathy, electrolyte imbalance, medication adverse effects, infection, hematologic abnormalities, nutritional deficiencies, and paraneoplastic syndromes (Breitbart, et al., 2004). Of note, opioid toxicity, benzodiazepines, and anticholinergic drugs may all cause or aggravate delirium in patients with advanced cancer (Bruera & Neumann, 1998). Lanken et al. (2008) suggest that agitation in a delirious patient may be a sign of pain that would justify a trial of pain medication. Delirium and agitation may also be caused by urinary retention and constipation (Matzo & Sherman, 2006).

Palliative care practitioners advocate use of a standardized assessment tool to evaluate cognition in the person with suspected delirium. The Mini-Mental State Examination (MMSE), Memorial Delirium Assessment Scale (MDAS), Delirium Rating Scale (DRS), and Neecham Confusion Scale (NCS) are all useful tools for assessing and diagnosing delirium (Kuebler, et al., 2006).

Treatment

Treatment is selected based on the underlying cause of delirium. Haloperidol or midazolam may be used to temporarily control acute symptoms while other reversible causes are determined and treated. Clozapine (Clozaril), risperidone, and olanzapine are newer antipsychotic drugs that are effective in delirium. In one study, olanzapine resolved delirium in 76% of 82 hospitalized patients with advanced cancer (Breitbart, Tremblay, & Gibson, 2002). Other approaches include changing the type of opioid, increasing hydration, and managing metabolic and infectious complications (Bruera & Neumann, 1998). Support and protection of the patient during delirium is paramount. Should the patient be hyperactive, protection from falls, self-inflicted harm, or other safety hazards is a key nursing responsibility. Patients should not be physically restrained; rather a calm, respectful approach to reorientation is preferred (Campbell, 1998). Environmental stimulation (noise, lights) should be minimized until the acute phase of delirium passes. In the event a patient experiences unrelenting terminal restlessness and delirium that does not respond to all possible pharmacologic therapy in the final days or hours of life, sedation to the point of unresponsiveness may be warranted (see also Palliative Sedation under the Ethical Issues at the End of Life section of this chapter).

Complementary and Alternative Methods for Symptom Management

Complementary and alternative methods (CAMs) are a broad spectrum of practices and therapies that may be employed by persons with cancer. Persons with end-stage lung cancer may have several reasons for initiating CAMs at this point on their illness trajectory. Pam, Morrison, Ness, Fugh-Berman, and Leipzig (2000) suggest that dying patients experience a heavy symptom burden for which traditional medical treatment may produce adverse side effects. CAMs may have fewer troublesome effects and, if effective, be useful as alternatives to traditional treatments or complementary to traditional methods for symptom relief.

Persons who are told there is no traditional medical cure for their advanced cancer are vulnerable to the lure of unproven alternate methods. They are at risk for trying heavily promoted alternative therapies that may be harmful and also delay or impair beneficial treatment. An important recommendation by the American College of Chest Physicians (ACCP) Evidence-Based Clinical Practice Guidelines is to inquire about CAM use at each patient contact (Cassileth, et al., 2007). Patients then can be provided with evidence-based advice about the advantages and disadvantages of various CAMs. An excellent presentation of alternative and complementary therapies and evidence-based complementary therapies for symptom management is found in Berenson (2006).

Wendy Harpham, a physician with incurable non-Hodgkin lymphoma, was pressured about alternative treatment by well-meaning friends and relatives when she first was diagnosed (Harpham, 2001). Having complete confidence in her oncologist's recommendations for treatment, she dismissed the various other theories of healing suggested by her friends and family. After her conventional medicine treatment, she channeled her fears of recurrence into time-honored measures to promote physical, emotional, and spiritual recovery, such as eating well, exercise, counseling, a support group, and prayer. When her disease progressed and later recurred for a second time, she found herself motivated to evaluate the science behind the unproven alternative therapies she had been assured were safer or more effective than conventional treatment. She, like other patients who are worn out by treatment and discouraged when cancer progresses, wanted to believe the promises of proponents of unproven alternative therapies and felt tremendous personal and social pressure to be "open to notions of healing based on unproven theories" (Harpham, 2001, p. 135). Harpham offers several suggestions (see Table 8–4) that nurses can use while working with persons with advanced lung cancer and their families who are exploring or using CAMs. Patients are advised to avoid any therapy that is promoted as an "alternative" to conventional treatment.

Theory behind the concept of complementary therapies indicates that these methods enhance the effects of conventional medical therapy either directly, through interaction with the conventional therapy, or indirectly, by putting the body in better shape to use internal factors to fight the cancer. Increasing or decreasing certain foods in one's diet to enhance the effects of radiation, chemotherapy, or even surgery is an example of intending an interactive effect. An example of the second use of a complementary method is to increase physical activity to maintain lung function and decrease disability from fatigue. Following are descriptions of several clinical trials of complementary methods that can be used in conjunction with conventional methods to control symptoms (see also Table 8–5). Using these methods may also enhance the beliefs of patients that there are choices they can make about what will help them feel better.

Table 8–4 Guidelines for Working with Patients and Families Who Are Exploring CAMs

- Patients want to get well. Assure patients and their families that your number-one goal is to help them to feel better.
- Patients want to avoid distress, uncertainty, and poverty. First, reassure patients that although there may be discomforts and uncertainties to conventional treatment, you will work with them to prevent, minimize, or deal with any difficulties encountered. Then refer patients and their families to resources that describe the problems and uncertainties of the complementary or unproven alternative method.
- Patients want to enhance their own healing. Encourage their efforts. Refer them to accurate information about nutrition, exercise, hopefulness, prayer, and other factors that may facilitate self-healing.
- Patients want to feel empowered. Encourage patients to participate actively in their treatment to the degree that they wish.
- Patients want the best possible treatment. Emphasize the strengths of the scientific method; acknowledge the limitations of science; dedicate yourself to trying to narrow the gap between the quality of care patients want and what they actually receive.
- Patients want hope. Share success stories. Help patients and their families understand that there may be more hope in a conventional treatment with a small chance of cure than in an unproven therapy.

Source: Summarized from Harpham, 2001.

Table 8–5 Recommended Complementary Therapies[a]

Symptom	Therapy
Dyspnea	Relaxation promotion therapies
	A trial of acupuncture
Pain	Muscle relaxation
	Muscle relaxation/guided imagery
	Transcutaneous electrical nerve stimulation
	Massage
	Acupuncture
	Hypnosis
Nausea and vomiting	Small amounts of carbohydrates and water
	Decrease ingestion of protein and lipids

[a]See text for references and strength of evidence.

Dyspnea

Complementary therapies that promote relaxation, including imagery, massage, therapeutic touch, Reiki, music, and aromatherapy may be useful adjuncts to pharmacologic treatments (Berenson, 2006; Kazanowski, 2006). Corner, Plant, and Warner (1995) identified and evaluated nursing strategies for managing breathlessness in lung cancer. An intervention was developed in which a nurse practitioner provided 1-hour sessions of breathing retraining, counseling, simple relaxation techniques, and teaching of coping and adaptation (e.g., activity pacing) strategies over the course of 3–6 weeks to manage the emotional experience of breathlessness (Corner, Plant, A'Hern, & Bailey, 1996).

After 3 months, the 11 patients in the intervention group showed significant improvement over the nine control group patients in worst breathlessness, distress caused by breathlessness, and in functional capacity. A second randomized, multicenter study evaluated the effect of the intervention on a larger sample of 103 patients with advanced lung cancer (Bredin, et al., 1999). Patients who received the intervention experienced improvement in breathlessness, performance status, and physical and emotional status. A third study in 30 palliative care patients supported the preceding findings (Hately, Laurence, Scott, Baker, & Thomas, 2003). Intervention strategies used in the preceding studies were described as commonly used with patients for chronic lung disease but not routinely used with persons with lung cancer.

Acupuncture was used to relieve breathlessness in three studies. Filshie, Penn, Ashley, and Davis (1996) reported that acupuncture treatments lowered respiratory rates in 20 cancer patients who were breathless at rest, gave them maximal symptomatic relief from breathlessness and anxiety, and produced feelings of relaxation 90 minutes posttreatment compared to pretreatment levels. DiSalvo et al. (2008) noted that a nurse remained with each subject during the intervention, potentially influencing the positive acupuncture treatment results. A second study, using the Filshie et al. (1996) intervention with 24 COPD patients, by Lewith, Prescott, and Davis (2004), failed to find a difference between standardized acupuncture treatments and placebo treatments, both administered by a nurse. Vickers, Feinstein, Deng, and Cassileth (2005), comparing true and placebo acupuncture treatments in 47 advanced lung and breast cancer patients, found no significant difference in dyspnea scores between the two treatments. However, Cassileth et al. (2007) recommend a trial of acupuncture for lung cancer dyspnea.

Pain

Devine and Westlake's (1995) meta-analysis of the effects of psychoeducational interventions on cancer care in adults supported the use of muscle relaxation and the combination of muscle relaxation/guided imagery for relief of both pain and anxiety. Although subjects had various types of cancer and the length of time since diagnosis was not reported in many of the studies, the large and homogeneous effect sizes indicated that relaxation techniques may be effective for pain relief in end-stage lung cancer. A more recent review of CAMs by Pam et al. (2000) suggested the potential usefulness of relaxation and guided imagery, as well as transcutaneous electrical nerve stimulation (TENS) and massage for pain relief in dying patients. Because no well-designed research was found for music therapy, biofeedback, hypnosis, or aromatherapy with such patients, no recommendations were made for those methods. A review of relaxation interventions by Kwekkeboom and Gretarsdottir (2006) provided support for the use of progressive muscle relaxation for both acute and chronic pain. The ACCP guidelines recommend massage therapy as part of multimodality therapy for anxiety and pain. Acupuncture also is strongly recommended when pain is poorly controlled, when side effects from other modalities are significant, or when wishing to reduce the amount of pain medicine used (Cassileth, et al., 2007). Cassileth et al. also suggest that hypnosis is beneficial in reducing pain.

Nausea and Vomiting

No large-scale CAM research has been reported on treating nausea and vomiting in persons who are terminally ill (Pam, et al., 2000; Rhodes & McDaniel, 2001). Rhodes and McDaniel suggest that, in terminally ill persons with cancer, large amounts of protein and lipids may induce nausea and vomiting because of cachexia-associated changes in metabolism. They suggest that small amounts of carbohydrates and water may be the most appropriate diet for terminally ill persons with nausea. Acupuncture, acupressure, progressive relaxation, guided imagery, hypnosis, and biofeedback have been associated with positive results in chemotherapy-related nausea and vomiting (Berenson, 2006; Cassileth, et al., 2007; King, 2006). These therapies also may be helpful for persons with end-stage lung cancer.

Nutrition

Because fruit and vegetable intake is associated with lowered risk for lung cancer, some patients believe that increased intake of such foods may have some benefit even in late-stage lung cancer. Little research has been conducted that would indicate that foods and physical activity greater than that normally recommended to promote health will enhance chances of survival. For persons who have difficulty eating, help in the form of nutritional supplements or multivitamin–mineral supplements may be suggested. Although there has been no reported research on either the harmful or beneficial effects of nutritional supplements on the progression of lung cancer, use of high doses of vitamins and minerals is not supported scientifically and should be avoided (Brown, et al., 2001; Whitman, 2001).

Because nutritional supplements, vitamins, minerals, and herbal products may interact with cancer therapies, it is important that the healthcare provider be informed if they are being used. Cassileth et al. (2007) recommend that botanical agents be used only in the context of a clinical trial and only if patients do not respond to or refuse other therapies.

Ethical Issues at the End of Life

Ethical issues associated with end-of-life care in lung cancer patients arise due to the poor prognosis associated with the diagnosis, potentially debilitating treatments that may or may not pose substantial benefit to patients, and difficulty that may arise in managing intractable physical or existential suffering. The purpose of this second section is to explore the use of advance directives to express treatment preferences, issues associated with palliative chemotherapy and withholding or withdrawing life-sustaining measures, use of sedation at the end of life, and desire for assisted dying.

Advance Directives

Many individuals believe that a well-prepared advance directive assures that their current wishes regarding end-of-life decisions will be followed and that having an advance directive will reduce stress on themselves, family members, and healthcare providers. Although advance directives can facilitate implementation of a person's wishes for care at the end of life, evidence from the SUPPORT study indicated that often there was a discrepancy between the wishes of hospitalized patients and their family members and physicians (SUPPORT Principal Investigators, 1995). The SUPPORT study triggered numerous efforts to improve communication and procedures of end-of-life care. Simplification and standardization of advance directive forms has made the understanding and completion of such documents easier. Healthcare providers are becoming better educated to help patients determine important values related to their quality of living before they become seriously ill, to be sure that the appropriate persons are aware of their wishes related to those values, and that advance directive documents are in place.

An important point to consider is that a legal advance directive is only one part of end-of-life planning. Indeed, advance directives may not be sufficient to guide clinical decision making when patients are no longer able to speak for themselves (Perkins, 2007). First, an advance directive may not contain enough specific detail to guide many clinical decisions that may need to be made (Nishimura, et al., 2007). Second, individuals' wishes may change when they are actually within the dying situation. Even in the presence of an advance directive, the role of the oncology nurse is to assist patients and family members to recognize thoughts and emotions that drive their decisions and to communicate their feelings and desires over the course of the dying process. The nurse can help all persons involved identify treatment goals related to prolongation of life and subsequent quality of life. The nurse also can help to ensure that implications of treatment decisions are understood. The nurse may serve as team leader and as a liaison to keep physicians in touch with what may be day-to-day changes in patient status and in patient and family concerns (Coyle, 2006). For example, hospice nurses have provided leadership in this area and often function as team leaders for the patient and family's caregivers and volunteers.

Palliative Chemotherapy

When advance directives are discussed, decisions related to palliative chemotherapy and to withholding or withdrawing life-sustaining therapy must be addressed. Palliative chemotherapy may be initiated to relieve specific symptoms (such as superior vena cava syndrome) and may lead to prolonged survival. Administration of chemotherapy to persons with lung cancer is not uncommon in the last year of life. In a national study of chemotherapy given to advanced non-small cell lung cancer patients in community oncology settings, 43% of the patients received chemotherapy within 1 month of death (Murillo & Koeller, 2006). The researchers observed that their findings may be indicative of increased use of chemotherapy near the time of death. Possible explanations include an increase in aggressive care at the end of life; newer, targeted drug therapies for advanced disease; greater patient access to drug information about new treatments; and difficulty with predicting life expectancy in this group of patients.

However, patient age may be an important consideration when evaluating palliative chemotherapy as a treatment option. In a retrospective review of elderly patients treated with chemotherapy for advanced non-small cell lung cancer, O'Brien and colleagues (2008) concluded that there has been no substantial improvement in survival rates for this group in the past 13 years. For patients with recurrent small cell lung cancer, Schneider (2008) recommends a focus on improvement of quality of life.

Patients with a good performance status might benefit from further treatment, such as single-agent topotecan, whereas patients with a poor performance status may not benefit from further chemotherapy. To date, there is no agreement on the best chemotherapeutic regimens for patients who fail first-line treatment. Unfortunately, many patients who do receive second-line treatment often receive agents that are not consistent with FDA labeling or clinical studies (Ramsey, et al., 2008). Clearly, more studies that compare chemotherapy and best supportive care are warranted. Such studies must address quality of life and cost analyses of resources expended to provide such care. The challenge in deciding about palliative chemotherapy is achieving a balance between prolonging survival and improving symptoms and quality of life without unacceptable drug toxicity.

Withholding/Withdrawing Life-Sustaining Therapies

For persons with lung cancer, decisions to withhold/withdraw treatment are likely to be related to mechanical ventilation and artificial nutrition and hydration.

Mechanical Ventilation

Mechanical ventilation is used to support respiration in patients with acute or chronic respiratory failure. Patients with lung cancer who are admitted to intensive care settings and require mechanical ventilation have a high hospital mortality rate (Soares, et al., 2007). Although mechanical ventilation can be used to control dyspnea in terminal illness, it should only be considered as a temporary measure for a severe reversible condition (NCCN, 2008). Both patients and family members should be helped to understand that terminal dyspnea can be effectively decreased even if artificial ventilation is not chosen or if it is withdrawn.

Withdrawal of mechanical ventilation with the probability that death will ensue is an ethically justifiable decision. This justification is based on the right that patients or their surrogates have to refuse or discontinue other forms of treatment. Should a mechanically ventilated patient or his surrogate decide to discontinue such support, compassionate, humane processes are available to guide the process. The term "terminal weaning" is used to describe a step-by-step process of withdrawal of ventilator support (from a patient who is not expected to survive) (Knight, Espinosa, & Bruera, 2006). Extubation may or may not follow terminal weaning. Although institutions vary in the specific approaches used, a gradual reduction of ventilator settings is typically used and accompanied by administration of medications to alleviate patient discomfort. The rate of withdrawal will vary, depending on the level of remaining brain function (if any) and physiologic responses to reduction in ventilatory support. Campbell (2007) recommends several processes for terminal weaning that include use of a common measure to monitor the patient for respiratory distress, premedication or medication during ventilator withdrawal via opioids and benzodiazepines, and extubation after ventilator withdrawal unless contraindicated. Terminal weaning requires skillful management of any indications of patient discomfort and intensive family support. Should family members choose to remain at the patient's bedside during the procedure, staff should remain in constant attendance to care for both patient and family.

Nutrition and Hydration

Controversy exists about the use of nutrition and hydration in persons who are dying, perhaps because of the caregiving symbolism associated with provision of food and water (Ersek, 2003). Consensus exists regarding the notion that a highly personalized approach should be taken to nutrition and hydration decisions at the end of life. Food and fluid by mouth (if appropriate) always should be offered, but ethical decision analyses are required when considering the use or withdrawal of mechanical methods of providing nutrition and hydration. The Hospice and Palliative Nurses Association Position Statement on Artificial Nutrition and Hydration (2003) states that "decision-making regarding the use of artificial nutrition and hydration must occur in the context of an open discussion and incorporate the patient's values and goals for care" (p. 2). If a patient is not competent to make decisions, surrogate decision makers and advance directives must be consulted. Hence, nurses must respect a patient's or patient surrogate's decisions regarding these interventions. In situations where a patient's wishes are unknown, family members and the healthcare team collaborate to decide if artificial nutrition and hydration is in the patient's best interest. Such decisions are made by balancing the risk of discomfort from progressive dehydration (e.g., fatigue, delirium, restlessness, renal failure, and pressure ulcers) with discomforts associated with administration of artificial hydration (e.g., need for physical restraints, symptoms of fluid overload) for a person who is close to death (Bruera, et al., 2005). Although few randomized controlled clinical trials have been conducted to assess the potential usefulness of parenteral hydration in terminal illness, Bruera and colleagues suggest that parenteral hydration may be useful in alleviating levels of sedation and myoclonus in some patients.

Patients who wish to control the timing of death may chose to voluntarily stop eating and drinking. Although this is a legal action, families and healthcare providers may find this to be an ethically troubling choice. Because little is known about the quality of the dying experience under these circumstances, Ganzini et al. (2003) surveyed hospice nurses' experiences with patients who refused food and fluids to hasten death. According to the nurses' reports, most patients died within 15 days of stopping food and fluids; on a scale of 0 (very bad death) to 9 (very good death), the median score for the quality of death was 8. More research in this area should reveal additional insights regarding the quality of dying under these circumstances.

Palliative Sedation

Despite intensive efforts to relieve physical and existential suffering when death is imminent, an occasional patient will present with intractable problems that cannot be adequately managed. Use of palliative (sometimes termed "terminal") sedation may be an answer for some patients and practitioners. According to De Graeff and Dean (2007), palliative sedation therapy refers to "the use of specific sedative medications to relieve intolerable suffering from refractory symptoms by a reduction in patient consciousness" (p. 68). Usually, other life-prolonging interventions are withheld or withdrawn because they could prolong dying without adding to comfort or quality of life. The practice of palliative sedation is ethically supported under the principle of double effect, provided that it is practiced with the intent of relieving suffering and not of hastening death (Luce & Luce, 2001). However, because death is a foreseeable outcome, some pa-

tients, families, and practitioners may not support this option. The frequency of use of palliative sedation varies widely; differences are likely due to variations in the use of the term and differing practice patterns (De Graeff & Dean, 2007). Intractable symptoms that may prompt consideration of terminal sedation include delirium, terminal restlessness, pain, dyspnea, and nausea/vomiting (De Graeff & Dean, 2007). The use of palliative sedation for intolerable existential or spiritual suffering remains highly controversial. A variety of medications may be used including midazolam, propofol, and barbiturates (Lo & Rubenfeld, 2005).

Assisted Suicide

Despite growing interest in the United States to improve care of the dying, public, patient, and professional opinion studies reveal some support for the right to assisted suicide and euthanasia (Masci, 2007; Miller, et al., 2004; Wilson, et al., 2007). Assisted suicide is defined as "making a means of suicide available to a patient (e.g., providing pills, weapon) with knowledge of the patient's intention. The patient who is physically capable of suicide subsequently acts to end his or her own life" (American Nurses Association [ANA], 1994, p. 1). To date, Oregon is the only state to have legalized the practice of physician-assisted suicide. Because terminally ill patients with lung cancer may experience distressing symptoms at the end of life, nurses who care for these patients may receive requests for assisted suicide.

The nursing profession has taken a clear stand on how nurses should respond to patient requests for assisted suicide. The ANA (1994) issued a position statement on assisted suicide that outlines the ethical role of nurses in end-of-life care but articulates prohibition against participating in assisted suicide. However, ANA's Code of Ethics for Nurses (2001) emphasizes the advocacy role of nursing, stating that "the nurse promotes, advocates for, and strives to protect the health, safety, and rights of the patient" (p. 12). Whether this statement supports a nurse's role as advocate for a patient's ethical or legal right to assisted suicide is open to debate.

The Oncology Nursing Society (ONS) (2007) issued a position statement, "Nurses' Responsibility to the Patient Requesting Assistance in Hastening Death," recognizing that terminal illness may include intense physical symptoms, existential suffering, and fear of loss of control at the end of life. ONS (pp. 763–764) recommends that nurses respond to requests for assisted suicide by:

- Assessing the patient's rationale for the request and engaging in a nonjudgmental multidisciplinary evaluation of unmet needs.
- Promptly attending to unrecognized and unmet needs with intensive interventions.
- Maintaining a nonjudgmental approach or language with the patient, family, significant others, and colleagues.
- Resisting any inclination to withdraw physically or emotionally from the patient.
- Reaffirming nonabandonment to the patient. However, if the nurse chooses to withdraw from that patient's care, continuing care must be provided until an appropriate replacement can be determined.

In Oregon, where assisted suicide is legal, nurses may choose to continue to care for the patient or withdraw, provided the patient is not abandoned. It is ethically permissible for a nurse to choose to remain with a patient who engages in assisted suicide, provided both the nurse and the patient are comfortable with this action (Oregon Nurses Association, 1995).

Regardless of individual opinions about the acceptability of assisted suicide, healthcare providers support the goal of universal access to expert symptom management and psychosocial support that successfully alleviates suffering for all terminally ill people. Even if such care is available, a subset of individuals may experience an end-of-life situation that is incompatible with their values about life, death, and the dying process. Should such individuals request assistance with suicide, the options of terminal sedation or voluntarily stopping eating and drinking may be acceptable legal alternatives (Quill, Lee, & Nunn, 2000). Regardless, a healthcare professional must carefully weigh the ethical and legal ramifications of a request for assisted suicide and ultimately make a decision that is compatible with personal values or morals about the end-of-life experience.

Conclusion

This chapter focused on issues related to symptom management and ethical decision making for persons with terminal-stage lung cancer. Expert symptom management is the mainstay of successful care of terminally ill people with lung cancer. Care is focused on comfort and alleviation of dyspnea, pain, cough, anorexia, fatigue, neurocognitive disorders, and any other symptoms that may arise due to disease or treatment sequelae. In addition to medications, oxygen therapy, and other supportive practices, the use of complementary therapies may enhance the quality of the end-of-life experience for patients with lung cancer and their families. Pharmacological and nonpharmacological measures were reviewed for management of commonly experienced symptoms. Guidelines were presented for working with patients and families who are considering or using CAMs to prolong survival or to improve quality of life.

Several ethical issues that may confront persons with end-stage lung cancer, their families, and professional caregivers were discussed. The need for ethical decision making is prompted by the poor prognosis of persons with advanced lung cancer, potentially debilitating treatments that may provide little benefit in terms of length of survival, and difficulty managing intractable physical and existential suffering.

Nurses who provide care to patients and families prior to and during the dying trajectory need knowledge and skills in palliative care. Nurses must have an ability to foster appropriate and continuing communication among patients, families, and healthcare professionals to successfully resolve conflicts regarding the needs and desires of all involved. The provision of compassionate end-of-life care requires that nurses have a complete understanding of symptom management at the end of life and give full attention to the needs of all who face this difficult time.

References

American Nurses Association. (1994). *Position statement on assisted suicide*. Washington, DC: Author.

American Nurses Association. (2001). *Code of ethics for nurses with interpretive statements*. Washington, DC: Author.

American Pain Society. (2005). *Guideline for the management of cancer pain in adults and children*. Retrieved May 22, 2008, from http://www.guideline.gov/summary/summary.aspx?ss=15&doc_id=7297&nbr=4341#s25

Ashburn, M., & Rice, L. J. (Eds.). (1998). *The management of pain*. New York: Churchill Livingstone.

Bekar, A., Kocaeli, H., Abas, F., & Bozkurt, M. (2007). Bilateral high-level percutaneous cervical cordotomy in cancer pain due to lung cancer: A case report. *Surgical Neurology, 67*(5), 504–507.

Berenson, S. (2006). Complementary and alternative therapies in palliative care. In B. F. Ferrell & N. Coyle (Eds.), *Textbook of palliative nursing* (2nd ed., pp. 491–509). New York: Oxford University Press.

Berger, A. M., Shuster, J., & Von Roenn, J. (2006). *Principles and practice of palliative care and supportive oncology* (3rd ed.). Philadelphia: Lippincott-Raven.

Booth, S., Kelly, M. J., Cox, N. P., Adams, L., & Guz, A. (1996). Does oxygen help dyspnea in patients with cancer? *American Journal of Respiratory & Critical Care Medicine, 153*(5), 1515–1518.

Bredin, M., Corner, J., Krishnasamy, M., Plant, H., Bailey, C., & A'Hern, R. (1999). Multicentre randomised controlled trial of nursing intervention for breathlessness in patients with lung cancer. *British Medical Journal, 318*(7188), 901–904.

Breitbart, W., Chochinov, H., & Passik, S. (2004). Psychiatric symptoms in palliative medicine. In D. Doyle, G. Hanks, N. Cherny, & K. Calman (Eds.), *Oxford textbook of palliative medicine* (3rd ed., pp. 746–771). New York: Oxford University Press.

Breitbart, W., & Cohen, K. (2000). Delirium in the terminally ill. In H. M. Chochinov & W. Breitbart (Eds.), *Handbook of psychiatry in palliative medicine* (pp. 75–90). New York: Oxford University Press.

Breitbart, W., Tremblay, A., & Gibson, C. (2002). An open trial of olanzapine for the treatment of delirium in hospitalized cancer patients. *Psychosomatics, 43*, 175–182.

Brown, J., Byers, T., Thompson, K., Eldridge, B., Doyle, C., & Williams, A. (2001). Nutrition during and after cancer treatment: A guide for informed choices by cancer survivors. *CA: A Cancer Journal for Clinicians, 51*(3), 153–181.

Bruera, E., Kuehn, N., Miller, M., Selmser, P., & Macmillan, K. (1991). The Edmonton Symptom Assessment System (ESAS): A simple method for assessment of palliative care patients. *Journal of Palliative Care, 7*(2), 6–9.

Bruera, E., & Neumann, C. (1998). Management of specific symptom complexes in patients receiving palliative care. *Canadian Medical Association Journal, 158*(13), 1717–1726.

Bruera, E., Sala, R., Rico, M., Moyano, J., Centeno, C., Willey, J., et al. (2005). Effects of parenteral hydration in terminally ill cancer patients: A preliminary study. *Journal of Clinical Oncology, 23*(10), 2366–2371.

Bruera, E., Schmitz, B., Pither, J., Neumann, C., & Hanson, J. (2000). The frequency and correlates of dyspnea in patients with advanced cancer. *Journal of Pain & Symptom Management, 19*(5), 357–362.

Bruera, E., Sweeney, C., Willey, J., Palmer, J., Strasser, F., Morice, R., et al. (2003). A randomized controlled trial of supplemental oxygen versus air in cancer patients with dyspnea. *Palliative Medicine, 17*(8), 659–663.

Campbell, M. L. (1998). *Forgoing life-sustaining therapy: How to care for the patient who is near death.* Aliso Viejo, CA: AACN.

Campbell, M. L. (2007). How to withdraw mechanical ventilation: A systematic review of the literature. *AACN Advanced Critical Care, 18*(4), 397–403.

Cassileth, B., Deng, G., Gomez, J., Johnstone, P., Kumar, N., & Vickers, A. (2007). Complementary therapies and integrative oncology in lung cancer: ACCP evidence-based clinical practice guidelines (2nd ed.). *Chest, 132*(Suppl. 3), 340S–354S.

Chan, K., Shan, M., Tse, D., & Thorsen, A. (2004). Palliative medicine in malignant respiratory diseases. In D. Doyle, G. Hanks, N. Cherny, & K. Calman (Eds.), *Oxford textbook of palliative medicine* (3rd ed., pp. 587–618). New York: Oxford University Press.

Chochinov, H. M., & Breitbart, W. (Eds.). (2000). *Handbook of psychiatry in palliative medicine.* New York: Oxford University Press.

Claessens, M. T., Lynn, J., Zhong, Z., Desbiens, N. A., Phillips, R. S., Wu, A. W., et al. (2000). Dying with lung cancer or chronic obstructive pulmonary disease: Insights from SUPPORT. *Journal of the American Geriatric Society, 48*(Suppl. 5), S146–S153.

Cleeland, C. S., Mendoza, T. R., Wang, X. S., Chou, C., Harle, M. T., Morrissey, M., et al. (2000). Assessing symptom distress in cancer patients: The M.D. Anderson Symptom Inventory. *Cancer, 89*(7), 1634–1646.

Cooley, M. E. (2000). Symptoms in adults with lung cancer: A systematic research review. *Journal of Pain and Symptom Management, 19*(2), 137–153.

Cooley, M. E., Short, T., & Moriarty, H. (2003). Symptom prevalence, distress, and change over time in adults receiving treatment for lung cancer. *Psycho-Oncology, 12*(7), 674–708.

Corner, J., Plant, H., A'Hern, R., & Bailey, C. (1996). Non-pharmacological interventions for breathlessness in lung cancer. *Palliative Medicine, 10*(4), 299–305.

Corner, J., Plant, H., & Warner, L. (1995). Developing a nursing approach to managing dyspnea in lung cancer. *International Journal of Palliative Nursing, 1*(1), 5–10.

Coyle, N. (2006). Introduction to palliative nursing care. In B. F. Ferrell & N. Coyle (Eds.), *Textbook of palliative nursing* (2nd ed., pp. 5–11). New York: Oxford University Press.

De Graeff, A., & Dean, M. (2007). Palliative sedation therapy in the last weeks of life: A literature review and recommendations for standards. *Journal of Palliative Medicine, 10*(1), 67–85.

Devine, E., & Westlake, S. (1995). The effects of psychoeducational care provided to adults with cancer: Meta-analysis of 116 studies. *Oncology Nursing Forum, 22*(9), 1369–1381.

DiMaio, M., Gridelli, C., Gallo, C., Manzione, L., Brancaccio, L., Barbera, S., et al. (2004). Prevalence and management of pain in Italian patients with advanced non-small-cell lung cancer. *British Journal of Cancer, 90*(12), 2288–2296.

DiSalvo, W., Joyce, M., Tyson, L., Culkin, A., & MacKay, K. (2008). Putting evidence into practice: Evidence-based interventions for cancer-related dyspnea. *Clinical Journal of Oncology Nursing, 12*(2), 341–352.

Doyle, D., Hanks, G., Cherny, N., & Calman, K. (Eds.). (2004). *Oxford textbook of palliative medicine* (3rd ed.). New York: Oxford University Press.

Dudgeon, D. (2006). Dyspnea, death rattle, and cough. In B. F. Ferrell & N. Coyle, (Eds.), *Textbook of palliative nursing* (2nd ed., pp. 249–264). New York: Oxford University Press.

Ersek, M. (2003). Artificial nutrition and hydration: Clinical issues. *Journal of Hospice and Palliative Nursing, 5*(4), 221–230.

Ferrell, B. F., & Coyle, N. (Eds.). (2006). *Textbook of palliative nursing* (2nd ed.). New York: Oxford University Press.

Filshie, J., Penn, K., Ashley, S., & Davis, C. (1996). Acupuncture for the relief of cancer-related breathlessness. *Palliative Medicine, 10*(2), 145–150.

Gallo-Silver, L., & Pollack, B. (2000). Behavioral interventions for lung cancer-related breathlessness. *Cancer Practice, 8*(6), 268–273.

Ganzini, L., Goy, E., Miller, L., Harvath, T., Jackson, A., & Delorit, M. (2003). Nurses' experiences with hospice patients who refuse food and fluids to hasten death. *New England Journal of Medicine, 349*(4), 359–365.

Gift, A., Jablonski, A., Stommel, M., & Given, W. (2004). Symptom clusters in elderly patients with lung cancer. *Oncology Nursing Forum, 31*(2), 203–210.

Gift, A., Stommel, M., Jablonski, A., & Given, W. (2003). A cluster of symptoms over time in patients with lung cancer. *Nursing Research, 52*(6), 393–400.

Griffin, J., Koch, K., Nelson, J., & Cooley, M. (2007). Palliative care consultation, quality-of-life measurements, and bereavement for end-of-life care in patients with lung cancer: ACCP evidence-based clinical practice guidelines (2nd ed.). *Chest, 132*(Suppl. 3), 404S–422S.

Griffin, J., Nelson, J., Koch, K., Niell, H., Ackerman, T., Thompson, M., et al. (2003). End-of-life care in patients with lung cancer. *Chest, 123*(Suppl. 1), 312S–331S.

Harpham, W. (2001). Alternative therapies for curing cancer: What do patients want? What do patients need? *CA: A Cancer Journal for Clinicians, 51*(2), 131–141.

Hately, J., Laurence, V., Scott, A., Baker, R., & Thomas, P. (2003). Breathlessness clinics within specialist palliative care settings can improve the quality of life and functional capacity of patients with lung cancer. *Palliative Medicine, 17*(5), 410–417.

Hoffman, A., Given, B., von Eye, A., Gift, A., & Given, C. (2007). Relationships among pain, fatigue, insomnia, and gender in persons with lung cancer. *Oncology Nursing Forum, 34*(4), 785–792.

Hopwood, P., & Stephens, R. J. (2000). Depression in patients with lung cancer: Prevalence and risk factors derived from quality-of-life data. *Journal of Clinical Oncology, 18*(4), 893–903.

Hoskin, P. J. (2004). Radiotherapy in symptom management. In D. Doyle, G. Hanks, N. Cherny, & K. Calman (Eds.), *Oxford textbook of palliative medicine* (3rd ed., pp. 239–255). New York: Oxford University Press.

Hospice and Palliative Nurses Association. (2003). *Position statement: Artificial nutrition and hydration in end-of-life care.* Retrieved May 22, 2008, from http://www.hpna.org/pdf/PositionStatement_ArtificialNutritionAndHydration.pdf

Hospice and Palliative Nurses Association. (2007). *Hospice and palliative nursing: Scope and standards of practice.* New York: American Nurses Association.

Irick, N., & Hostetter, M. B. (2000). Interpleural analgesia for analgesia due to metastatic lung cancer. *Journal of Pharmaceutical Care in Pain and Symptom Control, 8*(3), 61–67.

Jennings, A., Davies, A., Higgins, J., Gibbs, J., & Broadley, K. (2002). A systematic review of the use of opioids in the management of dyspnea. *Thorax, 57,* 939–944.

Joyce, M., McSweeney, M., Carrieri-Kohlman, V., & Hawkins, J. (2004). The use of nebulized opioids in the management of dyspnea: Evidence synthesis. *Oncology Nursing Forum, 31*(3), 551–559.

Kazanowski, M. (2006). Symptom management in palliative care. In M. L. Matzo & D. W. Sherman (Eds.), *Palliative care nursing: Quality care to the end of life* (pp. 319–344). New York: Springer.

Kemp, C. (1999). *Terminal illness: A guide to nursing care* (2nd ed.). Philadelphia: Lippincott.

King, C. (2006). Nausea and vomiting. In B. F. Ferrell & N. Coyle (Eds.), *Textbook of palliative nursing* (2nd ed., pp. 177–194). New York: Oxford University Press.

Knight, P., Espinosa, L., & Bruera, E. (2006). Sedation for refractory symptoms and terminal weaning. In B. R. Ferrell & N. Coyle (Eds.), *Textbook of palliative nursing* (2nd ed., pp. 467–483). New York: Oxford University Press.

Krech, R., Davis, J., Walsh, D., & Curtis, E. (1992). Symptoms of lung cancer. *Palliative Medicine, 6*(4), 309–315.

Kuebler, K., Heidrich, D., Vena, C., & English, N. (2006). Delirium, confusion, agitation, and restlessness. In B. F. Ferrell & N. Coyle (Eds.), *Textbook of palliative nursing* (2nd ed., pp. 401–420). New York: Oxford University Press.

Kurtz, M. E., Kurtz, J. C., Stommel, M., Given, C., & Given, B. (2000). Symptomatology and loss of physical functioning among geriatric patients with lung cancer. *Journal of Pain and Symptom Management, 19*(4), 249–256.

Kvale, P., Selecky, P., & Prakash, U. (2007). Palliative care in lung cancer: ACCP evidence-based clinical practice guidelines (2nd ed.). *Chest, 132*(Suppl. 3), 368S–403S.

Kvale, P., Simoff, M., & Prakash, U. (2003). Palliative care. *Chest, 123*(Suppl. 1), 284S–311S.

Kwekkeboom, K., & Gretarsdottir, E. (2006). Systematic review of relaxation interventions for pain. *Journal of Nursing Scholarship, 38*(3), 269–277.

Lanken, P., Terry, P., DeLisser, H., Fahy, B., Hansen-Flaschen, J., Heffner, J., et al. (2008). An official American Thoracic Society clinical policy statement: Palliative care for patients with respiratory diseases and critical illnesses. *American Journal of Respiratory Critical Care Medicine, 177*(8), 912–927.

LeGrand, S. B., & Walsh, D. (1999). Palliative management of dyspnea in advanced cancer. *Current Opinion in Oncology, 11*(4), 250–254.

Lewith, G., Prescott, P., & Davis, C. (2004). Can a standardized acupuncture technique palliate disabling breathlessness. *Chest, 125*(5), 1783–1790.

Lin, A., & Ray, M. (2006). Targeted and systemic radiotherapy in the treatment of bone metastasis. *Cancer Metastasis Reviews, 25*(4), 669–675.

Lo, B., & Rubenfeld, G. (2005). Palliative sedation in dying patients. *Journal of the American Medical Association, 294*(14), 1810–1816.

Luce, J. M., & Luce, J. A. (2001). Management of dyspnea in patients with far-advanced lung disease. *Journal of the American Medical Association, 285*(10), 1331–1337.

Masci, D. (2007, October 7). *The right-to-die debate and the tenth anniversary of Oregon's Death With Dignity Act. The Pew Forum on Religion & Public Life.* Retrieved June 7, 2008, from http://pewforum.org/docs/?DocID=251

Matzo, M. L., & Sherman, D. (2006). *Palliative care nursing: Quality care to the end of life* (2nd ed.). New York: Springer Pub.

McCarthy, E. P., Phillips, R. S., Zhong, Z., Drews, R. E., & Lynn, J. (2000). Dying with cancer: Patients' function, symptoms, and care preferences as death approaches. *Journal of the American Geriatric Society, 48*(5), S110–S121.

McCorkle, R., & Young, K. (1978). Development of a symptom distress scale. *Cancer Nursing, 1*(5), 373–378.

McGuire, D. B., Yarbro, C. H., & Ferrell, B. F. (Eds.). (1995). *Cancer pain management* (2nd ed.). Sudbury, MA: Jones and Bartlett.

Mercadante, S., Casuccio, A., & Fulfaro, F. (2000). The course of symptom frequency and intensity in advanced cancer patients followed at home. *Journal of Pain and Symptom Management, 20*(2), 104–112.

Miller, L., Harvath, T., Ganzini, L., Goy, E., Delorit, M., & Jackson, A. (2004). Attitudes and experiences of Oregon hospice nurses and social workers regarding assisted suicide. *Journal of Palliative Medicine, 18*(8), 685–691.

Murillo, J., & Koeller, J. (2006). Chemotherapy given near the end of life by community oncologists for advanced non-small cell lung cancer. *The Oncologist, 11*(10), 1095–1099.

National Comprehensive Cancer Network (NCCN). (2008). *NCCN clinical guidelines in oncology: Palliative care.* Retrieved April 14, 2008, from www.nccn.org/professionals/physician-gls/PDF/palliative.pdf

National Consensus Project for Quality Palliative Care. (2004). *Clinical practice guidelines for quality palliative care.* Retrieved April 15, 2008, from http://nationalconsensusproject.org

Nishimura, A., Mueller, P., Evenson, L., Downer, L., Bowron, C., Thieke, M., et al. (2007). Patients who complete advance directives and what they prefer. *Mayo Clinic Proceedings, 82*(12), 1480–1486.

O'Brien, M., Yau, T., Coward, J., Hughes, S., Papadopoulos, P., Popat, S., et al. (2008). Time and chemotherapy treatment trends in the treatment of elderly patients (age ≥ 70 years) with non-small cell lung cancer. *Clinical Oncology, 20*(2), 142–147.

Oncology Nursing Society. (2007). Nurses' responsibility to the patient requesting assistance in hastening death. *Oncology Nursing Forum, 34*(4), 763–764.

Oregon Nurses Association. (1995). ONA provides guidance on RN's dilemma. Position statement on nurses' role in the Death with Dignity Act. *Oregon Nurse, 60*(2), 12–13.

Paice, J. A., & Fine, P. G. (2006). Pain at the end of life. In B. F. Ferrell & N. Coyle (Eds.), *Textbook of palliative nursing* (2nd ed., pp. 131–153). New York: Oxford University Press.

Pam, C., Morrison, R. S., Ness, J., Fugh-Berman, A., & Leipzig, M. (2000). Complementary and alternative medicine in the management of pain, dyspnea, and nausea and vomiting near the end of life: A systematic review. *Journal of Pain and Symptom Management, 20*(5), 374–387.

Payne, D. K., & Massie, M. J. (2000). Anxiety in palliative care. In H. M. Chochinov & W. Breitbart (Eds.), *Handbook of psychiatry in palliative medicine* (pp. 63–74). New York: Oxford University Press.

Perkins, H. S. (2007). Controlling death: The false promise of advance directives. *Annals of Internal Medicine, 147*(1), 51–57.

Portenoy, R., Thaler, H., Kornblith, A., Lepore, J., Friedlander-Klar, H., Kiyasu, E., et al. (1994). The Memorial Symptom Assessment Scale: An instrument for the evaluation of symptom prevalence, characteristics, and distress. *European Journal of Cancer, 30A*(9), 1326–1336.

Quill, T. E., Lee, B. C., & Nunn, S. (2000). Palliative treatments of last resort: Choosing the least harmful alternative. *Annals of Internal Medicine, 132*(6), 488–493.

Ramsey, S., Martins, R., Blough, D., Tock, L., Lubeck, D., & Reyes, C. (2008). Second-line and third-line chemotherapy for lung cancer: Use and cost. *American Journal of Managed Care, 14*(5), 297–306.

Rhodes, V., & McDaniel, R. (2001). Nausea, vomiting, and retching: Complex problems in palliative care. *CA: A Cancer Journal for Clinicians, 51*(4), 232–248.

Ripamonti, C. (1999). Management of dyspnea in advanced cancer patients. *Supportive Care in Cancer, 7*(4), 233–243.

Ripamonti, C., & Fusco, F. (2002). Respiratory problems in advanced cancer. *Supportive Care in Cancer, 10*(3), 204–216.

Sarna, L. (1998). Effectiveness of structured nursing assessment of symptom distress in advanced lung cancer. *Oncology Nursing Forum, 25*(6), 1041–1048.

Sarna, L., & Brecht, M. (1997). Dimensions of symptom distress in women with advanced lung cancer: A factor analysis. *Heart & Lung, 26*(1), 23–30.

Schneider, B. (2008). Management of recurrent small cell lung cancer. *Journal of the National Comprehensive Cancer Network, 6*(3), 323–331.

Silvestri, G. A. (2000). Palliation for the dying patient with lung cancer. *Respiratory Care, 45*(12), 1490–1496.

Smith, E. L., Hann, D., Ahles, T. A., Furstenberg, C. T., Mitchell, T. A., Meyer, L., et al. (2001). Dyspnea, anxiety, body consciousness, and quality of life in patients with lung cancer. *Journal of Pain and Symptom Management, 21*(4), 323–329.

Soares, M., Darmon, M., Salluh, J., Ferreira, C., Thiery, G., Schlemmer, B., et al. (2007). Prognosis of lung cancer patients with life-threatening complications. *Chest, 131*(3), 840–846.

Stiefel, F., Berney, A., & Mazzocato, C. (1999). Psychopharmacology in supportive care in cancer: A review for the clinician. *Supportive Care in Cancer, 7*(6), 379–385.

Strohl, R., & Hawkins, R. (2006). Bone metastasis. In D. Camp-Sorrell & R. Hawkins (Eds.), *Clinical manual for the oncology advanced practice nurse* (2nd ed., pp. 727–731). Pittsburgh: Oncology Nursing Press.

SUPPORT Principal Investigators. (1995). A controlled trial to improve care for seriously ill hospitalized patients: The study to understand prognoses and preferences for outcomes and risks of treatment. *Journal of the American Medical Association, 274*(20), 1591–1598.

Swarm, R., Karanikolas, M., & Cousins, M. (2004). Anaesthetic techniques for pain control. In D. Doyle, G. Hanks, N. Cherny, & K. Calman (Eds.), *Oxford textbook of palliative medicine* (3rd ed., pp. 378–396). New York: Oxford University Press.

Temel, J., Pirl, W., & Lynch, T. (2006). Comprehensive symptom management in patients with advanced-stage non-small-cell lung cancer. *Clinical Lung Cancer, 7*(4), 241–249.

Vainio, A., & Auvinen, A. (1996). Prevalence of symptoms among patients with advanced cancer: An international collaborative study. *Journal of Pain and Symptom Management, 12*(1), 3–10.

Vickers, A., Feinstein, M., Deng, D., & Cassileth, B. (2005). Acupuncture for dyspnea in advanced cancer: A randomized, placebo-controlled pilot trial. *BMC Palliative Care, 4*(5), 1–8.

Whitman, M. (2001). Understanding the perceived need for complementary and alternative nutraceuticals: Lifestyle issues. *Clinical Journal of Oncology Nursing, 5*(5), 190–194.

Wilson, K. G., Chochinov, H. M., McPherson, C. J., Skirko, M. G., Allard, P., Chary, S., et al. (2007). Desire for euthanasia or physician-assisted suicide in palliative cancer care. *Health Psychology, 26*(3), 314–323.

World Health Organization. (1990). *Cancer pain relief and palliative care* (Technical Report Series 804). Geneva, Switzerland: Author.

Zeppetella, G. (1998). The palliation of dyspnea in terminal disease. *American Journal of Hospice & Palliative Care, 15*(6), 322–330.

Zerwekh, J. (2006). *Nursing care at the end-of life: Palliative care for patients and families*. Philadelphia: F. A. Davis.

Chapter 9

Nutritional Issues Facing Lung Cancer Individuals

Gail M. Wilkes

Kelly M. Smallcomb

Nutrition is an important dimension of care for all individuals with lung cancer. In this chapter, factors that underscore the importance of nutrition as a critical element of care will be addressed. These factors include weight loss as a predictor of survival and response to treatment. It is well known that good nutrition is a basic survival need and that as patients experience nutritional impact symptoms, such as anorexia, nausea, vomiting, depression, and diarrhea, assuring adequate nutrition is one of the most challenging problems for oncology nurses, their cancer patients, and the patients' families. Lung cancer itself may be complicated by the paraneoplastic syndrome of cachexia, which is often associated with anorexia. Unfortunately, weight loss has been shown to be a poor prognostic finding, so early identification of nutritional imbalance is critical. Nutrition as a predictor of survival and the causes of nutritional deficits and malnutrition together with assessment and intervention strategies will be presented. While this chapter discusses the classic literature describing nutrition studies in patients with cancer, or specifically lung cancer, few recent studies have been done. Nursing or multidisciplinary studies on effective strategies for managing nutritional issues in patients with lung cancer is a fertile area for research.

Nutrition as a Predictor of Survival

Although it is clear that the most important factor in predicting survival in lung cancer is stage of disease, weight loss of greater than 5% at 3 months or greater than 10% of usual weight at 6 months is also an important predictor. Numerous older, classical studies have documented this and are included in this discussion (no recent studies exist). In 1980, Costa et al. found patients with lung cancer who did not lose weight survived significantly longer than those who lost weight. DeWys et al. (1980) retrospectively studied 3,047 patients with 11 tumor types, including lung cancer, who were enrolled in 12 different Eastern Cooperative Oncology Group (ECOG) chemotherapy protocols and found that in nine protocols, patients who lost weight had significantly shorter survival. Other similar results have been documented. Blackburn and colleagues (1977) documented the significance of weight loss over time, as shown in Table 9–1.

Table 9–1 Weight Loss Over Time: Significant or Severe

Weight Loss Over Time	Significant Weight Loss	Severe Weight Loss
1 week	≤ 2% of usual weight	< 2% of usual weight
1 month	≤ 5%	> 5%
	≤ 7.5%	> 7.5%
	≤ 10%	> 10%

Source: Blackburn, Bistrian, Maini, Schlamm, & Smith, 1977.

Lanzotti et al. (1977) found that weight loss was the major prognostic indicator for survival in inoperable patients with limited-disease lung cancer, and for patients with extensive disease, symptom status, metastases, and percentage of weight loss were prognostic indicators. More recently, Scott et al. (1997) studied approximately 1,600 patients with unresectable non-small cell lung cancer (NSCLC) in four radiation clinical trials and found that weight loss greater than 5% was a significant predictor of survival. Skarin et al. (2001) reviewed the cases of 91 patients aged under 40 years old who were diagnosed with lung cancer. They found that the factors that adversely affected survival by multivariate analysis were advanced stage of disease and weight loss of 5% or greater. Tombolini and fellow authors (2000) studied 41 elderly patients who were medically inoperable with stage IIIA and IIIB NSCLC and who received radiotherapy alone. They found that patients who presented with weight loss greater than 10% had an overall 24-month survival of 14% as compared to 58% for patients without weight loss ($p = 0.0027$). Other studies looked at clinical survival predictors in 208 patients with advanced cancer and found that those with primary lung cancer, weight loss of greater than

8.1 kg in the prior 6 months, and serum albumin less than 3.5 mg/dL, among other factors, had significantly shorter survival (Vigano, et al., 2000).

Individuals who are well nourished tolerate cancer treatment with less morbidity, mortality, and increased response as compared to those who lose weight or who are malnourished (see Table 9–1). Smale et al. (1981) studied 159 patients undergoing cancer surgery and found that 66% of patients who were identified as malnourished had major complications, such as infection, delayed wound healing, pneumonia, and death, compared to 8% of patients who were identified as well nourished. This is not surprising when one recalls the immune defects related to malnutrition, as shown in Table 9–2. In addition, significant weight loss during treatment is likely to result in delays in treatment and decreased treatment dosage of either chemotherapy or radiation therapy, which may negatively influence response to treatment.

Other researchers found that patients with impaired nutrition had increased postoperative complications following lobectomy for lung cancer, compared to well-nourished patients (Jagoe, Goodship, & Gibson, 2001). Weight loss also is an important predictor of treatment response.

Table 9–2 Effects of Vitamin/Trace Element Deficiency and Malnutrition on Immune Function

Deficient Trace Element or Vitamin	Immune Dysfunction
Vitamin A	Loss of skin and mucous membrane integrity, along with alterations in lymphocyte function and proliferation
Vitamin C	Altered cell-mediated immunity and the ability of neutrophils and macrophages to kill bacteria
Vitamin E (severe)	Altered cell-mediated immunity
Selenium	Decreased antibody synthesis
Vitamin B^6 (pyridoxine)	Altered cellular and humoral immune function
Vitamin B^{12}	Altered lymphocyte responses and ability of neutrophils to kill bacteria
Zinc	Depressed cell-mediated immunity, altered B cell activity, altered neutrophil and macrophage function
Copper	Altered lymphocyte and neutrophil function
Iron	Impaired cellular and humoral immune responses
Chronic malnutrition	Decreased number of T lymphocytes Decreased natural killer cell activity and interleukin-2 production Diminished/delayed hypersensitivity response to known antigens Diminished B cell function (decreased secretory immunoglobulins, decreased complement activity) Altered cytokine production/activity and diminished T cell response to them Diminished ability of neutrophils to phagocytose and kill bacteria

Source: Chandra, 1990.

Choi et al. (2001) reported on the predictive factors for radiation response in NSCLC from the First International Workshop on Prognostic and Predictive Factors in Lung Cancer, where weight loss of more than 10% of body weight in the prior 6 months was a significant host-related factor.

Weight loss is an exclusionary factor for many clinical trials, because it has been well documented that patients with significant weight loss respond poorly in nonsurgical treatments (Bauer, Birch, & Paja, 1985). For example, in the inter-group phase III trial of regionally advanced unresectable NSCLC, which involved the Radiation Therapy Oncology Group (RTOG), Eastern Cooperative Oncology Group (ECOG), and Southwest Oncology Group (SWOG), patients who had a weight loss of greater than or equal to 5% for 3 months prior to the study were excluded (Sause, et al., 2000).

Quality of life is also influenced by nutritional status (Tchekmedyian, Cella, & Heber, 1999). The individual who is cured of lung cancer, or who is in remission, is usually able to maintain a good nutritional status, especially if counseled about a healthy diet. In contrast, the individual for whom anorexia or weight loss was an initial symptom fears disease recurrence when appetite begins to wane or weight begins to fall. For this individual, when disease recurs, attention to appetite and reversing weight loss with appetite stimulants, along with palliative treatment, can help decrease fear and disfigurement by cachexia. Ovensen et al. (1993) examined quality of life among 100 individuals newly diagnosed with NSCLC, ovarian cancer, and breast cancer who were in good physical condition at the time of diagnosis. They found that the individuals with greater than 5% weight loss over a 3-month time period rated significantly lower on the Quality of Life Index (QI-index) compared to those who were weight stable. The QI-index is a multi-dimensional tool that addresses physical, psychological, and social functioning; it was developed by Spitzer in 1981 to assess quality of life changes in patients with chronic illnesses (Spitzer et al., 1981).

Causes of Nutritional Deficits and Malnutrition in Lung Cancer

While a number of factors can influence nutritional status, primary factors include the malignancy itself, presence of nutritional impact symptoms, coping and response to illness, cultural factors, ability to purchase and prepare food, and concurrent medical problems. Table 9–3 describes the most common risk factors for malnutrition in the person with cancer.

First, it is estimated that about 50% of individuals who are diagnosed with lung cancer experience weight loss (DeWys, et al., 1980). Severe weight loss is often associated with advanced disease and can be associated with anorexia. Systemic symptoms, such as anorexia and weight loss, are more common with primary tumors that have advanced locally or regionally, such as to adjacent structures or to the mediastinum (Fretz & Peterson, 2001). As the

---

Table 9–3 Risk Factors in the Development of Malnutrition

Weight loss ≤ 5% in 1 month, ≤ 10% in 6 months

Inadequate oral intake for ≤ 7 days

Serum albumin < 3.5 g/dL

Recent surgery, severe infection

Recent radiation therapy or aggressive chemotherapy

Persistent system distress lasting more than 2 weeks, for example nausea and vomiting

Dysphagia, diarrhea, mucositis, depression, anorexia

Diminished self-care ability or lack of caretaker

Dementia

Poverty

Addiction (alcohol, drugs)

Source: Wilkes, 1999.

disease progresses further, individuals may develop cancer cachexia, the most common paraneoplastic syndrome, with skeletal muscle wasting. Characteristics associated with cancer cachexia are anorexia, early satiety, weight loss, weakness, fatigue, impaired immune function, skeletal muscle wasting, and poor performance status (Puccio & Nathanson, 1997). Cachexia is a complex phenomenon and appears to be orchestrated by the proinflammatory cytokines tumor necrosis factor, interleukin-1 and -6, and interferon gamma (Langstein & Norton, 1991; Laviano, et al., 2005; Morley, Thomas, & Wilson, 2006). These factors lead to increased release of the hormone leptin, which then results in decreased expression of neuropeptide Y (NPY), a substance related to appetite control. Increased levels of leptin and decreased NPY ultimately lead to decreased appetite and weight loss (Inui, 2002). There is abnormal metabolism of glucose, fats, and protein and preferential glucose synthesis. Skeletal muscle is catabolized or broken down to make glucose to a much greater degree than fat is broken down for energy, and the very inefficient anaerobic glycolysis replaces the usual efficient aerobic glycolysis. The person with cachexia may have glucose intolerance, in some cases, hyperglycemia and hyperlipidemia, along with wasting of skeletal muscle and loss of subcutaneous fat stores. The evidence is mixed as to whether cachexic individuals have increased energy expenditure. However, Russell et al. (1984) observed a 37% increase in basal energy expenditure (BEE) in patients newly diagnosed with small cell lung cancer (SCLC), followed by a decline in BEE following response to chemotherapy. Dietary protein needs in the adult cancer patient are estimated to be 25–200% greater than healthy individuals (Hurst & Gallagher, 2006).

Second, nutritional impact symptoms may result from treatment or disease. These, as defined by Ottery (1994), are symptoms that interfere with the adequate intake of nutrients, such as stomatitis, nausea, and vomiting. Grosvenor, Bulcavage, and Chebowski (1989) interviewed 254 patients to identify symptoms that could influence nutrition following surgery, chemotherapy, or radiation, and found the following symptoms were experienced: abdominal fullness (64%), taste changes (46%), constipation (41%), mouth dryness (40%), nausea (39%), and vomiting (27%). Table 9–4 describes potential adverse effects of cancer therapy on nutrition.

In addition, symptoms that increase metabolic rate, such as fever, also increase the need for calories and protein. For the person with advanced lung cancer, dyspnea may make the person anorexic, or the work of eating may increase the perceived breathlessness so that eating is avoided. Finally, a recent study demonstrated that albumin levels and malnutrition are associated with higher incidence of toxicity related to paclitaxel–cisplatin chemotherapy in patients with advanced NSCLC than in those who are not malnourished or who have a normal serum albumin (Sanchez-Lara, et al., 2008). Expert symptom management is a critical part of the nutritional care of the person with lung cancer. Management strategies are discussed in the following section.

Nutritional status is also influenced by affective factors, and the individual with lung cancer often experiences many emotions during the disease trajectory. Anxiety and depression are most common, and each may be associated with anorexia or loss of appetite. Helping the person explore past effective coping strategies and identify constructive strategies to deal with the perceived threat to his or her well-being is useful, as is providing referrals to mental health

Table 9–4 Selected Potential Adverse Effects of Cancer Therapy on Nutrition

Surgery (general and site specific)	• General catabolism secondary to fever, infection; short-term starvation due to NPO • Esophagus: postoperative decreased gastric motility with stasis
Chemotherapy (agent specific)	• Nausea and/or vomiting • Diarrhea • Mucositis (stomatitis, esophagitis, gastritis) • Anorexia • Taste alterations • Constipation • Infection
Radiation therapy (site specific)	• General: anorexia, fatigue • Esophagus/chest: esophagitis, dysphagia, stricture
Biotherapy	• Fatigue, flulike symptoms • Stomatitis • Taste distortions • Nausea, vomiting • Constipation, diarrhea • Smell distortions
Medications used in symptom management	• Analgesics, including hydromorphone, morphine • Antibiotics, such as aminoglycosides, cephalosporins, trimethoprim–sulfamethoxazole (Bactrim) • Antifungal agents, such as amphotericin B • Antiviral agents, such as ganciclovir • Antidepressants, such as paroxetine and sertraline

Source: Modified from Wilkes, 1999.

professionals as needed. The reader is directed to Chapter 12, Living with Hope with Lung Cancer, for a broader discussion. Nutrition is a basic human survival need, and if the individual has anorexia and is losing weight, this pattern can engender fear. Often family members continue to try to help by reminding and pleading with the patient to eat; the patient's inability to eat can lead to irritability and become a source of tension that pushes family members apart at a time when they need to be together.

People's eating habits are often derived from their cultural heritage. Eating has a dimension of socialization, when people eat together to socialize as well as to eat. Food itself may have intrinsic meaning and influence disease treatment. For example, in the Chinese culture, cancer may be considered a "cold" disease, and food, including water, must be "hot" so that yin and yang can be balanced and treatment can be successful. Patients who are hospitalized may lose weight when food is not culturally acceptable, and it is often the oncology nurse who works with the family to bring in food that can meet both nutritional and cultural requirements. Unfortunately, malnourished patients with cancer often have longer hospital stays than those who are well nourished (Ottery, 1994). Other important social factors that influence nutritional status are the ability to obtain, prepare, and consume food and water. Individuals who are on a fixed budget or limited income may not be able to purchase high-calorie, high-protein foods. Some individuals with lung cancer may be homeless, living in shelters, while others may live in a rooming house without cooking facilities. In addition, in an effort to take some control over a situation that feels controlled by disease and others, some individuals seek an anticancer diet as part of their therapy. Often these fad diets are not balanced, have too little protein and too few calories, and result in weight loss.

Lastly, concurrent medical problems can complicate nutritional care. Individuals who have lost weight and who may be anorexic, with diabetes mellitus or high cholesterol, may refuse to eat high-caloric, high-protein foods because of prior teaching. It is important to help them rethink nutritional goals and dietary rules during treatment for lung cancer.

Nutritional Assessment

Nutrition has been called the forgotten ingredient in cancer care (Wilkes, 2000). Some clinicians perceive that nothing can be done or it won't make any difference in the outcome. Others may think that a nutritional assessment means that a midarm circumference measurement to assess protein stores and a triceps skin fold measurement to assess fat stores must be done, and the clinician does not feel competent to do this. While this was true 20 years ago, it

is not the case today. The most common anthropometric measure is weight. Brown and Radke (1998), in a retrospective review of 93 patients with NSCLC treated either in a cancer center or its associated academic medical center, found that 97% of patients had a nutritional status assessment. The most common assessments were weight change (92%) and anorexia or decreased food intake (84%). The authors found that 60% of the assessments led to nutritional intervention, most commonly nutritional supplements (89%), followed by teaching to increase and monitor food intake (68%). Nutritional interventions were more common for patients with dysphagia or depression, as compared to patients with anorexia and weight loss. However, only 44% of patients who had nutritional interventions had a documented reassessment for effectiveness of the intervention. The authors concluded that weight loss was a common problem for patients with NSCLC from diagnosis to death, and there was great opportunity for nurses to broaden their nutritional assessment of patients to include both history of food intake, eating patterns, nutritional impact symptoms, and physical/laboratory evaluation of protein stores. In addition, the authors highlighted the need for regular evaluation of effectiveness after a nutritional intervention was made so that appropriate goals could be achieved: minimizing weight loss, stabilizing weight, and improving quality of life.

Today nurses are constantly challenged to do more with less. If nutritional problems need to be identified early, with consequent early intervention, how can nurses make this a priority? How can oncology nurses who care for patients with lung cancer perform a credible nutritional assessment that can then be done regularly to evaluate the effectiveness of intervention and need for revision of the nutritional plan? The most commonly used tools for nutrition assessment include the Mini Nutritional Assessment (MNA) and the Patient-Generated Subjective Global Assessment (PG-SGA). While the MNA is thought to be simpler and require less training (DiMaria-Ghalili & Guenter, 2008), the PG-SGA has been validated specifically for use in the oncology population and has shown a greater sensitivity and specificity in identifying malnutrition (Read, et al., 2005). The PG-SGA tool, shown in Figure 9–1, is currently preferred for use with cancer patients.

The MNA is validated for use in the elderly population. It can be found online with a User Guide at http://www.mna-elderly.com/mna_forms.html and is shown in Figure 9–2.

The PG-SGA was originally developed at Toronto General Hospital for a general medical patient population. Ottery (1994) modified it for use in an oncology patient population. This multidimensional assessment is a scored tool (Ottery, Walsh, & Strawford, 1998):

- 0 points reflects minimal impact on nutritional status
- 1 = mild impact
- 2 = moderate impact
- 3 = potentially severe impact
- 4 = potentially life threatening

The summed total correlates with nutritional risk:

- Stage A is well nourished (low score)
- Stage B is moderately malnourished or suspected of being malnourished
- Stage C is severely malnourished, with the highest score

The patient participates in the assessment by completing the top portion and by checking off boxes or providing short answers to the following: current weight and height, weight 6 and 3

months ago, and weight 2 weeks ago; food intake during the past month; nutrition impact symptoms that interfere with food intake; and functional capacity over the past month. Each response has a numerical weight, which is summed at the end. Weight loss over time is determined, with the highest score (4) for 10% in 1 month or 20% in 6 months. The second part is completed by the nurse, physician, or dietitian, and it captures diagnoses, metabolic demand, and results of a brief physical exam of fat stores, muscle, and fluid status. Again, a numerical rating is used. One point is given for each of the following diagnoses: cancer, AIDS, presence of pulmonary/cardiac cachexia, presence of decubitus or open wound, presence of trauma, and age greater than 65 years. Metabolic stress is numerically graded based on presence of fever and its duration or use of steroids and amount. The physical exam is rated, where there are no points if the patient has no deficits to three points for severe deficits. More specific grading is found on the reverse side of the tool.

Based on the total score, Ottery (1994) recommends the following nutritional triage, which is shown on the reverse side of the form:

0–1   No intervention; reassess on a regular basis

2–3   Patient/family teaching by nurse, dietitian, or other clinician; pharmacologic intervention as needed; laboratory assessment as needed

4–8   Dietitian intervention necessary, together with nurse or physician to manage nutritional impact symptoms

≥ 9   Critical need for improved symptom management and/or nutritional intervention

Figure 9–1 Patient-Generated Subjective Global Assessment Tool.

Scored Patient-Generated Subjective Global Assessment (PG-SGA)

Patient ID Information

History

1. Weight *(See Table 1 Worksheet)*

In summary of my current and recent weight:

I currently weigh about _____ pounds
I am about _____ feet _____ tall

One month ago I weighed about _____ pounds
Six months ago I weighed about _____ pounds

During the past two weeks my weight has:

□ decreased$_{(1)}$ □ not changed$_{(0)}$ □ increased$_{(0)}$

2. Food Intake: As compared to my normal, I would rate my food intake during the past mouth as:

□ unchanged$_{(0)}$
□ more than usual
□ less than usual$_{(1)}$
   I am now taking:
   □ normal food, but less than normal$_{(1)}$
   □ little solid food$_{(2)}$
   □ only liquids$_{(3)}$
   □ only nutritional supplements$_{(3)}$
   □ very little of anything$_{(4)}$
   □ only tube feedings or only nutrition by vein$_{(0)}$

3. Symptoms: I have had the following problems that have kept me from eating enough during the past two weeks (check all that apply):

□ no problems eating$_{(0)}$

□ no appetite, just did not feel like eating$_{(3)}$

□ nausea$_{(1)}$ □ vomiting$_{(3)}$
□ constipation$_{(1)}$ □ diarrhea$_{(3)}$
□ mouth sores$_{(2)}$ □ dry mouth$_{(1)}$
□ things taste funny or have no taste$_{(1)}$ □ smells bother me$_{(1)}$
□ problems swallowing$_{(2)}$ □ feel full quickly$_{(1)}$

□ pain; where?$_{(3)}$ _____

□ other**$_{(1)}$ _____

**Examples: depression, money, or dental problems

4. Activities and Function: Over the past month, I would generally rate my activity as:

□ normal with no limitations$_{(0)}$

□ not my normal self, but able to be up and about with fairly normal activities$_{(1)}$

□ not feeling up to most things, but in bed or chair less than half the day$_{(2)}$

□ able to do little activity and spend most of the day in bed or chair$_{(3)}$

□ pretty much bedridden, rarely out of bed$_{(3)}$

Additive Score of the Boxes 1-4 [_____] A

The remainder of this form will be completed by your doctor, nurse, or therapist. Thank you.

5. Disease and its relation to nutritional requirements *(See Table 2)*

All relevant diagnoses (specify) _____

Primary disease stage (circle if known or appropriate) I II III IV Other _____
Age _____

Numerical score from Table 2 [_____] B

6. Metabolic Demand *(See Table 3 Worksheet)*
□ no stress   □ low stress   □ moderate stress   □ high stress

Numerical score from Table 3 [_____] C

7. Physical *(See Table 4 Worksheet)*

Numerical score from Table 4 [_____] D

Global Assessment *(See Table 5 Worksheet)*
□ Well-nourished or anabolic (SGA-A)
□ Moderate or suspected malnutrition (SGA-B)
□ Severely malnourished (SGA-C)

Total numerical score of boxes A + B + C + D [_____]
(See triage recommendations below)

Clinician Signature _____ MD RN PA MD DO Other... Date_____

Nutritional Triage Recommendations: Additive score is used to define specific nutritional interventions including patient & family education, symptom management including pharmacologic intervention, and appropriate nutrient intervention (food, nutritional supplements, enteral, or parenteral triage). First-line nutrition intervention includes optional symptom management.

0-1   No intervention required at this time. Reassessment on routine and regular basis during treatment.
2-3   Patient & family education by dietitian, nurse, or other clinician with phamacologic intervention as indicated by symptom survey (Box 3) and laboratory values as appropriate.
4-8   Requires intervention by dietitian, in conjunction with nurse or physician as indicated by symptoms survey (Box 3).
≥9   Indicates a critical need for improved symptom management and/or nutrient intervention options.

© FD Ottery, 2000   Grateful acknowledgment is given to the Society for Nutritional Oncology Adjuvant Therapy (NOAT) & the Oncology Dietetic Practice Group of the American Dietetic Association, with special recognition of Suzanne Kasenic, Susan DeBolt, Paula McCallum & Christine Polisena.

continues

Figure 9–1 Patient-Generated Subjective Global Assessment Tool (continued).

Tables & Worksheets for PG-SGA Scoring
FD Ottery, 2000

The PG-SGA numerical score is derived by totaling the scores from boxes A-D of the PG-SGA on the reverse side. Boxes 1-4 are designed to be completed by the patient. The points assigned to items in boxes 1-4 are noted patenthetically after each item. The following worksheets are offered as aids for calculating scores of sections that are not so marked.

Table 1 - Scoring Weight (wt) Loss
Determined by adding points for subacute and acute wt change. Subacute: If information is available about weight loss during past 1 mouth, hold the point score to the points for acute wt change. Only include the wt loss over 6 months if the wt from 1 month is unavailable. Acute: refers to wt change during past two weeks. Add 1 point to subacute score if patient lost wt; add no points if patient gained or maintained wt during the past two weeks.

Wt loss in 1 month	Points	Wt loss in 6 months
10% or greater	4	20% or greater
5-9.9%	3	10-19.9%
3-4.9%	2	6-9.9%
2-2.9%	1	2-5.9%
0-1.9%	0	0-1.9%

Points for Box 1 = Subacute + Acute = ☐

Table 2 - Scoring criteria for disease &/or condition
Score is derived by adding 1 point for each of the conditions listed below that pertain to the patient.

Category	Points
Cancer	1
AIDS	1
Pulmonary or cardiac cachexia	1
Presence of decubitus, open wound, or fistula	1
Presence of trauma	1
Age greater than 65 years	1

Points for Box 2 = ☐ B

Table 3 Worksheet - Scoring Metabolic Stress
Score for metabolic stress is determined by a number of variables known to increase in points & caloric needs. The score is additive so that a patient who has a fever of > 102 degrees (3 points) who is on 10 mg of prednisone chronically (2 points) would have an additive score for this section of 5 points.

Stress	none (0)	low (1)	moderate (2)	high (3)
Fever	no fever	>99 and <101	≥101 and <102	≥102
Fever duration	no fever	<72 hrs	72 hrs	>72 hrs
Steroids	no steroids	low dose (<10mg prednisone equivalents/day)	moderate dose (≥10 and <30mg prednisone equivalents/day)	high dose steroids (≥30mg prednisone equivalents/day)

Points for Table 3 = ☐ C

Table 4 Worksheet - Physical Examination
Physical exam includes a subjective evaluation of 3 aspects of body composition: fat, muscle, & fluid status. Since this is subjective, each aspect of the exam is rated for degree of deficit. Muscle deficit impacts point score more than fat deficit. Definition of categories: 0 = no deficit, 1+ = mild deficit, 2+ = moderate deficit, 3+ = severe deficit. Rating of deficit in these categories are *not* additive but are used to clinically assess the degree of deficit (or presence of of excess fluid).

Fat Stores:				
orbital fat pads	0	1+	2+	3+
triceps skin fold	0	1+	2+	3+
fat overlying lower ribs	0	1+	2+	3+
Global fat deficit rating	0	1+	2+	3+

Field Status:				
ankle edema	0	1+	2+	3+
sacral edema	0	1+	2+	3+
ascites	0	1+	2+	3+
Global fluid status rating	0	1+	2+	3+

Muscle Status:				
temples (temporalis muscle)	0	1+	2+	3+
clavicles (pectoralis & deltoids)	0	1+	2+	3+
shoulders (deltoids)	0	1+	2+	3+
interosseous muscles	0	1+	2+	3+
scapula (latissimus dorsi, trapezius, deltoids)	0	1+	2+	3+
thigh (quadriceps)	0	1+	2+	3+
calf (gastrocnemius)	0	1+	2+	3+
Global muscle status rating	0	1+	2+	3+

Point score for the physical exam is determined by the overall subjective rating of total body deficit; again muscle deficit takes precedence over fat loss or fluid excess.

No deficit	score = 0 points
Mild deficit	score = 1 point
Moderate deficit	score = 2 points
Severe deficit	score = 3 points

Points for Worksheet 4 = ☐ D

Table 5 Worksheet - PG-SGA Global Assessment Categories

Category	Stage A	Stage B	Stage C
	Well-nourished	Moderately malnourished or suspected malnutrition	Severely malnourished
Weight	No wt loss **or** Recent non-fluid wt gain	~5% wt loss within 1 month (or 10% in 6 months) No wt stabilization or wt gain (i.e., continued wt loss)	a. >5% loss in 1 month (or >10% loss in 6 months) b. No wt stabilization or wt gain (i.e., continued wt loss)
Nutrient Intake	No deficit **or** Significant recent improvement	Definite decrease in intake	Severe deficit in intake
Nutrient Impact Symptoms	None **or** Significant recent improvement allowing adequate intake	Presence of nutrition impact symptoms (Box 3 of PG-SGA)	Presence of nutrition impact symptoms (Box 3 of PG-SGA)
Functioning	No deficit **or** Significant recent improvement	Moderate functional deficit **or** Recent deterioration	Severe functional deficit **or** recent significant deterioration
Physical Exam	No deficit **or** Chronic deficit but with recent clinical improvement	Evidence of mild to moderate loss of SQ fat &/or muscle mass &/or muscle tone on palpation	Obvious signs of malnutrition (e.g., severe loss of SQ tissues, possible edema)

Global PG-SGA rating (A, B, or C) = ☐

Source: © FD Ottery, 2000. Grateful acknowledgment is given to the Society for Nutritional Oncology Adjuvant Therapy (NOAT) & the Oncology Dietetic Practice Group of the American Dietetic Association, with special recognition of Suzanne Kasenic, Susan DeBolt, Paula McCallum & Christine Polisena.

Figure 9–2 A Guide to Completing the Mini Nutritional Assessment MNA®.

Nestlé Nutrition
INSTITUTE

Mini Nutritional Assessment
MNA®

Last name:	First name:	Sex:	Date:

Age:	Weight, kg:	Height, cm:	I.D. Number:

Complete the screen by filling in the boxes with the appropriate numbers.
Add the numbers for the screen; if score is 11 or less, continue with the assessment to gain a Malnutrition Indicator Score.

Screening

A Has food intake declined over the past 3 months due to loss of appetite, digestive problems, chewing or swallowing difficulties?
0 = severe loss of appetite
1 = moderate loss of appetite
2 = no loss of appetite ☐

B Weight loss during the last 3 months
0 = weight loss greater than 3 kg (6.6 lbs)
1 = does not know
2 = weight loss between 1 and 3 kg (2.2 and 6.6 lbs)
3 = no weight loss ☐

C Mobility
0 = bed or chair bound
1 = able to get out of bed/chair but does not go out
2 = goes out ☐

D Has suffered psychological stress or acute disease in the past 3 months
0 = yes   2 = no ☐

E Neuropsychological problems
0 = severe dementia or depression
1 = mild dementia
2 = no psychological problems ☐

F Body Mass Index (BMI) (weight in kg)/(height in m²)
0 = BMI less than 19
1 = BMI 19 to less than 21
2 = BMI 21 to less than 23
3 = BMI 23 or greater ☐

Screening score (subtotal max. 14 points) ☐ ☐
12 points or greater   Normal—not at risk—no need to complete assessment
11 points or below   Possible malnutrition—continue assessment

Assessment

G Lives independently (not in a nursing home or hospital)
0 = no   1 = yes ☐

H Takes more than 3 prescription drugs per day
0 = yes   1 = no ☐

I Pressure sores or skin ulcers
0 = yes   1 = no ☐

Ref: Vellas B, Villars H, Abellan G et al. Overview of the MNA® – Its history and challenges. J Nutr Health Aging 2006;10:455–465.
Rubenstein LZ, Harker JO, Salva A, Guigoz Y, Vellas B. Screening for Undernutrition in Geriatric Practice: Developing the Short-Form Nutritional Assessment (MNA-SF). J Geront 2001;56A:M366–377.
Guigoz Y. The Mini-Nutritional Assessment (MNA®) Review of the Literature—What does it tell us? J Nutr Healthy Aging 2006;10:466–487.
©Nestlé, 1994. Revision 2006. N67200 12/99 10M
For more information: www.mna-elderly.com

J How many full meals does the patient eat daily?
0 = 1 meal
1 = 2 meals
2 = 3 meals ☐

K Selected consumption markers for protein intake
• At least one serving of dairy products (milk, cheese, yogurt) per day   yes ☐   no ☐
• Two or more servings of legumes or eggs per week   yes ☐   no ☐
• Meat, fish or poultry every day   yes ☐   no ☐
0.0 = if 0 or 1 yes
0.5 = if 2 yes
1.0 = if 3 yes ☐ ☐

L Consumes two or more servings of fruits or vegetables per day?
0 = no   1 = yes ☐

M How much fluid (water, juice, coffee, tea, milk . . .) is consumed per day?
0.0 = less than 3 cups
0.5 = 3 to 5 cups
1.0 = more than 5 cups ☐ ☐

N Mode of feeding
0 = unable to eat without assistance
1 = self-fed with some difficulty
2 = self-fed without any problem ☐

O Self view of nutritional status
0 = views self as being malnourished
1 = is uncertain of nutritional state
2 = views self as having no nutritional problem ☐

P In comparison with other people of the same age, how does the patient consider his/her health status?
0.0 = not as good
0.5 = does not know
1.0 = as good
2.0 = better ☐ ☐

Q Mid-arm circumference (MAC) in cm
0.0 = MAC less than 21
0.5 = MAC 21 to 22
1.0 = MAC 22 or greater ☐ ☐

R Calf circumference (CC) in cm
0 = CC less than 31   1 = CC 32 or greater ☐

Assessment (max. 16 points)	☐ ☐ ☐
Screening score	☐ ☐
Total Assessment (max. 30 points)	☐ ☐ ☐

Malnutrition Indicator Score		
17 to 23.5 points	at risk of malnutrition	☐
Less than 17 point	malnourished	☐

continues

Figure 9–2 A Guide to Completing the Mini Nutritional Assessment MNA® (continued).

Mini Nutritional Assessment (MNA®)

The MNA® is a screening and assessment tool that can be used to identify elderly patients at risk of malnutrition. The User Guide will assist you in completing the MNA® accurately and consistently. It explains each question and how to assign and interpret the score.

Introduction:

While the prevalence of malnutrition in the freeliving elderly population is relatively low, the risk of malnutrition increases dramatically in the institutionalized and hospitalized elderly.[1] The prevalence of malnutrition is even higher in cognitively impaired elderly individuals and is associated with cognitive decline.[2]

Patients who are malnourished when admitted to the hospital tend to have longer hospital stays, experience more complications, and have greater risks of morbidity and mortality than those whose nutritional state is normal.[3]

By identifying patients who are malnourished or at risk of malnutrition either in the hospital or community setting, the MNA® allows clinicians to intervene earlier to provide adequate nutritional support, prevent further deterioration, and improve patient outcomes.[4]

Mini Nutritional Assessment MNA®

The MNA® provides a simple and quick method of identifying elderly patients who are at risk for malnutrition, or who are already malnourished. It identifies the risk of malnutrition before severe changes in weight or serum protein levels occur.

The MNA® may be completed at regular intervals in the community and in the hospital or long-term care setting.

The MNA® was developed by Nestlé and leading international geriatricians and remains one of the few validated screening tools for the elderly. It has been well validated in international studies in a variety of settings[5–7] and correlates with morbidity and mortality.

Instructions to Complete the MNA®

Before beginning the MNA®, please enter the patient's information on the top of the form:

— **Name**

— **Gender**

— **Age**

— **Weight (kg)**—To obtain an accurate weight, remove shoes and heavy outer clothing. Use a calibrated and reliable set of scales. If applicable: convert pounds (lbs) to kilograms (1 kg = 2.2 lbs).

— **Height (cm)**—Measure height without shoes using a stadiometer (height gauge) or, if the patient is bedridden, by knee height or demispan (see Appendices 4 or 5). Convert inches to centimeters (1 inch = 2.54 cm).

— **ID number** (e.g., hospital number)

— **Date of screen**

Screening (MNA®SF)

Complete the screen by filling in the boxes with the appropriate numbers. Then, add together the numbers to determine the total score of the screen. If the score is 11 or less, continue on with the assessment to determine the <u>Malnutrition Indicator Score</u>.

Key Points

Ask the patient to answer questions A – E, using the suggestions in the shaded areas. If the patient is unable to answer the question, ask the patient's caregiver to answer. Using the patient's medical record or your professional judgment, answer any remaining questions.

A. Has food intake declined over the past three months due to loss of appetite, digestive problems, chewing or swallowing difficulties?

Score 0 = Severe decrease in food intake

1 = Moderate decrease in food intake

2 = No decrease in food intake

Figure 9–2 A Guide to Completing the Mini Nutritional Assessment MNA®
(continued).

Ask patient

⇨ *"Have you eaten less than normal over the past three months?"*

⇨ *If so, "is this because of lack of appetite, chewing, or swallowing difficulties?"*

⇨ *If yes, "have you eaten much less than before or only a little less?"*

⇨ *If this is a re-assessment, then rephrase the question:*

⇨ *"Has the amount of food you have eaten changed since your last assessment?"*

B. Involuntary weight loss during the last 3 months?

Score 0 = Weight loss greater than 3 kg (6.6 pounds)

1 = Does not know

2 = Weight loss between 1 and 3 kg (2.2 and 6.6 pounds)

3 = No weight loss

Ask patient/patient medical record (if long-term or residential care)

⇨ *"Have you lost any weight without trying over the last 3 months?"*

⇨ *"Has your waistband gotten looser?"*

⇨ *"How much weight do you think you have lost? More or less than 3 kg (or 6 pounds)?"*

Though weight loss in the overweight elderly may be appropriate, it may also be due to malnutrition. When the weight loss question is removed, the MNA® loses its sensitivity, so it is important to ask about weight loss even in the overweight.

C. Mobility?

Score 0 = Bed or chair bound

1 = Able to get out of bed/chair, but does not go out

2 = Goes out

Ask patient/patient medical record/information from caregiver

⇨ *"Are you presently able to get out of the bed/chair?"*

⇨ *"Are you able to get out of the house or go outdoors on your own?"*

D. Has the patient suffered psychological stress or acute disease in the past three months?

Score 0 = Yes

1 = No

Ask patient/patient medical record/professional judgment

⇨ *"Have you suffered a bereavement recently?"*

⇨ *"Have you recently moved your home?"*

⇨ *"Have you been sick recently?"*

continues

Figure 9–2 A Guide to Completing the Mini Nutritional Assessment MNA®
(continued).

E. Neuropsychological problems?

Score 0 = Severe dementia or depression

1 = Mild depression

2 = No psychological problems

Review patient medical record/professional judgment/ask nursing staff or caregiver

The patient's caregiver, nursing staff, or medical record can provide information about the severity of the patient's neuropsychological problems (dementia).

If a patient cannot respond (i.e., one with dementia) or is severely confused, ask the patient's personal or professional caregiver to answer the following questions or check the patient's answers for accuracy (Questions A, B, C, D, G, J, K, L, M, O, P).

F. Body mass index (BMI)? (weight in kg / height in m²)

Score 0 = BMI less than 19

1 = BMI 19 to less than 21

2 = BMI 21 to less than 23

3 = BMI 23 or greater

Determining BMI

BMI is used as an indicator of appropriate weight for height. BMI is calculated by dividing the weight in kg by the height in m² (Appendix 1).

$$BMI = \frac{weight\ (kg)}{height\ (m^2)}$$

Before determining BMI, record the patient's weight and height on the MNA® form.

1. *Convert subject's weight to metric using formula 1kg = 2.2lbs*
   Convert subject's height to metric using formula 1inch = 2.54cm
2. *If height has not been measured, please measure using a stadiometer or height gauge (Refer to Appendix 3).*
3. *If the patient is unable to stand, measure height using indirect methods such as measuring demi-span (half arm span) or knee height (see Appendices 4 and 5). If height cannot be measured either directly or by indirect methods, use a verbal or historical height to calculate a BMI. Verbal height will be the least accurate, especially for bedridden patients and patients who have lost height over the years.*
4. *Using the BMI chart provided (Appendix 1), locate the patient's height and weight and determine the BMI. **It is essential that a BMI is included in the MNA®—without it the tool is not valid.***
5. *Fill in the appropriate box on the MNA® form to represent the BMI of the patient.*
6. *To determine BMI for a patient with an amputation, see Appendix 2.*

The screening section of the questionnaire is now complete. Add the numbers to obtain the screening score.

A score of 12 points or greater indicates:
Patient is not at nutrition risk. There is no need to complete the rest of the questionnaire.
Rescreen at regular intervals.

A score of 11 points or less indicates:
Patient may be at risk for malnutrition. Please complete the full MNA® assessment by answering questions G–R.

Figure 9–2 A Guide to Completing the Mini Nutritional Assessment MNA®
(continued).

Assessment (MNA®)

G. Lives independently (not in a nursing home)?

Score 0 = No

1 = Yes

Ask patient

This question refers to the normal living conditions of the individual. Its purpose is to determine if the person is usually dependent on others for care. For example, if the patient is in the hospital because of an accident or acute illness, where does the patient normally live?

⇨ *"Do you normally live in your own home, or in an assisted living, residential setting, or nursing home?"*

H. Takes more than 3 prescription drugs per day?

Score 0 = Yes

1 = No

Ask patient/patient medical record

Check the patient's medication record/ask nursing staff/ask doctor/ask patient

I. Pressure sores or skin ulcers?

Score 0 = Yes

1 = No

Ask patient/patient medical record

⇨ *"Do you have bed sores?"*

Check the patient's medical record for documentation of pressure wounds or skin ulcers, or ask the caregiver/nursing staff/doctor for details, or examine the patient if information is not available in the medical record.

J. How many full meals does the patient eat daily?

Score 0 = 1 meal

1 = 2 meals

3 = 3 meals

Ask patient/check food intake record if necessary

⇨ *"Do you normally eat breakfast, lunch, and dinner?"*

⇨ *"How many meals a day do you eat?"*

A full meal is defined as eating more than 2 items or dishes when the patient sits down to eat.

For example, eating potatoes, vegetable, and meat is considered a full meal; or eating an egg, bread, and fruit is considered a full meal.

continues

Figure 9–2 A Guide to Completing the Mini Nutritional Assessment MNA®
(continued).

K. Selected consumption markers for protein intake

⇨ At least one serving of dairy products per day? Yes ☐ No ☐

⇨ Two or more servings of legumes or eggs per week? Yes ☐ No ☐

⇨ Meat, fish, or poultry every day? Yes ☐ No ☐

0.0 = if 0 or 1 Yes answer(s)

0.5 = if 2 Yes answers

1.0 = if 3 Yes answers

Ask the patient or nursing staff, or check the completed food intake record

⇨ *"Do you consume any dairy products (a glass of milk/cheese in a sandwich/cup of yogurt/can of high protein supplement) every day?"*

⇨ *"Do you eat beans/eggs? How often do you eat them?"*

⇨ *"Do you eat meat, fish, or chicken every day?"*

L. Consumes two or more servings of fruits or vegetables per day?

Score 0 = No

1 = Yes

Ask the patient/check the completed food intake record if necessary

⇨ *"Do you eat fruits and vegetables?"*

⇨ *"How many portions do you have each day?"*

A portion can be classified as:

One piece of fruit (apple, banana, orange, etc.)

One medium cup of fruit or vegetable juice

One cup of raw or cooked vegetables

M. How much fluid (water, juice, coffee, tea, milk) is consumed per day?

Score 0.0 = Less than 3 cups

0.5 = 3 to 5 cups

1.0 = More than 5 cups

Ask patient

⇨ *"How many cups of tea or coffee do you normally drink during the day?"*

⇨ *"Do you drink any water, milk, or fruit juice? What size cup do you usually use?"*

A cup is considered 200–240ml or 7–8oz.

Figure 9–2 A Guide to Completing the Mini Nutritional Assessment MNA®
(continued).

N. Mode of feeding?

Score 0 = Unable to eat without assistance *

1 = Feeds self with some difficulty **

2 = Feeds self without any problems

Ask patient/patient medical record/information from caregiver

⇨ *"Are you able to feed yourself?"/"Can the patient feed himself/herself?"*

⇨ *"Do you need help to eat?"/"Do you help the patient to eat?"*

⇨ *"Do you need help setting up your meals (opening containers, buttering bread, or cutting meats)?"*

*Patients who must be fed or need help holding the fork would score 0.

**Patients who need help setting up meals (opening containers, buttering bread, or cutting meats), but are able to feed themselves would score 1 point.

Pay particular attention to potential causes of malnutrition that need to be addressed to avoid malnutrition (e.g., dental problems, need for adaptive feeding devices to support eating).

O. Self-View of Nutritional Status

Score 0 = Views self as being malnourished

1 = Is uncertain of nutritional state

2 = Views self as having no nutritional problems

Ask patient

⇨ *"How would you describe your nutritional state?"*

Then prompt   *"Poorly nourished?"*
"Uncertain?"
"No problems?"

The answer to this question depends upon the patient's state of mind. If you think the patient is not capable of answering the question, ask the caregiver/nursing staff for their opinion.

P. In comparison with other people of the same age, how does the patient consider his/her health status?

Score 0.0 = Not as good

0.5 = Does not know

1.0 = As good

2.0 = Better

Ask patient

⇨ *"How would you describe your state of health compared to others your age?"*
Then prompt: *"Not as good as others of your age?"*
"Not sure?"
"As good as others of your age?"
"Better?"

Again, the answer will depend upon the state of mind of the person answering the question.

---

continues

Figure 9–2 A Guide to Completing the Mini Nutritional Assessment MNA®
(continued).

Q. Mid-arm circumference (MAC) in cm

Score 0.0 = MAC less than 21

0.5 = MAC 21 to 22

1.0 = MAC 22 or greater

Measure the mid-arm circumference in cm as described in Appendix 6.

R. Calf circumference (CC) in cm

Score 0 = CC less than 31

1 = CC 31 or greater

Calf circumference should be measured in cm as described in Appendix 7.

*Measure the calf at the widest area. Take additional measurements above and below the widest point to ensure that
the first measurement was the largest.*

Final Score

⇨ Total the points from the assessment section of the MNA® (maximum 16 points).
⇨ Add the assessment and screening scores together to get the total <u>Malnutrition Indicator Score</u>
(maximum 30 points).
⇨ Check the appropriate box indicator.
⇨ If the score is greater than 23.5 points, the patient is in a normal state of nutrition and no further action is
required.
⇨ If the score is less than 23.5 points, refer the patient to a dietitian or nutrition specialist for nutrition intervention.

Until a dietitian is available, give the patient/caregiver some advice on how to improve nutritional intake such as:

⇨ Increase intake of energy/protein dense foods (e.g., puddings, milkshakes, etc.).
⇨ Supplement food intake with additional snacks and milk.
⇨ If diet alone does not improve the patient's nutritional intake, the patient may need oral nutritional supplements.
⇨ Ensure adequate fluid intake; 6–8 cups/glasses per day

Follow-up

⇨ Re-screen all patients every three months.
⇨ Please refer results of assessments & re-assessments to dietitian/doctor and record in medical record.

Figure 9–2 A Guide to Completing the Mini Nutritional Assessment MNA®
(continued).

Appendix 1

BODY MASS INDEX TABLE

Height (feet and inches)

Weight (pounds)	5'0"	5'1"	5'2"	5'3"	5'4"	5'5"	5'6"	5'7"	5'8"	5'9"	5'10"	5'11"	6'0"	6'1"	6'2"	6'3"	6'4"	Weight (kilograms)
100	20	19	18	18	17	17	16	16	15	15	14	14	14	13	13	12	12	45
105	21	20	19	19	18	18	17	16	16	16	15	15	14	14	13	13	13	47
110	21	21	20	19	19	18	18	17	17	16	16	15	15	15	14	14	13	50
115	22	22	21	20	20	19	19	18	17	17	17	16	16	15	15	14	14	52
120	23	23	22	21	21	20	19	19	18	18	17	17	16	16	15	15	15	54
125	24	24	23	22	21	21	20	20	19	18	18	17	17	16	16	16	15	57
130	25	25	24	23	22	22	21	20	20	19	19	18	18	17	17	16	16	59
135	26	26	25	24	23	22	22	21	21	20	19	19	18	18	17	17	16	61
140	27	26	26	25	24	23	23	22	21	21	20	20	19	18	18	17	17	63
145	28	27	27	26	25	24	23	23	22	21	21	20	20	19	19	18	18	66
150	29	28	27	27	26	25	24	23	23	22	22	21	20	20	19	19	18	68
155	30	29	28	27	27	26	25	24	24	23	22	22	21	20	20	19	19	70
160	31	30	29	28	27	27	26	25	24	24	23	22	22	21	21	20	19	72
165	32	31	30	29	28	27	27	26	25	24	24	23	22	22	21	21	20	75
170	33	32	31	30	29	28	27	27	26	25	24	24	23	22	22	21	21	77
175	34	33	32	31	30	29	28	27	27	26	25	24	24	23	22	22	21	79
180	35	34	33	32	31	30	29	28	27	27	26	25	24	24	23	22	22	82
185	36	35	34	33	32	31	30	29	28	27	27	26	25	24	24	23	23	84
190	37	36	35	34	33	32	31	30	29	28	27	26	26	25	24	23	23	86
195	38	37	36	35	33	32	31	31	30	29	28	27	26	26	25	24	24	88
200	39	38	37	35	34	33	32	31	30	30	29	28	27	26	26	25	24	91
205	40	39	37	36	35	34	33	32	31	30	29	29	28	27	26	26	25	93
210	41	40	38	37	36	35	34	33	32	31	30	29	28	28	27	26	26	95
215	42	41	39	38	37	36	35	34	33	32	31	30	29	28	28	27	26	98
220	43	42	40	39	38	37	36	34	33	32	32	31	30	29	28	27	27	100
225	44	43	41	40	39	37	36	35	34	33	32	31	31	30	29	28	27	102
230	45	43	42	41	39	38	37	36	35	34	33	32	31	30	30	29	28	104
235	46	44	43	42	40	39	38	37	36	35	34	33	32	31	30	29	29	107
240	47	45	44	43	41	40	39	38	36	35	34	33	33	32	31	30	29	109
245	48	46	45	43	42	41	40	38	37	36	35	34	33	32	31	31	30	111
250	49	47	46	44	43	42	40	39	38	37	36	35	34	33	32	31	30	114

| 150 | 152.5 | 155 | 157.5 | 160 | 162.5 | 165 | 167.5 | 170 | 172.5 | 175 | 177.5 | 180 | 182.5 | 185 | 187.5 | 190 |

Height (centimeters)

☐ Underweight ▦ Weight Appropriate ☐ Overweight ☐ Obese

Source: Adapted from Clinical Guidelines on the Identification, Evaluation, and Treatment of Overweight and Obesity in Adults: The Evidence Report. National Institute of Health, National Heart Lung and Blood Institute.

continues

Figure 9–2 A Guide to Completing the Mini Nutritional Assessment MNA®
(continued).

Appendix 2

Determining BMI for Amputees

⇨ To determine the BMI for amputees, first determine the patient's estimated weight including the weight of the missing body part.[8,9]

— Use a standard reference (see table) to determine the proportion of body weight contributed by an individual body part.

— Multiply patient's current weight by the percent of body weight of the missing body part to determine estimated weight of missing part.

— Add the estimated weight of the missing body part to patient's current weight to determine estimated weight prior to amputation.

⇨ Divide estimated weight by estimated body height^2 to determine BMI.

WEIGHT OF SELECTED BODY COMPONENTS
It is necessary to account for the missing body component(s) when estimating IBW.

Table
Percent of Body Weight Contributed by Specific Body Parts

Body Part	Percentage
Trunk w/o limbs	50.0
Hand	0.7
Forearm with hand	2.3
Forearm without hand	1.6
Upper arm	2.7
Entire arm	5.0
Foot	1.5
Lower leg with foot	5.9
Lower leg without foot	4.4
Thigh	10.1
Entire leg	16.0

References cited:
Malone A., Anthropometric Assessment. In Charney P., Malone E., eds. *ADA Pocket Guide to Nutrition Assessment.* Chicago, IL: American Dietetic Association; 2004:142–152.

Osterkamp L.K. Current perspective on assessment of human body proportions of relevance to amputees. *J Am Diet Assoc.* 1995;95:215–218.

Example: 80-year-old man, amputation of the left lower leg, 1.72 m, 58 kg

1. Estimate body weight: Current body weight + proportion for the missing leg

    58 (kg) + [58 (kg) × 0.059] = 61.4 kg

2. Calculate BMI: Estimated body weight / body height (m)^2
    61.4/1.72 ×1.72 = 20.8

3. Calculate energy intake:
    ⇨ Recommended energy intake − 5.9%
    ⇨ Empirical formula (30 kcal/kg/day):
       30 kcal/kg/d × [61.4 kg − (61.4 × 0.059)] = 1,832 kcal/day

Conclusion: Corrected BMI is 21, and estimated energy intake is 1,800–1,900 kcal/d

Figure 9–2 A Guide to Completing the Mini Nutritional Assessment MNA® (continued).

Appendix 3

Measuring Height Using a Stadiometer

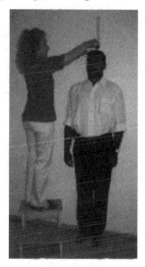

1. Ensure the floor surface is even and firm.
2. Have subject remove shoes and stand up straight with heels together, and with heels, buttocks, and shoulders pressed against the stadiometer.
3. Arms should hang freely with palms facing thighs.
4. Take the measurement with the subject standing tall, looking straight ahead with the head upright and not tilted backwards.
5. Make sure the subject's heels stay flat on the floor.
6. Lower the measure on the stadiometer until it makes contact with the top of the head.
7. Record standing height to the nearest centimeter.

Source: Accessed at: http://www.ktl.fi/publications/ehrin/product2/part_iii5.htm.

Appendix 4

Measurement of Demispan

⇨ **Demispan** *(half-arm span) is the distance from the midline at the sternal notch to the tip of the middle finger Height is then calculated from a standard formula.*[10]

1. Locate and mark the edge of the right collar bone (in the sternal notch) with the pen.
2. Ask the patient to place the left arm in a horizontal position.
3. Check that the patient's arm is horizontal and in line with shoulders.
4. Using the tape measure, measure distance from mark on the midline at the sternal notch to the tip of the middle finger.
5. Check that arm is flat and wrist is straight.
6. Take reading in cm.

Calculate height from the formula below:

Females

Height in cm =
$(1.35 \times$ demispan in cm$) + 60.1$

Males

Height in cm =
$(1.40 \times$ demispan in cm$) + 57.8$

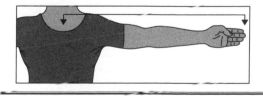

Source: http://www.rxkinetics.com/height_estimate.html. Accessed December 12, 2006.

continues

Figure 9–2 A Guide to Completing the Mini Nutritional Assessment MNA®
(continued).

Appendix 5

Measurement of Knee Height

⇨ **Knee height** is one method to determine stature in the bed- or chair-bound patient and is measured using a sliding knee height caliper. The subject must be able to bend the knee and the ankle to 90-degree angles.

1. Have the subject bend the knee and ankle of one leg at a 90-degree angle while lying supine or sitting on a table with legs hanging off the side of the table.
2. Place the fixed blade of the knee caliper under the heel of the foot in line with the ankle bone. Place the fixed blade of the caliper on the anterior surface of the thigh about 3.0 cm above the patella.
3. Be sure the shaft of the caliper is in line with and parallel to the long bone in the lower leg (tibia) and is over the ankle bone (lateral malleolus). Apply pressure to compress the tissue. Record the measurement to the nearest 0.1 cm.
4. Take two measurements in immediate succession. They should agree within 0.5 cm. Use the average of these two measurements and the person's chronologi-cal age in the country and ethnic group specific equations in the following table.
5. The value calculated from the selected equation is an estimate of the person's true stature. The 95 percent confidence for this estimate is plus and minus twice the SEE value for each equation.

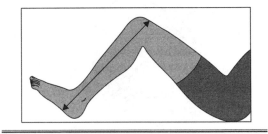

Source: http://www.rxkinetics.com/height_estimate.html. Accessed December 12, 2006.

Figure 9–2 A Guide to Completing the Mini Nutritional Assessment MNA® (continued).

Using population-specific formula, calculate height from standard formula:

Gender and ethnic group	Equation
Non-Hispanic white men (U.S.)[11] [SEE = 3.74 cm]	Stature (cm) = 78.31 + (1.94 × knee height) − (0.14 × age)
Non-Hispanic black men (U.S.)[11] [SEE = 3.80 cm]	Stature (cm) = 79.69 + (1.85 × knee height) − (0.14 × age)
Mexican-American men (U.S.)[11] [SEE = 3.68 cm]	Stature (cm) = 82.77 + (1.83 × knee height) − (0.16 × age)
Non-Hispanic white women (U.S.)[11] [SEE = 3.98 cm]	Stature (cm) = 82.21 + (1.85 × knee height) − (0.21 × age)
Non-Hispanic black women (U.S.)[11] [SEE = 3.82 cm]	Stature (cm) = 89.58 + (1.61 × knee height) − (0.17 × age)
Mexican-American women (U.S.)[11] [SEE = 3.77 cm]	Stature (cm) = 84.25 + (1.82 × knee height) − (0.26 × age)
Taiwanese men[12] [SEE = 3.86 cm]	Stature (cm) = 85.10 + (1.73 × knee height) − (0.11 × age)
Taiwanese women[12] [SEE = 3.79 cm]	Stature (cm) = 91.45 + (1.53 × knee height) − (0.16 × age)
Elderly Italian men[13] [SEE = 4.3 cm]	Stature (cm) = 94.87 − (1.58 × knee height) - (0.23 × age) +4.8
Elderly Italian women[13] [SEE = 4.3 cm]	Stature (cm) = 94.87 + (1.58 × knee height) − (0.23 × age)
French men[14] [SEE = 3.8 cm]	Stature (cm) = 74.7 + (2.07 × knee height) − (-0.21 × age)
French women[14] [SEE = 3.5 cm]	Stature (cm) = 67.00 + (2.2 × knee height) − (0.25 × age)
Mexican men[15] [SEE = 3.31 cm]	Stature (cm) = 52.6 + (2.17 × knee height)
Mexican women[15] [SEE = 2.99 cm]	Stature (cm) = 73.70 + (1.99 × knee height) − (0.23 × age)
Filipino men[16]	Stature (cm) = 96.50 + (1.38 × knee height) − (0.08 × age)
Filipino women[16]	Stature (cm) = 89.63 + (1.53 × knee height) − (0.17 × age)
Malaysian men[17] [SEE = 3.51 cm]	Stature (cm) = (1.924 × knee height) + 69.38
Malaysian women[17] [SEE = 3.40]	Stature (cm) = (2.225 × knee height) + 50.25

continues

Figure 9–2 A Guide to Completing the Mini Nutritional Assessment MNA®
(continued).

Appendix 6

Measuring Mid-Arm Circumference

1. Ask the patient to bend their non-dominant arm at the elbow at a right angle with the palm up.
2. Measure the distance between the acromial surface of the scapula (*bony protrusion surface of upper shoulder*) and the olecranon process of the elbow (*bony point of the elbow*) on the back of the arm.
3. Mark the mid-point between the two with the pen.
4. Ask the patient to let the arm hang loosely by his/her side.
5. Position the tape at the mid-point on the upper arm and tighten snugly. Avoid pinching or causing indentation.
6. Record measurement in cm.
7. If MAC is less than 21, score = 0.
   If MAC is 21–22, score = 0.5.
   If MAC is 22 or greater, score = 1.0.

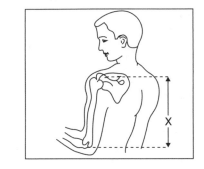

Source: Moore, M.C. *Pocket Guide to Nutrition and Diet Therapy.* 1993.

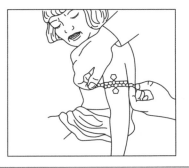

Source: PEN Group. *A pocket guide to clinical nutrition: Assessment of nutritional status.* British Dietetic Association. 1997.

Appendix 7

Measuring Calf Circumference

1. The subject should be sitting with the left leg hanging loosely or standing with their weight evenly distributed on both feet.
2. Ask the patient to roll up their trouser leg to uncover the calf.
3. Wrap the tape around the calf at the widest part and note the measurement.
4. Take additional measurements above and below the point to ensure that the first measurement was the largest.
5. An accurate measurement can only be obtained if the tape is at a right angle to the length of the calf, and should be recorded to the nearest 0.1 cm.

Figure 9–2 A Guide to Completing the Mini Nutritional Assessment MNA® (continued).

References

1. Guigoz Y, Vellas B. Garry PJ. Assessing the nutritional status of the elderly: The Mini Nutritional Assessment as part of the geriatric evaluation. Nutr Rev 1996;54:S59–S65.
2. Fallon C, Bruce I, Eustace A, et al. Nutritional status of community dwelling subjects attending a memory clinic. J Nutr Health Aging 2002;6(Supp):21.
3. Kagansky N, Berner Y, Koren-Morag N, Perelman L, Knobler H, Levy S. Poor nutritional habits are predictors of poor outcomes in very old hospitalized patients. Am J Clin Nutr 2005;82:784–791.
4. Vellas B, Villars H, Abellan G et al. Overview of the MNA®—It's history and challenges. J Nutr Health Aging 2006;10:455–465.
5. Guigoz Y, Vellas J, Garry P (1994). Mini Nutritional Assessment: A practical assessment tool for grading the nutritional state of elderly patients. Facts Res Gerontol 4 (supp. 2):15–59.
6. Guigoz Y. The Mini-Nutritional Assessment (MNA®) review of the literature—what does it tell us? J Nutr Health Aging 2006;10:465–487.
7. Murphy MC, Brooks CN, New SA, Lumbers ML. The use of the Mini Nutritional Assessment (MNA) tool in elderly orthopaedic patients. Eur J Clin Nutr 2000;54:555–562.
8. Malone A. Anthropometric Assessment. In Charney P, Malone E, eds. *ADA Pocket Guide to Nutrition Assessment.* Chicago, IL: American Dietetic Association; 2004:142–152.
9. Osterkamp LK. Current perspective on assessment of human body proportions of relevance to amputees. J Am Diet Assoc. 1995;95:215–218.
10. Hickson M, Frost G. A comparison of three methods for estimating height in the acutely ill elderly population. J Hum Nutr Diet 2003;6:1–3.
11. Chumlea WC, Guo SS, Wholihan K, Cockram D, Kuczmarski RJ, Johnson CL. Stature prediction equations for elderly non-Hispanic white, non-Hispanic black, and Mexican-American persons developed from NHANES III data. J Am Diet Assoc 1998;98:137–142.
12. Cheng HS, See LC, Sheih. Estimating stature from knee height for adults in Taiwan. Chang Gung Med J. 2001;24:547–556.
13. Donini LM, de Felice MR, De Bernardini L, et al. Prediction of stature in the Italian elderly. J Nutr Health Aging. 2004;8:386–388.
14. Guo SS, Wu X, Vellas B, Guigoz Y, Chumlea WC. Prediction of stature in the French elderly. Age & Nutr. 1994;5:169–173.
15. Mendoz-Nunez VM, Sanchez-Rodriguez MA, Cervantes-Sandoval A, et al. Equations for predicting height for elderly Mexican-Americans are not applicable for elderly Mexicans. Am J Hum Biol 2002;14:351–355.
16. Tanchoco CC, Duante CA, Lopez ES. Arm span and knee height as proxy indicators for height. J Nutritionist-Dietitians' Assoc Philippines 2001;15:84–90.
17. Shahar S, Pooy NS. Predictive equations for estimation of statue in Malaysian elderly people. Asia Pac J Clin Nutr. 2003;12(1):80–84.

The Oncology Nursing Society (ONS) standards (Brant & Wickham, 2004) identify nutrition as a high-impact problem area that requires assessment, and when the cause of the problem is identified, intervention should follow quickly. ONS reinforces the need for oncology nurses to use evidence-based interventions and have developed Putting Evidence into Practice (PEP) cards on the following symptoms that patients with cancer may experience: anorexia, depression, nausea and vomiting, fatigue, sleep/wake cycle disturbance, constipation, dyspnea, mucositis, pain, anxiety, and diarrhea. The nurse who administers chemotherapy to the patient with lung cancer is aware of weight changes, because the dose is determined by body surface area and weight. If the patient is losing weight due to nausea and vomiting, this nutritional impact symptom requires more aggressive antiemesis for control, along with teaching the person who prepares meals to cook foods in a Ziploc bag that can be boiled to minimize food odors. If the patient assessment reveals the patient cannot eat due to a metallic taste in food related to cisplatin chemotherapy, then the intervention will include teaching the patient to use plastic utensils rather than metal silverware to eat and to use spices, if the patient likes them, to minimize the taste of metal.

Changes in body composition due to nutritional deficits or malnutrition result in the loss of subcutaneous fat and lean body mass (skeletal muscle such as the intercostal muscles that are necessary for respiration). This leads to fatigue, weakness, skin breakdown, atrophy of skeletal muscles, and increased respiratory effort. Research by Ferrigno and Buccheri (2001) showed that anthropometric measurements in patients with NSCLC did not independently predict survival, but that together with other prognostic factors, survival may be predicted.

Body composition can be tested with bioelectrical impedance analysis. In this process, a machine calculates the percentage of lean body mass, fat, and water. Other easier tests include the following (Klein, 1997; Hill, 1995):

- Grip (muscle) strength: Ask the patient to squeeze your index and middle fingers for 10 seconds and assess the strength of the grip.
- Respiratory muscle strength: Hold a piece of paper 4 inches away from the patient and ask the patient to blow. If the paper barely moves, there is likely nutritional deficiency.
- Tendon bone test (muscle): Inspect then palpate the patient's face, back, upper arms, and back of hands. If tendon(s) and bone(s) are visible, then the patient has likely lost at least 30% of total protein stores.
- Positive thumb test (fat): Use your thumb and index finger to gently pinch the skin of the patient's upper arm; if the triceps or biceps muscle is felt, then the patient's body fat stores are probably greater than 10%.

Laboratory assessment of nutritional parameters may also be helpful. Serum albumin is most commonly used, although a number of factors can affect this value, such as decreased rate of synthesis and losses in the urine and/or feces. In addition, because the half-life is 21 days, it is slow to reflect changes. In contrast, prealbumin (transthyretin) has a half-life of 2 days, is unaffected by hydration, and may be a better indicator for early monitoring. Tayek (1999) calls serum albumin an "excellent" predictor of survival in cancer, because it is most influenced by protein reserves and severity of metabolic threat (e.g., cancer). In a study by Reinhardt et al. (1980), of 2,060 patients in Veterans Affairs hospitals, it was found that a 1 g drop in serum albumin levels (e.g., 3.5 g/dL to 2.5 g/dL) resulted in a 33% increase in mortality, thus illustrating the importance of monitoring changes in protein status and implementing dietary strategies to prevent depletion.

It is also important to assess whether the patient is taking any complementary therapies, such as herbal preparations. If so, assess tolerance, side effects (such as early satiety, nausea, or vomiting), and impact on appetite and food intake. For example, herbal formulations are available on the Internet for the management of cancer symptoms, such as nausea, diarrhea, and anorexia. There are usually no regulations governing their production or scientific evidence to support their use. When herbs are purchased in the community, they often contain fillers or other substances that may be detrimental. The oncology nurse should help the patient and family discuss their interest and what they want to try, teach them to buy from a reputable source if the herbs will not interact with current therapy or management, introduce one agent at a time, use the herbs cautiously, and find credible resources.

Nutritional Care Planning

Early intervention to try to prevent malnutrition is easier than trying to reverse it after it occurs (Ottery, 1994). If the patient is well nourished, a brief review of a balanced diet may be sufficient. The goals are to reinforce the importance of nutrition, and the patient will be more likely to report any changes in appetite or weight. For those patients undergoing combined chemotherapy and radiation therapy or radiation alone and who are at risk for developing dysphagia from the esophagitis that commonly develops, assessment prior to beginning therapy and systematically during therapy should be done. The plan should include strategies to maximize oral intake to stabilize or reverse weight loss. Interventions include managing nutritional impact symptoms, such as nausea, vomiting, diarrhea, dysphagia, early satiety, and fatigue (see Table 9–5 for symptom management strategies). For example, if the patient has early satiety, using a drug such as metoclopramide (Reglan) may increase gastric emptying and gastric transit time. In addition, the nurse can teach the patient nonpharmacologic strategies, such as eating foods rich in calories and protein in the smallest amount (calorie and protein dense) rather than eating junk food, using a small plate instead of a large one, eating small amounts of food frequently throughout the day, keeping small cups of custards or puddings in the refrigerator so they can be eaten easily, and making certain to have a bedtime snack.

In addition, a review of the patient's eating pattern, cultural factors, favorite foods, and ability to buy and prepare foods is important before recommending foods or fluids with higher caloric and protein density per given volume. Many oral supplements are available; the optimal supplement is one that gives the most calories and protein per unit volume. In addition, products may be purchased in the grocery store, such as Carnation Instant Breakfast, that give equal calories and protein, especially when mixed with whole milk. Calories can be added by making a frappé with the addition of ice cream. Most liquid nutritional supplements are lactose free; however, clear liquid juice-based nutrition supplements are available for individuals with milk protein allergies and those who

Table 9–5 Symptom Management Strategies

Symptom	Management Strategies

Anorexia	• Manage symptoms causing decreased appetite (such as pain, nausea, diarrhea, fever, taste alterations)
	• Assess and intervene if depression or emotional issues are involved
	• Teach patient:
	  1. Eat small, frequent, high-calorie, high-protein portions with snacks between and at bedtime; use small portions on small plates; add 1 tablespoon of dry powdered milk to foods made with milk (e.g., mashed potatoes, custard) to get extra protein
	  2. Drink calorie-dense oral supplements as adjuncts or sole nutrition
	  3. Have someone make your favorite foods ahead of time and store in the refrigerator
	  4. Try to eat as much as you can at breakfast (e.g., one-third of daily calories) because your appetite is probably best in the morning
	  5. Try gentle exercise for 5–10 minutes 30 minutes before eating
	  6. Make eating area attractive, play music if desired
	  7. Eat favorite desserts that contain lots of calories
	• Review medication profile to identify drug–nutrition interactions; discuss changes with physician
	• Consider use of agents to stimulate appetite and weight gain, as well as other medications to manage unresolved symptoms
	• Continue to monitor symptom severity and weekly weight, as well as dietary intake diaries

Early satiety	• Teach patient:
	  1. Eat foods that are high in calories and proteins; don't fill up with empty foods, such as lettuce, diet soda, and bouillon
	  2. Drink calorie-dense liquids, such as milk, milk shakes, juice, or fruit punch
	  3. Try not to drink much liquid with food because this will fill you up; drink coffee, tea, water, or milk after you eat
	  4. Use a small plate, and serve or have served small amounts of each food on the plate; eat small, frequent portions throughout the day, including a bedtime snack
	  5. Keep high-calorie, high-protein snacks that are ready to eat throughout the day, such as custard, rice pudding
	• Possible cause may be delayed gastric emptying; discuss with physician use of metoclopramide (Reglan) 10 mg q.i.d., 30 minutes prior to eating

Taste changes	• Teach patient:
	  1. Taste changes are usually temporary and include a bitter or metallic taste for meat or other high protein foods; foods may have less taste
	  2. Eat foods that look and smell attractive to you

Table 9–5 Symptom Management Strategies (continued)	
Symptom	**Management Strategies**
	3. Use plastic eating utensils rather than metal silverware
	4. If meat tastes or smells strange, eat foods with neutral odor and flavor, such as cheeses, eggs, fish
	5. Increase the flavor of meat, chicken, and fish by marinating with sweet fruit juices, sweet and sour sauce, or sweet wine
	6. Try different seasonings, such as Jane's Krazy Mixed-Up Seasonings, salt and pepper, basil, oregano, or rosemary
	7. Try tart foods made with citrus, such as lemon custard (as long as you do not have a sore mouth or throat)
	8. Eat foods at room temperature
	9. Eat a few pineapple chunks to get rid of bad taste or to change taste sensation between eating different foods
Nausea, vomiting	• Aggressive management of nausea, vomiting with antiemetics (single or in combination)
	• Teach patient:
	1. Eat small, frequent meals in an attractive environment away from smells of cooking
	2. Eat foods that are cold or at room temperature, soft and salty (yogurt, pretzels, skinned chicken that is baked or broiled, soft and bland fruits and vegetables, such as canned pears; avoid foods that are greasy, spicy, or rich; avoid foods with strong odors)
	3. Cook foods that are available in a plastic pouch for boiling or microwave use to eliminate smells of cooking
	4. Separate solid foods and liquids by about an hour
	5. Drink cold liquids; try ginger ale
	6. Avoid the sight and smell of foods when not eating
	7. Stay up 1–2 hours after eating, and keep head elevated
	8. Relax between eating, and do not think of food
	9. Take antinausea pill 30–60 minutes before eating; if nauseated, try saltines or toast
	10. When you feel well, try to eat or drink high-calorie, high-protein milkshakes or supplements
	11. Avoid favorite foods when you feel nauseated because you may develop a distaste for them
	12. Wear loose clothes; try to get outside for fresh air
Dry mouth	• Teach patient:
	1. Frequent mouth care (rinses or brushing teeth) every 2–4 hours
	2. Avoid citrus and dry foods

continues

Table 9–5 Symptom Management Strategies (continued)

Symptom	Management Strategies
	3. Increase saliva by drinking liquids with meals or sucking sour candy
	4. Drink 2–3 quarts of fluid per day
	5. Moisten and lubricate mouth and lips frequently
	6. Suck sugarless candy
	• Discuss use of pilocarpine with physician to increase salivation, or patient may try artificial saliva or other mouth lubricants
Stomatitis and esophagitis	• Discuss topical analgesics with physician (e.g., benzocaine, dyclonine hydrochloride, viscous lidocaine) and teach patient to use 15 minutes before eating
	• Teach patient:
	1. Cleanse mouth with recommended mouth rinse (e.g., sodium bicarbonate, salt) before eating
	2. Avoid acidic foods and juices (orange, pineapple) and use of spices
	3. Avoid hot or cold foods, hard or irritating foods
	4. Eat chilled food and fluids, chilled oral supplements
	5. Eat foods that are soft and tender (e.g., milk shakes, mashed potatoes, macaroni and cheese, custards, scrambled eggs, pureed meats)
	6. Mix foods with butter, thin gravy, or sauce so foods are easier to swallow
	7. Use a blender to puree foods
	8. Use a straw to drink liquids
	9. Eat frequent small meals of high-calorie, high-protein foods
	10. Try frozen Popsicles, or freeze favorite drink in ice cubes and suck
	11. Brush teeth with a soft toothbrush b.i.d., if recommended by your nurse
	12. Rinse mouth with recommended mouth rinse after meals and at bedtime
	13. Follow provider's directions for treating infection, if needed
Dysphagia	• Teach patient:
	1. Eat small meals high in calories and proteins frequently
	2. Modify consistency of foods to prevent aspiration; texture should facilitate swallowing; use thickeners if liquids are difficult to swallow
	3. Avoid temperature extremes and foods that are spicy, acidic, or irritating; choose foods that are cool
	4. Supplement diet with high-protein, high-calorie supplements, puddings
	5. If aspiration is a risk, sit upright when eating, thicken liquids or eat soft solids, and practice breathing and swallowing techniques (e.g., inhale and place small amount of food on tongue; swallow, exhale, and/or cough; wait 1–2 minutes before next bite)
	6. Use a blender to puree meats and other foods for soft, solid consistency

---

Table 9–5 Symptom Management Strategies (continued)

Symptom	Management Strategies

Constipation	• Assess elimination pattern, use of cathartics, and modify plan as needed to assure bowel evacuation q 2 days (usually)
	• Teach patient:
	  1. Take recommended bowel regime daily
	  2. Use stool softener
	  3. Drink fluids frequently throughout the day, 2–3 quarts per day
	  4. Eat high-fiber diet, including fresh fruits, vegetables, prunes
	  5. Call provider if no bowel movement in 2 days, especially if on opioids

Diarrhea	• Assess bowel elimination pattern, discuss antidiarrheal medicines with physician (prescription or over-the-counter antidiarrheal medicines)
	• Teach patient:
	  1. Take antidiarrheal medicine as instructed
	  2. Notify provider if diarrhea persists more than 2 days, if diarrhea worsens, or if you feel weak or lightheaded
	  3. Eat small, frequent meals that are warm or at room temperature
	  4. Eat foods high in sodium and potassium (e.g., soups, bananas, potatoes, bouillon, Gatorade)
	  5. Eat foods high in soluble fiber (e.g., oatmeal, rice, apricots, banana, potatoes)
	  6. Eat boiled white rice, tapioca, or cream of rice cereal, as tolerated
	  7. Drink at least eight glasses of fluid per day; if tolerated, and add calories by diluting juice in water
	  8. Avoid foods that cause gas (e.g., beans, broccoli, soda)
	  9. Avoid fatty foods (e.g., bacon, cheeses, oils)
	  10. Avoid citrus fruits, juices, and alcohol
	  11. Avoid foods high in insoluble fiber (e.g., granola, bran cereal, nuts, seeds, vegetables)
	  12. Avoid alcohol- and caffeine-containing fluids
	  13. Use sitz baths as needed to provide comfort; use soft tissues or milk skin lotion on toilet tissue when cleaning yourself

Fever	• Teach patient:
	  1. Report fever over 100.5°F–101°F as directed by your physician or nurse
	  2. Drink increased volume of fluid (e.g., juices, ginger ale, ice water); try to drink one glass every hour
	  3. Take antipyretic medicine as directed
	  4. Try to eat even though you do not feel hungry; eat foods made ahead of time and stored in the refrigerator, such as custards, rice pudding

Source: Cunningham, 1997; Bristol-Myers Squibb, 1999; Wilkes, 1999.

are intolerant for other reasons. A combination of juice and milk-protein-based oral nutrition supplements may help prevent taste fatigue and improve long-term compliance with necessary supplementation. A list of commonly used oral nutrition supplements that are currently available can be found in Table 9–6. As a general rule, a patient with cancer needs 25–35 calories/kg/day or 13–15 calories per pound, and 1–2 g/kg/day with an average of 1.5 g/kg or 0.7 g/pound of protein per day (Wilkes, 1999). Most patients will require a daily multivitamin to protect against micronutrient deficiency.

Often, for many patients with lung cancer who are receiving treatment or who have advanced disease, fatigue is a difficult problem that can interfere with nutrition. Suggestions to improve energy and nutrition include making foods ahead of time and keeping them in the refrigerator, having friends or family do the shopping and meal preparation, using small plates and portions, and eating small amounts frequently throughout the day.

If the patient has anorexia, and despite dietary modifications the patient is still losing weight, then pharmacologic intervention is often appropriate (Ottery, et al., 1998), as shown in Table 9–7. The megestrol acetate oral solution (Megace OS) is indicated for the treatment of anorexia in HIV-infected patients who have lost weight, but it has been shown in a number of studies to increase appetite, oral intake, nonfluid weight, and to decrease nausea and vomiting in patients with cancer (Tchekmedyian, Hickman, & Siau, 1992; Loprinzi, Shaid, & Dose, 1993). Maximal weight gain responses with a daily dose of Megace OS 800 mg occur in about 8–12 weeks, although appetite usually improves within 2 weeks of starting the drug. In a study by Loprinzi and colleagues (1999), megestrol ac-

etate OS (800 mg q.d.) was compared with dexamethasone (0.75 mg q.i.d.) and the anabolic steroid fluoxymesterone in terms of appetite stimulation and weight gain. Both megestrol acetate and dexamethasone were found to stimulate appetite and nonfluid weight gain significantly more than fluoxymesterone. The patients who received dexamethasone had more drug side effects, and 36% discontinued the drug as compared to 25% who took megestrol acetate. Megestrol acetate OS was well tolerated and has been shown to improve quality of life, but it is expensive and also slightly increases the risk of deep vein thrombosis (DVT). Patients should be taught the signs and symptoms of DVT and report them right away.

Corticosteroids have been studied extensively and shown to improve appetite; however, they also can cause myopathy with long-term use, along with hyperglycemia and difficulties sleeping. Corticosteroids are, in general, reserved for patients with advanced disease with limited life expectancy (Jatoi, 2006).

Cannabinoids, such as dronabinol (Marinol) and nabilone (Cesamet), have been shown to stimulate the appetite via the hypothalamic cannabinoid-1 receptors in some studies (Inui, 2002), but in other studies cannabinoids are not likely to be effective (Adams, Cunningham, Caruso, Norling, & Shepard, 2008). However, the effects of these drugs are less reliable and result in side effects such as euphoria, dizziness, drowsiness, and mood changes that make compliance challenging. While further research is needed to establish therapeutic dosages, recent research from Jatoi et al. (2002) indicates that 800 mg megestrol (Megace) is more effective than either 2.5 mg of dronabinol given twice daily alone or the combination of the two medications.

Table 9–6 Commonly Used Commercial Oral Nutrition Supplements

Nutrition Supplement	Manufacturer	Calories (svg)	Protein (g/svg)	Characteristics
Ensure	Ross	250	9	lactose and gluten free; low residue; milk and soy protein based
Ensure Plus	Ross	350	13	lactose and gluten free; low residue; milk and soy protein based; concentrated calories and protein; omega-3 marine oils
Ensure High Protein	Ross	230	12	lactose and gluten free; low residue; milk protein based; additional protein for wound healing and protein-calorie malnutrition
Ensure Fiber	Ross	250	9	lactose and gluten free; milk protein based; fiber for digestive health
Glucerna Shakes	Ross	200	10	reduced sugar content; for people with diabetes; milk protein based;
Enlive!	Ross	250	9	juice based; fat free for patients with malabsorption; low residue
Boost	Nestlé	240	10	lactose and gluten free; low residue; milk protein based
Boost High Protein	Nestlé	240	15	lactose and gluten free; low residue; milk protein based; additional protein for wound healing and protein-calorie malnutrition
Boost Glucose Control	Nestlé	250	14	reduced sugar content; for people with diabetes; milk protein based;
Resource Breeze	Nestlé	250	9	juice based; fat free for patients with malabsorption; low residue
Resource Support	Nestlé	360	21	lactose free; concentrated calories and protein; omega-3 marine oils;
Carnation Instant Breakfast (powder)	Nestlé	220	13	mix with 8 oz milk; economical price and available in grocery stores

continues

Table 9-6 Commonly Used Commercial Oral Nutrition Supplements (continued).

Nutrition Supplement	Manufacturer	Calories (svg)	Protein (g/svg)	Characteristics
Carnation Instant Breakfast No Added Sugar (powder)	Nestlé	150	13	mix with 8 oz milk; for people with diabetes; economical price and available in grocery stores
Carnation Instant Breakfast Lactose Free	Nestlé	250	8.75	lactose and gluten free; low residue; milk protein based
Carnation Instant Breakfast Lactose Free Plus	Nestlé	357	13.1	lactose and gluten free; low residue; milk protein based; concentrated calories and protein
Carnation Instant Breakfast Lactose Free VHC	Nestlé	560	22.5	lactose and gluten free; low residue; milk protein based; very concentrated calories and protein for fluid/volume sensitivity; high fat content
Juven (powder)	Ross	75	0	"Mix with 8 to 10 oz of water; contains HMB, arginine and glutamine; prevent muscle catabolism"

Table 9–7 Drugs Used in the Management of Anorexia

Agent/Dose	Side Effects	Comments
Dexamethasone 0.75 mg q.i.d.	Exacerbates progressive muscle wasting, weakness, immunosuppression, hyperglycemia, mood swings, osteoporosis, delirium	Indicated for bed-bound patients with advanced cancer for whom lean body mass is not a concern; inexpensive
Megestrol acetate 800 mg q.d. Megace ES 625 mg, 5 cc q.d.	Edema rare, thrombophlebitis 5% incidence, hyperglycemia, hypogonadism	Has been shown to increase appetite, oral intake resulting in nonwater weight gain; decreases nausea, and associated with increases in quality of life; expensive; megestrol acetate (Megace OS) is 20% more bioavailable than tablets, so they should be used; may be able to lower dose after appetite and oral intake have increased
Dronabinol 2.5 mg b.i.d.	Euphoria, dizziness, confusion	Has FDA indication for anorexia and weight loss in patients with cancer; increases appetite, decreases nausea, but weight gain is not statistically significant
Thalidomide 100 mg t.i.d. (investigational)	Drowsiness; fetal malformation so pregnancy must be ruled out	In studies with HIV-infected patients, results in weight gain (lean body mass)

Source. Modified from Wilkes, G., 1999.

Selected patients may benefit from oxandrolone (Oxandrin), an anabolic steroid that is indicated as an adjunctive therapy to help patients regain weight lost from extensive surgery, chronic infections, or severe trauma (Tchekmedyian, 2006).

Other appetite stimulants include Eldertonic, a supplement that is available over the counter. Each 45 mL (3 tablespoons) of Eldertonic contains the water-soluble vitamins thiamine, riboflavin, niacinamide, dexpanthenol, pyridoxine HCl, and cyanocobalamin, as well as the minerals zinc, manganese, and magnesium. The solution has an alcohol content of 13.5%. Eicosapentaenoic acid (EPA) has been studied as well. EPA in fish oil capsules showed no significant differences in appetite or weight, while EPA (energy dense) in supplement form showed an increase in weight gain (Adams, et al., 2008).

Unfortunately, today there is still no treatment to reverse the anorexia/cachexia syndrome (Tchekmedyian, 2006). Continued prospective research into both the pathophysiology and the treatment of cachexia is needed (Baracos, 2006).

Along with the appetite stimulant, it is important for the patient to do gentle resistive exercises so that the weight gained becomes lean muscle instead of fat (Evans, Roubenoff, & Shevitz, 1998; Tchekmedyian, 2006). In a review of the literature, patients who received dietary counseling and oral supplements reported improved caloric intake (Adams, et al., 2008).

In addition, Juven, a lower-calorie, powder-based nutrition supplement, has been shown to increase lean body mass in cachexic cancer and HIV patients. Juven contains L-arginine, L-glutamine, and beta-hydroxy-beta-methyl-butyrate (HMB), nutrients known to increase protein synthesis and reverse protein catabolism. In a study by Eubanks et al. (2002), cachexic patients with solid tumors who supplemented with Juven daily for 24 weeks gained an average of 0.95 kg at 4 weeks versus the control group, who lost an average of 0.26 kg. At 24 weeks, the treatment group gained an average of 1.6 kg. The therapeutic dosage of Juven is two packets daily mixed with 8–10 oz of water or juice.

The use of antidepressants and sleep aids with known appetite-stimulating side effects, such as mirtazapine (Remeron), should also be considered when appropriate.

Patients may be unable to take food orally, and the enteral route may be necessary until healing occurs. Total parenteral nutrition (TPN) has a role in providing nutritional support to patients who receive aggressive, potentially curative therapy. Unfortunately, however, the use of TPN in support of patients with advanced cancer does not impact survival time, and, in general, it is not appropriate in this setting (Cunningham & Huhmann, 2005). In addition, it may diminish quality of life by adding one more complicated task that consumes family time, rather than preserving the time for high-quality personal interaction.

Conclusion

Nutrition is a basic human need and provides the energy for life and the important work of breathing, healing, and for social interaction. Weight loss and nutritional deficits often accompany the diagnosis of lung cancer, and they may confer a poor prognosis. These factors may limit entry into a clinical trial and may decrease tolerance and response to aggressive treatment approaches. For others, lung cancer treatment may cause symptoms that interfere with nutrition and result in anorexia, weight loss, and malnutrition. Finally, for those who are not cured of their disease, advanced lung cancer can bring with it cachexia and anorexia. The oncology nurse is the catalyst who can bring attention to the importance of nutrition in the care plan of the person with lung cancer, regardless of where the person is on the disease trajectory. Initial assessment should be done early and should be tailored to the individual patient depending upon treatment goals. Two patient assessment tools were discussed: the Patient-Generated Subjective Global Assessment (PG-SGA) tool and the Mini Nutritional Assessment (MNA) tool. The PG-SGA provides a quick, valid, and reliable assessment upon which a plan can be generated. The MNA is easier to use but has not been validated in the oncology patient population. The oncology nurse collaborates with other members of the healthcare team to use evidence-based interventions to aggressively manage nutritional impact symptoms. Patient/family teaching is critical to empower patients and their families to maximize calories and proteins in an acceptable way. The oncology nurse helps to bring the process full circle by evaluating the patient's response to interventions and making revisions as needed. Finally, nursing and multidisciplinary research are needed to identify more effective measures in the management of nutritional issues of patients with lung cancer.

References

Adams, L., Cunningham, R., Caruso, R. A., Norling, M., & Shepard, N. (2008). *Anorexia PEP card*. Pittsburgh, PA: Oncology Nursing Society.

Baracos, V. E. (2006). More research needed on the treatment of the cancer anorexia/cachexia syndrome. *The Journal of Supportive Oncology, 4*(10), 508–509.

Bauer, M., Birch, R., & Paja, K. (1985). Prognostic factors in cancer of the lung. In J. D. Cox (Ed.), *Syllabus: A categorical course in radiation therapy; Lung cancer* (pp. 116–117). Oak Brook, IL: Radiological Society of North America Publications.

Blackburn, G., Bistrian, B., Maini, B., Schlamm, H., & Smith, M. (1977). Nutritional and metabolic assessment of the hospitalized patient. *Journal of Parenteral and Enteral Nutrition, 1*(1), 11–22.

Brant, J. M., & Wickham, R. S. (2004). *Statement on the scope and standards of oncology nursing practice*. Pittsburgh, PA: Oncology Nursing Society and American Nurses Association.

Bristol-Myers Squibb. (1999). *Nutrition for health tips*. Princeton, NJ: Bristol-Myers Squibb Oncology.

Brown, J., & Radke, K. (1998). Nutritional assessment, interventions, and evaluation of weight loss in patients with non-small cell lung cancer. *Oncology Nursing Forum, 25*(3), 547–553.

Chandra, R. (1990). Micronutrients and immune function: An overview. *Annals of the New York Academy of Science, 587*, 9–16.

Choi, N., Baumann, M., Flentjie, M., Kellokumpu-Lehtinen, P., Senan, S., Zamboglou, N., et al. (2001). Predictive factors in radiotherapy for non-small cell lung cancer: Present status. *Lung Cancer, 31*(1), 43–56.

Costa, G., Lane, W. W., Vincent, R. G., Siebold, J. A., Aragon, M., & Bewley, B. T. (1980). Weight loss and cachexia in lung cancer. *Nutrition in Cancer, 2*, 98–103.

Cunningham, R. (1997). *Tips and tools. Supportive solutions to pain, fatigue, and nutrition*. Princeton, NJ: Bristol-Myers Squibb Oncology.

Cunningham, R. S., & Huhmann, M. B. (2005). Nutritional disturbances. In C. H. Yarbo, M. H. Frogge, & M. Goodman (Eds.), *Cancer nursing: Principles and practice* (2nd ed., pp. 761–791). Sudbury, MA: Jones and Bartlett.

DeWys, W., Begg, D., Lavin, P., Band, P., Bennett, J., Bertino, J., et al. (1980). Prognostic effect of weight loss prior to chemotherapy in cancer patients. *American Journal of Medicine, 69*(4), 491–497.

DiMaria-Ghalili, R. A., & Guenter, P. A. (2008). The Mini Nutritional Assessment. *The American Journal of Nursing, 108*(2), 50–59.

Eubanks, P., Barber, A., D'Olimpio, J. T., Hourichane, A., & Abumrad, N. N. (2002). Reversal of cancer-related wasting using oral supplementation with a combination of β-hydroxy-β-methylbutyrate, arginine and glutamine. *American Journal of Surgery, 183*(4), 471–479.

Evans, W., Roubenoff, R., & Shevitz, A. (1998). Exercise and treatment of wasting: Aging and the human deficiency virus infection. *Seminars in Oncology, 25*(Suppl. 6), 112–122.

Ferrigno, D., & Buccheri, G. (2001). Anthropometric measurements in non-small-cell-lung cancer. *Support Care in Cancer, 10*(5), 522–527.

Fretz, P., & Peterson, M. (2001). Clinical signs and symptoms. In Fretz, P. C., & Peterson, M. W. (Eds.) *Lung tumors: A multidisciplinary database, clinical presentation and initial evaluation*. Virtual Hospital. Retrieved October 7, 2008, from http://lib.cpums.edu.cn/jiepou/tupu/atlas/www.vh.org/adult/provider/radiology/LungTumors/ClinicalPresentation/Text/ClinicalPresentation.html

Grosvenor, M., Bulcavage, L., & Chebowski, R. (1989). Symptoms potentially influencing weight loss in a cancer population. Correlations with primary site, nutritional status, and chemotherapy administration. *Cancer, 63*(2), 330–334.

Hurst, J. D., & Gallagher, A. L. (2006). Energy, macronutrient, micronutrient and fluid requirements. In L. Elliot, L. L. Molseed, P. D. McCallum, & B. Grant

(Eds.), *The clinical guide to oncology nutrition* (2nd ed., pp. 54–71). Chicago: American Dietetic Association.

Inui, A. (2002). Cancer anorexia-cachexia syndrome: Current issues in research and management. *CA: A Cancer Journal for Clinicians, 52*(2), 72–91.

Jagoe, R., Goodship, T., & Gibson, G. (2001). The influence of nutritional status on complications after operations for lung cancer. *Annals of Thoracic Surgery, 71*(3), 766–768.

Jatoi, A. (2006). Pharmacologic therapy for the cancer anorexia/weight loss syndrome: A data driven, practical approach. *The Journal of Supportive Oncology, 4*(10), 499–502.

Jatoi, A., Windschitl, H. E., Loprinzi, C. L., Sloan, J. A., Dahkil, S. R., Mailliard, J. A., et al. (2002). Dronabinol versus megesterol acetate versus combination therapy for cancer associated anorexia: A North Central Cancer Treatment Group study. *Journal of Clinical Oncology, 20*(2), 567–573.

Klein, S., Kinney, J., Jeejeebhoy, K., Alpers, D., Hellerstein, M., Murray, M., et al. (1997). Nutritional support in clinical practice: Review of published data, and recommendations for future research directions. *Journal of Parenteral and Enteral Nutrition, 21*(3), 133–156.

Langstein, H., & Norton, J. (1991). Mechanisms of cancer cachexia. *Hematology Oncology Clinics of North America, 5*(1), 103–123.

Lanzotti, V., Thomas, D., Boyle, L., Smith, T., Gehan, E., & Samuels, M. (1977). Survival with inoperable lung cancer: An integration of prognostic variables based on simple clinical criteria. *Cancer, 39*(1), 303–313.

Laviano, A., Meguid, M. M., Inui, A., Muscaritoli, M., & Rossi-Fanelli, F. (2005). Therapy insight: Cancer anorexia-cachexia syndrome: When all you can eat is yourself. *Nature Clinical Practice: Oncology, 2*(3), 158–165.

Loprinzi, C., Kugler, J., Sloan, J., Mailliard, J., Krook, J., Wilwerding, M., et al. (1999). Randomized comparison of megestrol acetate versus dexamethasone versus fluoxymesterone for the treatment of cancer anorexia/cachexia. *Journal of Clinical Oncology, 17*(10), 3299–3306.

Loprinzi, C., Schaid, D., Dose, A., Burnham, N., & Jensen, M. (1993). Body composition changes in patients who gain weight receiving megestrol acetate. *Journal of Clinical Oncology, 11*(1), 152–154.

Morley, J. E., Thomas, D. R., & Wilson, M. M. G. (2006). Cachexia: Pathophysiology and clinical relevance. *The American Journal of Clinical Nutrition, 83*(4), 735–743.

Ottery, F. (1994). Rethinking nutritional support in the cancer patient. *Seminars in Oncology, 21*(6), 770–778.

Ottery, F., Walsh, D., & Strawford, A. (2001). Pharmacological management of anorexia/cachexia. *Seminars in Oncology, 25*(2, Suppl. 6), 35–44.

Ovensen, L., Hannibal, J., & Mortensen, E. (1993). The interrelationship of weight loss, dietary intake and quality of life in ambulatory patients with cancer of the lung, breast and ovary. *Nutrition Cancer, 19*(2), 159–167.

Puccio, M., & Nathanson, L. (1997). The cancer cachexia syndrome. *Seminars in Oncology, 24*(3), 277–287.

Read, J. A., Crockett, N., Volker, D. H., MacLennan, P., Choy, B., Beale, P., et al. (2005). Nutritional assessment in cancer: Comparing the Mini Nutritional Assessment (MNA) with the scored Patient-Generated Subjective Global Assessment (PG-SGA). *Nutrition and Cancer, 53*(1), 51–56.

Reinhardt, G., Myscofski, J., Wilkens, D., Dobrin, D., Mangan, J., Jr., & Stannard, R. (1980). Incidence and mortality of hypoalbuminemic patients in hospitalized veterans. *Journal of Parenteral and Enteral Nutrition, 4*(4), 357–359.

Russell, D., Shike, M., Marliss, E., Detsky, A., Shepherd, F., Feld, R., et al. (1984). Effects of total parenteral nutrition and chemotherapy on metabolic derangements in small cell lung cancer. *Cancer Research, 44*(4), 1706–1711.

Sanchez-Lara, K., Diaz-Romero, C., Motola-Kuba, D., Rodriguez, C., Sosa Sanchez, R., Ceron, T., et al. (2008). Albumin serum levels and malnutrition are associated with toxicity secondary to paclitaxel-cisplain chemotherapy in patients with advanced non-small cell lung cancer: A prospective study. *Journal of Clinical Oncology, 26*(Suppl. May 20, Abstract No. 9623).

Sause, W., Kolesar, P., Taylor, S., IV, Johnson, D., Livingston, R., Komaki, R., et al. (2000). Final results of phase III trial in regionally advanced unresectable non-small cell lung cancer. Radiation Therapy Oncology Group, Eastern Cooperative Oncology Group, and Southwest Oncology Group. *Chest, 117*(2), 358–364.

Scott, C., Sause, W., Byhardt, R., Marcial, V., Pajak, T., Herskovic, A., et al. (1997). Recursive partitioning analysis of 1592 patients on four RTOG studies in inoperable non-small cell lung cancer. *Lung Cancer, 17*(Suppl. 1), S59–S74.

Skarin, A., Herbst, R., Leong, T., Bailey, A., & Sugarbaker, D. (2001). Lung cancer in patients under age 40. *Lung Cancer, 32*(3), 255–264.

Smale, B., Mullen, J., Buzby, G., & Rosato, E. (1981). The efficacy of nutritional assessment and support in cancer surgery. *Cancer, 47*(10), 2375–2381.

Spitzer, W. O., Dobson, A. J., Hall, J., Chesterman, E., Levi, J., Shepherd, R., et al. (1981). Measuring the quality of life of cancer patients: A concise QL-index for use by physicians. *J Chronic Dis, 34*(12), 585–597.

Tayek, J. (1999). Nutrition and biochemical aspects of the cancer patient. In D. Heber, G. L. Blackburn, & V. L. W. Go (Eds.), *Nutritional oncology* (pp. 515–536). San Diego, CA: Academic Press.

Tchekmedyian, N., Cella, D., & Heber, D. (1999). Nutritional support and quality of life. In D. Heber, G. L. Blackburn, & V. L. W. Go (Eds.), *Nutritional oncology* (pp. 587–592). San Diego, CA: Academic Press.

Tchekmedyian, N., Hickman, M., Siau, J., Greco, F., Keller, J., Browder, H., et al. (1992). Megestrol acetate in cancer anorexia and weight loss. *Cancer, 69*(5), 1268–1274.

Tchekmedyian, N. S. (2006). Treating the anorexia/cachexia syndrome. *The Journal of Supportive Oncology, 4*(10), 506–507.

Tombolini, V., Bonanni, A., Donato, V., Raffetto, N., Santarelli, M., Valeriani, M., et al. (2000). Radiotherapy alone in elderly patients with medically inoperable stage IIIA and IIIB non-small cell lung cancer. *Anticancer Research, 20*(6C), 4829–4833.

Vigano, A., Bruera, E., Jhangri, G., Newman, S., Fields, A., & Suarez-Almazor, M. (2000). Clinical survival predictors in patients with advanced cancer. *Archives of Internal Medicine, 160*(6), 861–868.

Wilkes, G. (1999). *Cancer and HIV clinical nutrition pocket guide.* Sudbury, MA: Jones and Bartlett.

Wilkes, G. (2000). Nutrition: The missing link in cancer care. *American Journal of Nursing, 100*(4), 46–51.

Chapter 10

Dyspnea Management: A Biopsychosocial Approach

Doris Howell

"If I sometimes get out of bed too quick, or even to reach over and take the phone up, I'm out of breath . . ."

Dyspnea is a distressing and complex symptom of lung cancer that develops early in about 60% of patients (Muers & Round, 1993). This is likely due to the advanced presentation of lung cancer (Sarna & Brecht, 1997). Reported prevalence rates of dyspnea vary depending on disease stage with ranges reported as low as 21% (Dudgeon, Kristjanson, Sloan, Lertzman, & Clement, 2001a) to 89% (Hollen, et al., 1999) and as high as 99% in seriously ill community samples (Skaug, Eide, & Gulsvik, 2007). Dyspnea is typically a chronic symptom that gradually worsens in severity with progressive disease (Bruera & Neumann, 1998).

The complexity of dyspnea has profound affects on multiple dimensions of quality of life, as depicted in Figure 10–1 (Sarna, et al., 2005; Sarna, et al., 2004). As noted in the figure, dyspnea affects individuals' functional abilities, restricting their ability to work and participate in leisure activities. This also affects social roles and relationships, which may lead to significant meaning being assigned to this symptom. Certainly dyspnea provokes profound fear and anxiety in both patients and families (Tarzian, 2000). In advanced stages of lung cancer, dyspnea in combination with other symptoms predicts depression (Kurtz, Kurtz, Stommel, Given, & Given, 2000), correlates with existential distress (Bailey, 1995), and affects quality of dying (Lynn, Schuster, & Kabacenell, 2000). Dyspnea also influences the use of healthcare resources, such as emergency care (Escalante, et al., 1996), and can lead to acute care hospitalization at the end of life (Brazil, Howell, Bedard, Krueger, & Heidebrecht, 2005).

Nurses play a critical role in dyspnea management through early identification and comprehensive assessment of multidimensional causes using standardized measures and by applying a biopsychosocial approach to address the totality of dyspnea experience from a patient-centered perspective. This chapter will provide a brief overview of pathophysiology and causal mechanisms of dyspnea. Empirical evidence is also presented for standardized comprehensive assessment of dyspnea and the need to capture the dyspnea experience of this symptom from a patient-centered perspective. Finally, evidence supporting components that should be combined in a biopsychosocial intervention approach are highlighted.

Figure 10–1 Impact of dyspnea on quality of life.

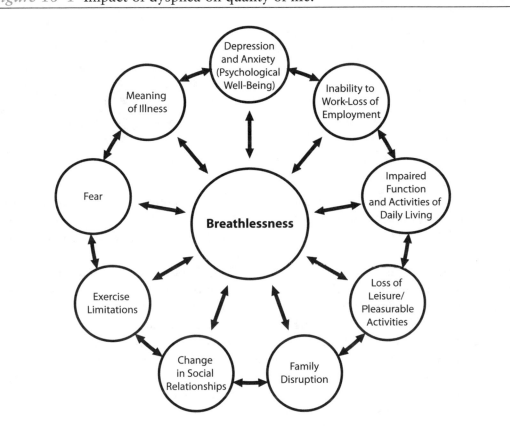

Dyspnea versus Breathlessness

Dyspnea is defined as a subjective, multidimensional experience of breathing discomfort, comprised of qualitatively distinct sensations that vary in intensity (American Thoracic Society [ATS], 1999, 2005). This discomfort is not necessarily related to exertion that compels an individual to increase his ventilation or decrease his activity (Ahmedzai, 1998). Dyspnea should not be con-

fused with tachypnea (increased rate of breathing due to metabolic causes, such as fever), hyperpnea (increased ventilation through metabolic acidosis), nor hyperventilation (psychologically induced increased respiration) (Ahmedzai, 1998).

Dyspnea is a combination of a "sensation" (neural activation resulting from stimulation of a receptor) and a "perception" (reaction of an individual to that sensation) (American Thoracic Society, 1999). The sensory dimension denotes the nociceptive bodily change and its intensity, whereas perception is the patient's evaluation and affective response to the sensation. Patients convey their perception of being short of breath with descriptors such as, "tightening in the chest," "I am afraid and feel like I am drowning," and "part of the way toward choking" (Howell, Fitch, & Velgi, 2008; O'Driscoll, Corner, & Bailey, 1999).

The terms "dyspnea" and "breathlessness" are often used interchangeably. The term "dyspnea" is most often used to denote the sensation or physical response to this bodily change, whereas the term "breathlessness" captures the unpleasant awareness or affective aspect (Dudgeon, 2002). The term "breathlessness" was coined to capture the subjective nature of dyspnea and the inseparability of physiological and emotional responses (Corner, Plant, & Warner, 1995). Patients describe this symptom not only as a physical bodily reaction but also in terms of how it feels interwoven with its impact on their lives (O'Driscoll, et al., 1999).

Pathophysiology and Causal Mechanisms

Breathing is under involuntary control and may be influenced by both physiological and psychological influences (Guyton, 1986) that are not clearly understood (Thomas & von Gunten, 2003). The major physiological influences are chemical, neural, and muscular (Whipp, 1987), innervated by a number of receptors (Figure 10–2). If any of these inputs are disturbed, an uncomfortable awareness of breathing and perception of breathlessness occurs (Interview, 2006, p. 63). Psychological factors also play a role in alterations in breathing by stimulating the respiratory center through the higher brain center (Quinn, 1999).

Chemical Receptors

Breathing is under the control of chemical receptors in the medulla and pons in the brain stem, and controls are regulated by the blood pH, CO_2, oxygen level, central processes in the brain cortex, as well as mechanoreceptors in the lung and respiratory muscles (Ripamonti & Bruera, 1997). Chemical control mechanisms that are important in the regulation of breathing include peripheral and central receptors. Peripheral chemoreceptors that are found in the arch of the aorta and at the bifurcation of the common carotid arteries are innervated by cranial nerves (IX and X) and are sensitive to changes in the level of oxygen in the arterial blood. Central chemical receptors that are situated in the medulla of the brain are connected to other neural centers and influence the pattern and rate of breathing, responding to very small changes in the acidity or pH of blood or cerebrospinal fluid (McCloskey, 1978). The pH is related to the pressure of carbon dioxide in the blood, which reflects the level of ventilation in the lungs. Even a minute increase in carbon dioxide, representing a decrease in blood pH, signifies a major reduction in ventilation, stimulating the respiratory center to increase ventilation to excrete this excess gas.

Neural Mechanisms

The neural mechanisms include airway stretch receptors that appear to control the breathing cycle. These receptors include (1) lung parenchymal receptors, which detect rises in the capillary pressure (e.g., pulmonary congestion); and (2) sensory receptors in the respiratory muscles (skeletal and diaphragm muscle receptors), which modulate breathing (Ahmedzai, 1998).

Figure 10–2 Factors impacting the need to breathe and perception of breathlessness.

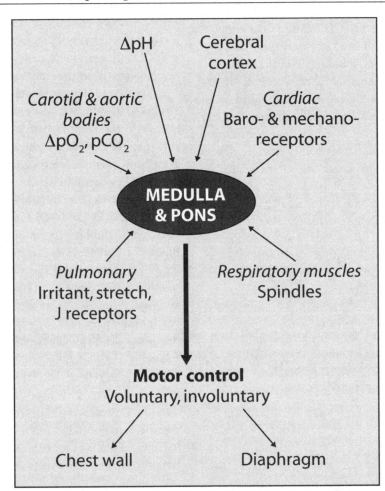

Source: From *Journal of Supportive Oncology, Volume 4(2),* "Dyspnea in Cancer Research Needs More Attention," p. 63–64. Copyright Elsevier, 2006.

Also, respiratory muscle receptors, both within the skeleton and diaphragm, may be involved in the modulation of breathing (Estenne, Ninane, & De Troyer, 1988). Stretching and, more importantly, muscle fatigue significantly affect overall strength and sensations that are perceived by the individual (Paintal, 1983). This gives the feeling of breathlessness perception (Campbell & Howell, 1963).

A differential effect of medications on the rib cage and diaphragm suggests that these muscles act independently (Ahmedzai, 1998). For example, opioids appear to inhibit rib cage movement, whereas benzodiazepines, such as midazolam, reduce tidal volume and depress ventilation by affecting thoracoabdominal muscles (Morel, Forster, Bachman, & Suter, 1984).

Upper airways and facial receptors also modify the sensation of dyspnea (Manning & Schwartzstein, 1998). Airflow over the face and inhalation of warm, humidified air through nasal passages or oral mucosa reduces stimulation of flow or temperature receptors, reducing dyspnea (Simon, et al., 1991). Mechanoreceptors on the face or a decrease in the temperature of the facial skin may alter afferent feedback to the brain through the trigeminal nerve, thus modifying the perception of dyspnea (ATS, 1999). In clinical practice, the movement of cool air with a fan has been shown to reduce breathlessness perception.

Emotional Stimulation

Physiological mechanisms alone do not explain the varied circumstances that lead to the perception of breathlessness (Tanaka, Akechi, Okuyama, Nishiwaki, & Uchitomi, 2002). Breathlessness can also be modified by the patient's affective response to the sensation of breathlessness that is likely linked to the "meaning" of the symptom, based on the patient's evaluation of its seriousness (Corner, et al., 1995; O'Neill, 2002; Dodd, et al., 2001). The affective dimension of dyspnea is more vulnerable to emotional influences than the sensory experience (von Leupoldt, Mertz, Kegat, Burmester, & Dahme, 2006). Emotional influences act on the higher brain center to stimulate the respiratory center, which in turn regulates breathing pattern (Quinn, 1999). Emotional distress, such as anxiety and depression, can perpetuate episodes of breathlessness dispro-

portionate to the extent of underlying disease (Cherniack & Altrose, 1987; Kellner, Samet, & Pathak, 1992).

Multidimensional Causative Factors

The experience of dyspnea is derived from a complex interplay among multiple physical, psychological, social, and environmental factors that influence perception of breathlessness (O'Driscoll, et al., 1999; ATS, 1999; Krishnasamy, Corner, Bredin, Plant, & Bailey, 2001). These factors are inseparable and in combination induce secondary physiological and behavioral responses to breathlessness (Tanaka, et al., 2002).

Physical causes of dyspnea in lung cancer are summarized in Table 10–1 (Thomas & von Gunten, 2003). Direct causes are those considered to occur as a result of tumor mass infiltration in the lungs, such as airway obstruction. Patients can experience periods of acute shortness of breath as a result of sudden events, such as upper airway obstruction, spontaneous pneumothorax, pulmonary emboli or edema, or cardiac episodes (Brown, Carrieri, Janson-Bjerklie, & Dodd, 1986; McDermott, 2000). Indirect causes are considered to be those that are secondary to the effects of cancer or its treatment, such as anemia.

Causative factors have been simplified as controller or gas exchange problems and pump problems or a combination of these (Dudgeon, 2001; Interview, 2006). Controller or gas exchange problems occur in the lungs and bronchial airways. Pulmonary damage can occur directly related to the cancer or from the oncology treatment. Pulmonary interstitial and pulmonary vascular injuries are well-recognized complications of many chemotherapeutic agents

Table 10-1 Causes of Dyspnea

Directly related to cancer
Primary/metastatic parenchymal lung involvement
Airway obstruction (intrinsic or extrinsic tumor)
Carcinomatous lymphangitis
Pleural tumor
Malignant pleural effusion
Pericardial effusion
Superior vena cava syndrome
Tumor microemboli
Phrenic nerve paralysis
Atelectasis
Tracheal esophageal fistula
Chest-wall invasion (carcinoma en cuirasse)
Pathologic chest-wall fractures
Indirectly related to cancer
Pneumonia
Cachexia
Anemia
Electrolyte abnormalities
Pulmonary embolus
Paraneoplastic syndromes
Ascites
Related to cancer therapy
Surgery (postlobectomy/pneumonectomy)
Radiation pneumonitis
Chemotherapy-induced pulmonary fibrosis
Chemotherapy-induced cardiomyopathy
Unrelated to cancer
Chronic obstructive pulmonary disease
Asthma
Congestive heart failure
Cardiac ischemia
Arrhythmias
Pulmonary vascular disease
Obesity
Neuromuscular disorders
Aspiration
Anxiety
Pneumothorax
Interstitial lung disease
Psychosocial/spiritual pain

Source: From *Journal of Supportive Oncology, Volume 1.* Thomas, J.R. & von Gunten, C.F. 23–24. Copyright Elsevier, 2003.

(Stover & Kaner, 2001). Thoracic irradiation can cause radiation pneumonitis in a small percentage of patients (5–15%) occurring 2 to 3 months following radiotherapy. This can lead to permanent lung fibrosis (Hood & Harwood, 2004).

Respiratory problems can be compounded by other conditions. Surgical dissection for lung cancer, especially for those with preexisting cardiopulmonary risk factors such as chronic obstructive pulmonary disease (COPD), can lead to pulmonary compromise (Dudgeon, et al., 2001a). Individuals with a current or long-term smoking history usually present with preexisting comorbidities, such as chronic obstructive pulmonary disease (ATS, 1999) that worsens the controller or gas exchange. Lung cancer and pulmonary disease share some causative mechanisms, including reduction of airflow and gas exchange, because of airway obstruction and destruction of lung parenchyma (Jantarakupt & Porock, 2005). Anemia, infection, or cardiomyopathy can also indirectly cause dyspnea (Hood & Harwood, 2004).

The second physical cause is pump problems. Systemic effects of cancer and chemotherapy can lead to wasting or myopathy of peripheral muscles, respiratory muscles, or the myocardium. This dysfunction occurs through a mismatch between the central respiratory motor output and ventilation (ATS, 1999); however, the effects are not well understood (Travers, et al., 2007). This problem appears to result from an impairment of maximal inspiratory pressure due to muscle wasting in patients with anorexia-cachexia syndrome (Dudgeon & Lertzman, 1998; Ripamonti & Bruera, 1997). Respiratory muscle weakness was a significant causal factor of dyspnea in a prospective study of 100 advanced cancer patients with dyspnea (Dudgeon & Lertzman, 1998). Older populations are also at risk for this problem due to the effects of aging on chest wall stiffness, decrease in skeletal muscle, and loss of elasticity of alveoli (Derby & O'Mahony, 2001).

Besides the physical factors that influence dyspnea sensation at the mechano- and chemoreceptor level, psychosocial factors, such as emotional distress, also impact the perception of breathlessness (Tanaka, et al., 2002). Anxiety and depression coexist with breathlessness in lung cancer patients (Lavoie, et al., 2001; Tanaka, et al., 2002; Bruera, Schmitz, Pither, Neumann, & Hanson, 2000; Dudgeon, Lertzman, & Askew, 2001b). Emotional distress can prolong the duration and perceived severity of breathlessness (McCarley, 1999). Anxiety is higher in this population than other cancer populations (Heedman & Strang, 2001). This emotional response to breathlessness is likely related to the physical and emotional burden of advanced lung cancer and the symbolic meaning of this symptom. Breathlessness is equated with impending death and an overwhelming fear of suffocating (Cooley, Short, & Moriarty, 2002; O'Driscoll, et al., 1999; Tishelman, Degner, & Mueller, 2000).

Social and environmental factors are also considered to be important causative factors in lung cancer breathlessness. Similar to those with chronic obstructive pulmonary disease, lung cancer patients report more severe breathlessness depending on environmental factors, such as extremely hot or cold weather. Inadequate social support and family conflict has been shown to influence shortness of breath (Brown, et al., 1986). There is limited evidence regarding the role of these factors in lung cancer-related breathlessness. Patients may respond to these changes by limiting their outside activities to avoid exacerbating breathlessness.

Assessment of Breathlessness

The identification of underlying treatable causes of dyspnea to target interventions is a prime motivator for assessment of breathlessness when lung cancer patients begin to experience this symptom. A comprehensive assessment also includes an understanding of breathlessness from the perspective of the patient on a number of dimensions. Gift (1990) describes five components to this evaluation. These include: (1) the sensation (physiological mechanisms); (2) perception of dyspnea (individual perception of level of distress, ability to adapt); (3) dyspnea distress (psychological aspects); (4) dyspnea response (coping style of patient); and (5) reporting of symptom (influenced by past health experience, culture, patient reporting method).

Dyspnea Sensation (Physiological Mechanisms)

Dyspnea sensation includes the mechanisms that trigger breathing (Gift, 1990). This definition has been expanded here to include the nociceptive aspects of dyspnea that trigger the sensation of dyspnea that should be included in a comprehensive assessment. The components of an evaluation of physical causes of dyspnea sensation are summarized in Table 10–2.

Table 10–2 **Evaluation of Dyspnea**

- History and physical examination
- Pulmonary function tests if appropriate
- Chest radiograph
- Ultrasound (localize pleural effusion)
- Perfusion lung scan (suspected embolism)
- Complete blood count
- Skin oxygen saturation
- Nutritional assessment

A complete history of the symptom, including its temporal onset (acute or chronic), aggravating and alleviating factors, qualities or word descriptors offered by the patient, effect of medications, past history of smoking, and chronic pulmonary or cardiac disease should be documented. A physical examination should follow the medical history to assess for potential indirect causes. Laboratory studies are used to detect blood abnormalities that can contribute to gas exchange problems, such as anemia. Radiological examinations show abnormalities that can possibly explain dyspnea. Pulse oximetry to assess for hypoxia is also important. However, its continued use is considered of limited value in advanced disease because it will unlikely result in changes to the clinical management (Thomas & von Gunten, 2003).

Dyspnea Perception

According to Gift (1990), the patient's perception of breathing discomfort and his or her thought processes regarding the meaning of breathlessness are important components of the dyspnea experience. Symptom perception is an attribution process that incorporates ways in which persons identify and evaluate symptoms and makes interpretations about their causes and consequences (ATS, 1999). A cognitive-psychological view of symptoms as an outcome of perceptual processes has replaced traditional views of symptoms as a direct outcome of biological processes (Dodd, et al., 2001; Teel, Meek, McNamara, & Watson, 1997). Patients' own thoughts and beliefs about symptoms (illness representation) may contribute to the meaning of symptoms (Donovan & Ward, 2001; Wenger, 1993; Turk & Okifuji, 2001). Questions that can be used to understand breathlessness perception from a patient-centered perspective are summarized in Table 10–3.

Table 10–3 Patient-Centered Assessment Questions

- What is being breathless like for you?
- What makes you feel less or more breathless?
- What does it feel like (meaning)?
- How does being breathless affect your life?
- What do you do to manage or cope with breathlessness?

Dyspnea Distress

The distress component involves the psychological or emotional aspects of dyspnea (Gift, 1990). A patient's interpretation of symptoms in the context of their illness experience (Downe-Wamboldt, Butler, & Coulter, 2006; Sarna, et al., 2005; Farncombe, 1997) and emotional distress can modify dyspnea perception (Ripamonti & Bruera, 1997). Dyspnea symptom scales, such as the Memorial Symptom Assessment Scale, that capture both the intensity and perceived distress (affective response) are recommended (Portenoy, et al., 1994). Valid measures to assess depression and anxiety are also important given their significance in breathlessness. A short valid measure to assess anxiety and dyspnea in cancer populations, such as the Hospital Anxiety and Depression Scale (Zigmond & Snaith, 1983), is recommended. Self-report scales are best used in conjunction with qualitative methods, such as interviews, which may help to uncover the extent of patient and family psychosocial distress (Bausewein, Farguhar, Booth, Gysels, & Higginson, 2007).

Dyspnea Response

Responses to dyspnea are influenced by the coping style (emotion focused or problem-solving focused) and the patients' view of their resources to manage stressful situations as part of an appraisal process (Gift, 1990). Responses to symptoms include physiological, psychological, sociocultural, and behavioral components (Dodd, et al., 2001). The physiological and psychological responses specific to dyspnea were described earlier in the chapter. Behavioral responses to breathlessness are also very important because they can impact positively or negatively on well-being. In clinical practice, patients may describe not feeling confident to leave the house, or they may severely limit their activities so as not to trigger episodes of breathlessness. This response may occur because they have little understanding of strategies they can use to minimize dyspnea severity and distress (Carrieri & Janson-Bjerklie, 1986; Kitely & Fitch, 2006). They may also believe that they are unable to exert control over symptoms (Donovan & Ward, 2001).

Symptom Reporting

As noted by Gift (1990), societal norms derived from culture or ethnicity may influence reporting of symptoms and the descriptors used. This view is supported by Hood and Harwood (2004), who suggest that patients' reporting of symptoms may vary due to different meanings of words and numbers according to language and culture. Studies have shown that ethnic differences in the descriptors used to describe breathlessness differ between patients, providers, and different racial groups (Hardie, et al., 2000). Patients may also have difficulty making the abstract connection between a quantitative scale and the perception of breathlessness (Thomas & von Gunten, 2003). As noted by Thorne (1999), the current tradition of quantifying human experience, such as pain or distress, into numerical form may decontextualize the meaning of individual experience that is fundamental to understanding these responses.

Standardized Reporting and Measurement

Patient self-report is the only reliable indicator of dyspnea because reliable objective measures do not exist (ATS, 1999). Respiratory rate, oxygen saturation, and arterial blood gas values do not correlate nor measure dyspnea (Thomas & von Gunten, 2003). Although it is subjective, its effects on function and multiple domains of activities of daily living and quality of life are objectively observed and can be measured (Ahmedzai, 1998; O'Driscoll, et al., 1999). Tools with sound psychometric properties, if they are clinically relevant, are most appropriate. Bausewein and colleagues (2007), in a systematic review of breathlessness measurement, concluded that one scale could not capture the many effects of breathlessness on patients. Consequently, they recommended combining one-dimensional scales with breathlessness-specific and disease-specific multidimensional quality of life scales or a generic quality of life instrument. Psychometric properties for different instruments for assessment of dyspnea were also identified in a review conducted by the Oncology Nursing Society (Joyce & Beck, 2005).

One-Dimensional Measures

Single-dimension numeric, verbal, or visual analog scales (VAS) capture severity and distress of breathlessness while facilitating rapid screening for dyspnea (Ahmedzai, 1998). The most common VAS (see Figure 10–3) that measures dyspnea intensity can be found in the literature. One VAS has a 100 mm vertical line with opposing anchors, such as "no dyspnea" at one end to "dyspnea as bad as it can be" at the other end (Mancini & Body, 1999). Another VAS has used anchors of "not breathless at all" to "extremely

Figure 10–3 Breathlessness scales.

Please rate how breathless you have felt in the last 24 hours:

When your breathing has been at its best?	When your breathing has been at its worst?	In general, how much distress does your breathlessness cause you?
10 Extreme Breathlessness	**10** Extreme Breathlessness	**10** Extreme Distress
9	**9**	**9**
8	**8**	**8**
7	**7**	**7**
6	**6**	**6**
5	**5**	**5**
4	**4**	**4**
3	**3**	**3**
2	**2**	**2**
1 No Breathlessness	**1** No Breathlessness	**1** No Distress

Source: Courtesy of the Interactive Education Unit, The Institute of Cancer Research.

breathless" (Mahler, et al., 2004). The VAS-D is recommended for daily assessment of dyspnea intensity (Mancini & Body, 1999) and strongly correlates with verbal rating scales of dyspnea (Dudgeon, et al., 2001b).

Several other VASs are reported in clinical practice. The Borg Scale is a variant of the VAS and uses numbers anchored with corresponding text (Borg, 1976). Patients find this less abstract to interpret than numbers along a line or scale. Another VAS is the Oxygen Cost Diagram (OCD). This VAS rates activities and their corresponding oxygen requirements along a continuum with "sleeping" at the lower end of the scale to "brisk walking uphill" at the top end of the scale (McGavin, Artvinli, & Naoe, 1978). Disease-specific VASs, such as the Lung Cancer Symptom Scale (Hollen, Gralla, Kris, & Potanovich, 1993), have the advantage of capturing other common lung cancer symptoms, such as cough, hemoptysis, and insomnia, that usually cluster with dyspnea and influence distress (Gift, Jablonski, Stommel, & Given, 2004).

Multidimensional Dyspnea Scales

Several multidimensional dyspnea scales are available for clinicians to choose and utilize in practice. The Baseline Dyspnea Index (BDI) measures the impact of dyspnea on activities of daily living and magnitude of effort to perform activities (Mahler, et al., 2004). The Transitional Dyspnea Index (TDI) was developed to assess changes from a single point in time (baseline) score obtained in the BDI. Both scales have demonstrated sensitivity to a range of clinical interventions (Mancini & Body, 1999). Shuttle walking tests (Booth & Adams, 2001) or the 6-minute walk test (Woo, 2000) are also useful measures of functional capacity.

Comprehensive multidimensional respiratory assessment instruments specific to breathlessness have also been developed. The University of California at San Diego's instrument, entitled the Shortness of Breath Questionnaire (SOBQ), asks patients to rate dyspnea during the past week on a six-point scale while performing different activities (Eakin, Resnikoff, Prewitt, Reis, & Kaplan, 1998). The Breathlessness Assessment Guide (Corner & O'Driscoll, 1999) is another comprehensive multidimensional assessment tool specific to dyspnea. However, its psychometric properties have not yet been evaluated.

Other commonly used generic quality of life multidimensional instruments for respiratory problems are: the American Thoracic Society Standardized Questionnaire (ATS-DLD-78) (American Thoracic Society, 1978); the Chronic Respiratory Disease Questionnaire (CRQ) (Guyatt, Berman, Townsend, Pugsley, & Chambers, 1987); and the St. George's Respiratory Questionnaire (SGRQ) (Jones, Quirk, Baveystock, & Littlejohns, 1992). Lung-cancer-specific quality of life measures, such as the Lung Cancer Symptom Scale (LCSS), which includes nine items for self-report of symptoms and quality of life (Hollen, et al., 1993), may also be important to capture the multidimensional impact of breathlessness.

Management of Breathlessness

Physical causes of breathlessness are rarely separable from the complex interplay between the psychological, social, emotional, spiritual, and functional dimensions of "total dyspnea" (Ahmedzai, 1998; O'Driscoll, et al., 1999). Consequently, strategies to manage breathlessness should be based on an understanding of the inseparability of the physical and psychological aspects of breathlessness as denoted by Corner and colleagues (1995) in Figure 10–4. This model emphasizes the need for an integrated biopsychosocial approach to breathlessness management. Biopsychosocial approaches emphasize the affective and other psychological states of the patient as a human person, as well as the significant relationships that surround the person, not just the biological basis of patient problems (Engel, 1997). While the empirical evidence is presented here for singular strategies, it is imperative that they are combined based on a biopsychosocial management approach and a patient-centered perspective to be most effective.

Figure 10–4 The integrated model of breathlessness scales.

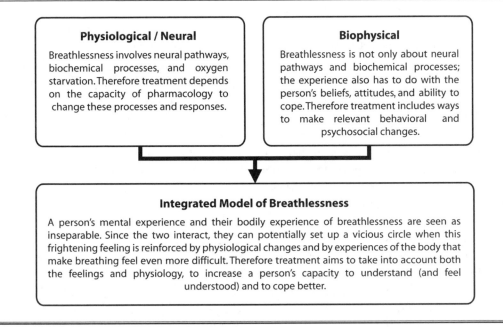

Physiological / Neural

Breathlessness involves neural pathways, biochemical processes, and oxygen starvation. Therefore treatment depends on the capacity of pharmacology to change these processes and responses.

Biophysical

Breathlessness is not only about neural pathways and biochemical processes; the experience also has to do with the person's beliefs, attitudes, and ability to cope. Therefore treatment includes ways to make relevant behavioral and psychosocial changes.

Integrated Model of Breathlessness

A person's mental experience and their bodily experience of breathlessness are seen as inseparable. Since the two interact, they can potentially set up a vicious circle when this frightening feeling is reinforced by physiological changes and by experiences of the body that make breathing feel even more difficult. Therefore treatment aims to take into account both the feelings and physiology, to increase a person's capacity to understand (and feel understood) and to cope better.

Source: Adapted from the *International Journal of Palliative Nursing* 1995, 1(1). Corner, Plant, & Warner, "Developing a Nursing Approach to Managing Dyspnea in Lung Cancer," 5–11. Reprinted courtesy of the Interactive Education Unit, The Institute of Cancer Research.

Biomedical Strategies

A number of general principles should be followed prior to the selection of biomedical management strategies (Ahmedzai, 1998). First, determine and treat the underlying cause(s). Second, do not add new problems to the experience of breathlessness, for example, medication side effects or social or financial burden. Third, consider if the treatment is worthwhile and feasible for patients. Finally, discuss all reasonable treatment options with the patient and family.

Biomedical strategies based on these principles emphasize: (1) tumor reduction with radiotherapy and chemotherapy, depending on tumor responsiveness and stage of disease; (2) treatment of disease complications, such as pleural or pericardial effusions or pneumonias if appropriate to prognosis; and (3) pharmacologic measures to reduce the effects of underlying comorbidities, such as chronic obstructive pulmonary disease (Ahnedzai, 1998; Houlihan, Inzeo, Joyce, & Tyson, 2004) or using short- or long-acting bronchodilators (Dudgeon & Rosenthal, 2000). Temporary control of dyspnea can often be achieved by managing underlying causes, such as pulmonary infection, chronic pulmonary disease, congestive heart failure, arrhythmias, atelectasis, and effusions (Jennings, Davies, Higgins, Gibbs, & Broadley, 2002).

Pharmacologic Measures

Pharmacologic measures are targeted to treatment of underlying causes of dyspnea or to reduce the sensation of breathlessness by altering the central perception of dyspnea. In advanced stages of lung cancer when dyspnea is likely to be moderate to severe, pharmacologic agents usually include opiates to reduce breathlessness perception, anxiolytics to reduce anxiety or associated panic symptoms, or corticosteroids to reduce inflammatory processes that induce dyspnea.

Opioids are first-line therapy for symptomatic control of dyspnea (Prommer & Casciato, 2004; Thomas & von Gunten, 2003) even though the mechanism by which they relieve dyspnea is not well understood. A number of randomized trials (Abernethy, et al., 2003; Bruera, et al., 2003), systematic reviews (Viola, et al., 2008), and a meta-analysis of 13 trials (Jennings, et al., 2002) show a moderate effect of morphine on dyspnea. The optimal type, dose, and mode of administration of opioids are less clear, but doses as low as 5 mg of subcutaneous morphine have been shown to be effective for dyspnea control in opioid-naïve patients for about 4 hours (Mazzacato, Buclin, & Rapin, 1999). Increases of 25% in baseline doses of opioids usually improve relief for patients who are already receiving opioids (Allard, et al., 1999). Opioid administration guidelines are outlined in Table 10–4. Nebulized morphine has been shown to be ineffective in controlling dyspnea (Jennings, et al., 2002) despite the presence of opioid receptors throughout the bronchial tree, particularly in the alveolar walls (Zebraski, Kochenash, & Raffa, 2000).

While opioids can be utilized effectively, antianxiety medications have been shown in clinical practice to be helpful. Benzodiazepines,

Table 10–4 Opioid Therapy for Dyspnea

Opioid-naïve patients

Mild dyspnea
- Hydrocodone 5 mg PO q4h or codeine 30 mg PO q4h
- For breakthrough symptom management, give an equivalent dose q1–2h, as needed

Severe dyspnea
- Morphine sulfate 5 mg PO q4h, oxycodone 5 mg PO q4h, or hydromorphone 1 mg PO q4h
- For breakthrough symptom management, give an equivalent dose q1–2h, as needed
- Titrate up in increments of 50%–100% every 24 hours, as needed.
  Note: For patients with severe pulmonary disease, such as COPD, start at 50% of the above doses and titrate more conservatively, with increments of 25% every 24 hours, as needed.

Opioid-tolerant patients
Increase baseline opioid dose by 25%–50% and titrate as above.

Source: From *Journal of Supportive Oncology, Volume 1.* Thomas, J.R. & von Gunten, C.F. 23-24. Copyright Elsevier, 2003.

such as lorazepam and diazepam, are commonly used to treat dyspnea that is exacerbated by panic disorder or concurrent severe anxiety (Cowcher & Hanks, 1990; Dudgeon & Rosenthal, 2000). However, only one of five randomized controlled trials found significant benefit from these agents (Thomas & von Gunten, 2003). When patients are highly anxious, these agents may offer some benefit in inducing sedation and may provide temporary relief, allowing patients and families to rally their coping responses. Dosing guidelines for anxiolytics are summarized in Table 10–5.

Table 10–5 Anxiolytic Therapy for Dyspnea

Lorazepam
0.5–1 mg PO q1h until dyspnea is settled, then dose routinely q4–6h to keep settled

Diazepam
5–10 mg PO q1h until dyspnea is settled, then dose routinely q6–8h

Clonazepam
0.25–2 mg PO q12h

Midazolam
0.5 mg IV every 15 min until dyspnea is settled, then give by continuous SC or IV infusion

Source: From *Journal of Supportive Oncology, Volume 1.* Thomas, J.R. & von Gunten, C.F. 23-24. Copyright Elsevier, 2003.

Other medications, such as bronchodilators and corticosteroids, may also help in managing breathlessness. Bronchodilators are most useful for treating underlying COPD causes of breathlessness but are also used for symptomatic treatment of dyspnea (Dudgeon & Rosenthal, 2000). Corticosteroids may also play an important role in dyspnea management. Rapid responses from the administration of corticosteroids have helped patients with upper airway disease (Elsayem & Bruera, 2007). High-dose corticosteroids can relieve dyspnea that is caused by superior vena cava syndrome and inflammatory processes that are caused by radiation, chemotherapy, and chronic pulmonary disease (Le Grand & Walsh, 1999). Few controlled studies have been conducted in lung cancer dyspnea with corticosteroids, but doses of dexamethasone 4–8 mg twice daily have been recommended (Le Grand & Walsh, 1999; Rousseau, 1996).

Oxygen and Air

Pushed air through the use of fans can help alleviate dyspnea. Placing fans or having an open window reduces dyspnea through stimulation of mechanoreceptors on the face. Cool air reduces facial skin temperature, which alters afferent feedback to the brain and modifies the perception of dyspnea (Manning & Schwartzstein, 1998).

The role of oxygen in the management of dyspnea remains controversial except in patients with hypoxemia (Dudgeon, 2001; Thomas & von Gunten, 2003). In a systematic review, Qaseem et al. (2008) found only one study that showed better oxygen saturation, respiratory effort and rate, and relief of dyspnea with oxygen (Abernethy, et al., 2003). A second study showed no difference between oxygen and air on a 6-minute walking test (Bruera, et al., 2003). In a double-blind crossover trial of oxygen and air, both experimental and controls improved symptomatically (lower breathlessness severity scores), with no statistical difference between the two groups on severity (Philip, et al., 2006). In this study, hypoxia was not corrected even for those on oxygen. Additionally, oxygen may exert a placebo effect by altering the patient's perception that something can be done to control this devastating symptom.

Nonpharmacologic Measures

Nonpharmacologic interventions are recommended as an adjunct to dyspnea management (Corner, Plant, A'Hern, & Bailey, 1996). Many of these measures are based on their effectiveness in chronic obstructive pulmonary disease (ATS, 1999). There are many nonpharmacologic strategies that patients can employ. This can be as simple as breathing techniques to more complex measures. Many of these techniques are discussed later. Oncology nurses should take an active role in helping the patient to learn these interventions.

In a systematic review, Thompson et al. (2005) found evidence for effective nonpharmacologic interventions in reducing breathlessness as compared to standard care. Two pilot studies comprised of multisite trials (*n* = 143 patients) demonstrated statistically significant differences in breathlessness, improvement in functional status, and lower levels of symptom distress (Corner, et al., 1995; Bredin, et al., 1999). This complex tailored intervention, which was carried out by specialist nurses, was comprised of multiple components, as shown in Figure 10–5 (Bredin, et al., 1999). Empirical evidence in COPD and lung cancer supports the use of these as singular components, but when combined they have the potential to impact on cognitive, emotional, and physical factors, thus influencing dyspnea perception.

Figure 10–5 The intervention model for dyspnea.

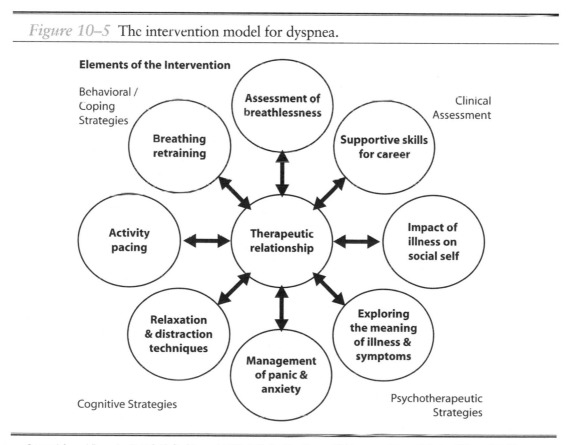

Source: Adapted from the *British Medical Journal* 1999, 318. Bredin, Corner, Krishnasamy, Plant, Bailey & A'Hern, "Multicentre Randomized Controlled Trial of Nursing Intervention for Breathlessness in Patients with Lung Cancer," 901–904. Reprinted courtesy of the Interactive Education Unit, The Institute of Cancer Research.

Breathing Techniques

Breathing techniques included in the Corner and colleagues (1995) intervention included pursed-lip breathing and diaphragmatic breathing, which are shown in COPD to be effective in decreasing the work of breathing (Jantarakupt & Porock, 2005). Pursed-lip breathing appears to work by slowing the respiratory rate and increasing intra-airway pressure that prevents the collapse of smaller airways (Thoman, Stoker, & Ross, 1966). Diaphragmatic breathing also helps the lungs to function more effectively and may promote relaxation (Gallo-Silver & Pollack, 2000). The efficacy of breathing techniques is highly variable across patients, and sustaining these skilled breathing techniques may be difficult (ATS, 1999), particularly at advanced stages of lung cancer. Therefore, simple positioning techniques, such as leaning over a bedside table to support the upper arms, can be helpful (Banzett, Lansing, & Brown, 1987).

Exercise Training

Patients often experience muscle deconditioning due to avoidance of activities that trigger breathlessness. However, exercise may be helpful to a lung cancer patient. Most of the studies about exercise training that have shown benefits are in the COPD population. Randomized trials in COPD have shown improvements in dyspnea, forced vital capacity, and exercise capacity after training (O'Donnell, McGuire, Semis, & Webb, 1995). Most of the programs that showed benefits combined weight training of upper and lower extremities and walking (Reis, Kaplan, Limberg, & Prewitt, 1995). Studies suggest that exercise training at least twice a week for 8 consecutive weeks is effective in improving physical endurance and reducing dys-

pnea in patients with COPD (ATS, 1999). Significant improvements were also noted in functional and peak exercise capacity in lung cancer patients following a standardized exercise program (Spruit, Janssen, Willemsen, Hochstenbag, & Wouters, 2006). The intervention in the study was comprised of cycling on stationary bikes for 20 minutes, treadmill walking for 20 minutes, weight training for upper and lower extremities, and stretching exercises. Because a patient's tolerance of exercise may vary according to factors such as disease stage, the appropriate level of intervention is best tailored to the individual patient.

Supportive Care and Psychological Interventions

Emotional support and counseling by specialized cancer nurses may also help improve distress of symptoms and promote a patient's sense of control. Nurse-led follow-up programs that incorporated specialized oncology nurses to deliver education and psychosocial support delayed an increase in symptom distress by about 6 weeks in lung cancer patients who were followed at home (McCorkle, et al., 1989). Significant improvements in breathlessness were also demonstrated in a nurse-led follow-up clinic compared to a standard care group (Moore, et al., 2002). Other specialized interventions that may alter central perception of breathlessness may also be effective in management of breathlessness. These are described in the following sections.

Cognitive-Behavioral Interventions

Dyspnea has cognitive and emotional components that contribute to dyspnea severity and distress. Cognitive-behavioral strategies modulate the effects of cognitive, emotional, and behavioral factors on conscious awareness of the demand to breathe, subsequently influencing the affective response to dyspnea (ATS, 1999). Cognitive strategies are designed to alter the patients' beliefs about symptoms and their view of being unable to exert control over symptoms. These interventions combine education and goal setting with active problem solving to increase patients' coping and self-management of symptoms. These strategies may also improve an individual's confidence in his or her ability to manage the consequences of dyspnea (Smoller, Polack, Otto, Rosenbaum, & Kradin, 1996).

Relaxation Therapy and Guided Imagery

Controlled breathing and other relaxation measures may help patients control dyspnea and decrease anxiety, thereby preventing emotional escalation of dyspnea (Cowcher & Hanks, 1990; Wickham, 1996). Guided imagery (Moody & McMillan, 2003) and relaxation has been found to be effective in COPD patients to reduce anxiety and the perception of dyspnea (Devine, 1996; Gift, Moore, & Soeken, 1992). These strategies may help to manage symptoms of panic that can be triggered in patients who are experiencing shortness of breath. Calming measures, such as relaxation breathing, controlled breathing (such as pursed-lip or diaphragmatic breathing), and thought stopping, may all be helpful to address panic breathing (Nathan, Corey, & Lim, 2004).

Psychoeducational Interventions

Psychoeducational interventions that provide information to patients about symptoms while building coping skills are effective in reducing emotional distress (Bottomley, 1997). These approaches may improve a patient's ability to cope with illness when combined with focused self-management strategies to manage breathlessness. The use of these interventions has not been examined for lung cancer dyspnea specifically. Psychotherapy combined with pharmacologic interventions by a psychiatrist or psychologist, depending on the stage of the disease, may be appropriate to manage anxiety and dyspnea.

Self-Management Interventions

Self-management education and support to improve knowledge and skills to manage illness are most effective if families are included in the learning process (Gibson, et al., 2003). Patients learn self-care management strategies through trial and error and may lack the comprehensive information necessary to minimize the impact of dyspnea (Carrieri & Janson-Bjerklie, 1986).

Behavioral changes that are necessary to improve self-management are seldom accomplished through educational programs alone. Self-management programs in chronic illness that are intensive and interactive, train patients to monitor themselves, and use patient-adjustable written action plans are shown to improve coping, symptom management, and overall quality of life and may be applicable to lung cancer (Lorig & Holman, 2003).

Conclusion

Dyspnea is a complex, multidimensional symptom that is devastating to individuals with lung cancer. A biopsychosocial intervention approach that targets the interrelated physical, psychological, social, environmental, and functional factors of both dyspnea sensation and perception is critical to its effective management. A patient-centered approach that addresses these multi-dimensional causes and the meaning of the symptom based on a patient-centered perspective has the greatest potential for reducing symptom suffering and optimizing quality of life.

References

Abernethy, A., Currow, D. C., Frith, P., Fazekas, B., McHugh, A., & Bui, C. (2003). Randomised double blind, placebo controlled crossover trial of sustained release morphine for the management of refractory dyspnea. *British Medical Journal, 327*(7414), 523–528.

Ahmedzai, S. (1998). Palliation of respiratory symptoms. In D. Doyle, G. W. C. Hanks, & N. MacDonald (Eds.), *Oxford textbook of palliative medicine* (2nd ed., pp. 583–616). London: Oxford Medical Publications.

Allard, P., Lamontagne, C., Bernard, P., & Tremblay, C. (1999). How effective are supplementary doses of opioids for dyspnea in terminally ill cancer patients? A randomized continuous sequential clinical trial. *Journal of Pain and Symptom Management, 17*(4), 256–265.

American Thoracic Society (ATS). (1978). Recommended respiratory disease questionnaires for use with adults and children in epidemiological research. *American Review Respiratory Disease, 14*, 7–53.

American Thoracic Society (ATS). (1999). Dyspnea: Mechanisms, assessment, and management: A consensus statement. *American Journal of Respiratory and Critical Care Medicine, 159*, 321–340.

American Thoracic Society (ATS). (2005). American Thoracic Society/European Respiratory Society statement on pulmonary rehabilitation. Retrieved October 1, 2008, from http://ajrccm.atsjournals.org/cgi/content/full/173/12/1390

Bailey, C. (1995). Nursing as therapy in the management of breathlessness in lung cancer. *European Journal of Cancer Care, 4*(4), 184–190.

Banzett, R. B., Lansing, R. W., & Brown, R. (1987). High-level quadriplegics perceive lung volume change. *Journal of Applied Physiology, 62*(2), 567–573.

Bausewein, C., Farguhar, M., Booth, S., Gysels, M., & Higginson, I. J. (2007). Measurement of breathlessness in advanced disease: A systematic review. *Respiratory Medicine, 101*(3), 399–410.

Booth, S., & Adams, L. (2001). The shuttle walking test: A reproducible method for evaluating the impact of shortness of breath on functional capacity in patients with advanced cancer. *Thorax, 56*(2), 146–150.

Borg, G. (1976). Simple rating methods for estimation of perceived exertion. *Wenner-Gren Center International Symposium Series 28*, 39–47.

Bottomley, A. (1997). Where are we now? Evaluating two decades of group interventions with adult cancer patients. *Journal of Psychiatric Mental Health Nursing, 4*(4), 251–265.

Brazil, K., Howell, D., Bedard, M., Krueger, P., & Heidebrecht, C. (2005). Preferences for place of care and place of death among informal caregivers of the terminally ill. *Palliative Medicine, 19*(6), 492–499.

Bredin, M., Corner, J., Krishnasamy, M., Plant, H., Bailey, C., & A'Hern, R. (1999). Multicentre randomized controlled trial of a nursing intervention for breathlessness in patients with lung cancer. *British Medical Journal, 318*(7188), 901–904.

Brown, M. L., Carrieri, V. K., Janson-Bjerklie, S., & Dodd, M. (1986). Lung cancer and dyspnea: The patient's perception. *Oncology Nursing Forum, 13*(5), 19–24.

Bruera, E., & Neumann, C. M. (1998). Management of specific symptom complexes in patients receiving palliative care. *Canadian Medical Association Journal, 158*(13), 1717–1726.

Bruera, E., Schmitz, B., Pither, J., Neumann, C. M., & Hanson, J. (2000). The frequency and correlates of dyspnea in patients with advanced cancer. *Journal of Pain and Symptom Management, 19*(5), 357–362.

Bruera, E., Sweeney, C., Willey, J., Palmer, J. L., Strasser, F., Morice, R. C., et al. (2003). A randomized control trial of supplemental oxygen versus air in cancer patients with dyspnea. *Palliative Medicine, 17*(8), 659–663.

Campbell, E. J. M., & Howell, J. B. L. (1963). The sensation of breathlessness. *British Medical Bulletin, 19*(1), 36–40.

Carrieri, V. K., & Janson-Bjerklie, S. (1986). Strategies patients use to manage the sensation of dyspnea. *Western Journal of Nursing Research, 8*(3), 284–305.

Cherniack, N. S, & Altrose, M. D. (1987). Mechanisms of dyspnea. *Clinical Chest Medicine, 8*(2), 207–214.

Cooley, M. E., Short, T. H., & Moriarty, H. J. (2002). Patterns of symptom distress in adults receiving treatment for lung cancer. *Journal of Palliative Care, 18*(3), 150–159.

Corner, J., & O'Driscoll, M. (1999). Development of a breathlessness assessment guide for use in palliative care. *Palliative Medicine, 13*(5), 375–384.

Corner, J., Plant, H., A'Hern, R., & Bailey, C. (1996). Non-pharmacological interventions for breathlessness in lung cancer. *Palliative Medicine, 10*(4), 229–305.

Corner, J., Plant, H., & Warner, L. (1995). Developing a nursing approach to managing dyspnea in lung cancer. *International Journal of Palliative Nursing, 1*(1), 5–11.

Cowcher, K., & Hanks, G. (1990). Long term management of respiratory symptoms in advanced cancer. *Journal of Pain and Symptom Management, 5*(5), 320–330.

Derby, S., & O'Mahony, S. (2001). Elderly patients. In B. R. Ferrell & N. Coyle (Eds.), *Textbook of palliative nursing* (pp. 435–449). New York: Oxford University Press.

Devine, E. C. (1996). Meta-analysis of the effects of psychoeducational care on patients in adults with asthma. *Respiratory Nursing Health, 19*(5), 367–376.

Dodd, M., Jansen, S., Facione, N., Faucett, J., Frolicher, J., Humphreys, J., et al. (2001). Advancing the science of symptom management. *Journal of Advanced Nursing, 33*(5), 668–676.

Donovan, H. S., & Ward, S. (2001). A representational approach to patient education. *Journal of Nursing Scholarship, 33*(3), 211–216.

Downe-Wamboldt, B., Butler, L., & Coulter, L. (2006). The relationship between meaning of illness, social support, coping strategies and quality of life of lung cancer patients and their family members. *Cancer Nursing, 29*(2), 111–119.

Dudgeon, D. (2001). Dyspnea, death rattle and cough. In B. R. Ferrell & N. Coyle (Eds.), *Textbook of palliative nursing* (pp. 20–38). New York: Oxford University Press.

Dudgeon, D. (2002). Managing dyspnea and cough. *Hematology/Oncology Clinics of North America, 16*(3), 557–577.

Dudgeon, D., & Lertzman, M. (1998). Dyspnea in the advanced cancer patient. *Journal of Pain and Symptom Management, 16*(4), 212–219.

Dudgeon, D., & Rosenthal, S. (2000). Pathophysiology and assessment of dyspnea in the patient with cancer. In R. K. Portenoy & E. Bruera (Eds.), *Topics in palliative care* (pp. 237–254). New York: Oxford University Press.

Dudgeon, D. J., Kristjanson, L., Sloan, J. A., Lertzman, M., & Clement, K. (2001a). Dyspnea in cancer patients: Prevalence and associated factors. *Journal of Pain and Symptom Management, 21*(2), 95–102.

Dudgeon, D. J., Lertzman, M., & Askew, G. R. (2001b). Physiological changes and clinical correlates of dyspnea. *Journal of Pain and Symptom Management, 21*(5), 373–379.

Eakin, E. G., Resnikoff, P. M., Prewitt, L. M., Reis, A. L., & Kaplan, R. M. (1998). Validation of a new dyspnea measure: The UCSD Shortness of Breath Questionnaire. University of Southern California, San Diego. *Chest, 113*(3), 625–632.

Elsayem, A., & Bruera, E. (2007). High-dose corticosteroids for the management of dyspnea in patients with tumor obstruction of the upper airway. *Supportive Care in Cancer, 15*(12), 1437–1439.

Engel, G. L. (1997). The need for a new medical model: A challenge for biomedicine. *Science, 196*(4286), 129–136.

Escalante, C., Martin, C., Elting, L., Cantor, S., Harle, T., Price, K., et al. (1996). Dyspnea in cancer patients. *Cancer, 78*(6), 1314–1319.

Estenne, M., Ninane, V., & De Troyer, A. (1988). Triangularis sterni muscle use during eupnea in humans: Effect of posture. *Respiratory Physiology, 74*(2), 151–162.

Farncombe, M. (1997). Dyspnea assessment and treatment. *Supportive Care in Cancer, 5*(2), 94–99.

Gallo-Silver, L., & Pollack, B. (2000). Behavioral interventions for lung cancer related breathlessness. *Cancer Practice, 8*(6), 268–273.

Gibson, P., Powell, H., Coughlan, J., Wilson, A., Abramson, M., Haywood, P., et al. (2003). Self management education and regular practitioner review for adults with asthma. *Cochrane Database of Systematic Reviews,* CD001117. DOI 10/1002/14651858.CD001117.

Gift, A., Moore, T., & Soeken, K. (1992). Relaxation to reduce dyspnea and anxiety in COPD patients. *Nursing Research, 41*(4), 242–246.

Gift, A. G. (1990). Dyspnea. *Nursing Clinics of North America, 25*(4), 955–965.

Gift, A. G., Jablonski, A., Stommel, M., & Given, W. (2004). Symptom clusters in elderly patients with lung cancer. *Oncology Nursing Forum, 31*(2), 203–210.

Guyatt, G. H., Berman, L. B., Townsend, M., Pugsley, S. O., & Chambers, L. W. (1987). A measure of quality of life for clinical trials in chronic lung disease. *Thorax, 42*(10), 773–778.

Guyton, A. C. (1986). *Textbook of medical physiology.* Philadelphia: W. B. Saunders.

Hardie, G. E., Janson, S., Gold, W., Carrieri-Kohlmann, V., & Boushey, H. (2000). Ethnic differences: Word descriptors used by African-American and white asthma patients during induced bronchoconstriction. *Chest, 117*(4), 935–943.

Heedman, P. A., & Strang, P. (2001). Symptom assessment in advanced palliative home care for cancer patients using the ESAS: Clinical aspects. *Anticancer Research, 21*(6A), 4077–4082.

Hollen, P. J., Gralla, R. J, Kris, M. G., Eberly, S., & Cox, C. (1999). Normative data and trends in quality of life from the Lung Cancer Symptom Scale (LCSS). *Supportive Care Cancer, 7*(3), 140–148.

Hollen, P. J., Gralla, R. J., Kris, M. G., & Potanovich, L. M. (1993). Quality of life assessment in individuals with lung cancer: Testing the Lung Cancer Symptom Scale (LCSS). *European Journal of Cancer, 29A*(Suppl. 1), S51–S58.

Hood, L. E., & Harwood, K. V. (2004). Dyspnea. In C. H. Yarbro, M. H. Frogge, & M. Goodman (Eds.), *Cancer symptom management* (3rd ed., pp. 100–150). Sudbury, MA: Jones and Bartlett.

Houlihan, N., Inzeo, D., Joyce, M., & Tyson, L. (2004). Symptom management of lung cancer. *Clinical Journal of Oncology Nursing, 8*(6), 645–652.

Howell, D., Fitch, M., & Velgi, K. (in press). A therapeutic nursing approach to breathlessness in lung cancer. *Canadian Oncology Nursing Journal.*

Interview with Deborah Dudgeon. (2006). Dyspnea in cancer patients needs more attention. *Supportive Care in Oncology, 4*(2), 63–64.

Jantarakupt, P., & Porock, D. (2005). Dyspnea management in lung cancer: Applying the evidence from chronic obstructive pulmonary disease. *Oncology Nursing Forum, 32*(4), 785–795.

Jennings, A. L., Davies, A. N., Higgins, J. P., Gibbs, J. S., & Broadley, K. E. (2002). A systematic review of the use of opioids in the management of dyspnea. *Thorax, 57*(11), 939–944.

Jones, P., Quirk, F., Baveystock, C., & Littlejohns, P. (1992). A self-complete measure of health status for chronic airflow limitation: The St. George's Respiratory Questionnaire. *The American Review of Respiratory Disease, 145*(6), 1321–1327.

Joyce, M., & Beck, S. L. (2005, April 13). Measuring oncology nursing-sensitive patient outcomes: Evidence-based summary. *Oncology Nursing Society.* Retrieved on October 22, 2008, from www.ons.org

Kellner, R., Samet, J., & Pathak, D. (1992). Dyspnea, anxiety, and depression in chronic respiratory impairment. *General Hospital Psychiatry, 14*(1), 20–28.

Kitely, C. A., & Fitch, M. (2006). Understanding the symptoms experienced by individuals with lung cancer. *Canadian Oncology Nursing Journal, 16*(1), 25–30.

Krishnasamy, M., Corner, J., Bredin, M., Plant, H., & Bailey, C. (2001). Cancer nursing practice development: Understanding breathlessness. *Journal of Clinical Nursing, 10*(1), 103–108.

Kurtz, M. E., Kurtz, J. C., Stommel, M., Given, C. W., & Given, B. A. (2000). Symptomatology and loss of physical functioning among geriatric patients with lung cancer. *Journal of Pain and Symptom Management, 19*(4), 249–256.

Lavoie, E. L., Hann, D. M., Ahles, T., Furstenberg, C. T., Mitchell, T. A., Meyer, L., et al. (2001). Dyspnea, anxiety, body consciousness and quality of life in patients with lung cancer. *Journal of Pain Symptom Management, 21*(4), 323–326.

Le Grand, S. B., & Walsh, D. (1999). Palliative management of dyspnea in advanced cancer. *Current Opinion in Oncology, 11*(4), 250–254.

Lorig, K. R., & Holman, H. (2003). Self-management education: History, definition, outcomes and mechanisms. *Annals of Behavioural Medicine, 26*(1), 1–7.

Lynn, J., Schuster, J. L., & Kabacenell, A. (2000). *Improving care for the end-of-life: A sourcebook for health care managers and clinicians.* New York: Oxford University Press.

Mahler, D. A., Ward, J., Fierro-Carrion, G., Waterman, L. A., Lentine, T., Mejia-Alfaro, R., et al. (2004). Development of self-administered versions of modified baseline and transitional dyspnea indexes in COPD. *Journal of COPD, 1*(2), 156–172.

Mancini, I., & Body, J. J. (1999). Assessment of dyspnea in advanced cancer patients. *Supportive Care in Cancer, 7*(4), 229–232.

Manning, H. L., & Schwartzstein, R. M. (1998). Mechanisms of dyspnea. In D. A. Mahler (Ed.), *Dyspnea* (pp. 63–95). New York: Marcel Dekker.

Mazzacato, C., Buclin, T., & Rapin, C. H. (1999). The effects of morphine on dyspnea and ventilatory function in patients with advanced cancer: A randomized double-blind controlled trial. *Annals of Oncology, 10*(12), 1511–1514.

McCarley, C. (1999). A model of chronic dyspnea. *Image: The Journal of Nursing Scholarship, 31*(3), 231–236.

McCloskey, D. I. (1978). Kinesthetic sensibility. *Physiology Review, 58*(4), 763–820.

McCorkle, R., Benoliel, J. Q., Donaldson, G., Georgiadou, F., Moinpour, C., & Goodell, B. (1989). A randomized clinical trial of home nursing care for lung cancer patients. *Cancer, 64*(6), 1375–1382.

McDermott, M. K. (2000). Dyspnea. In D. Camp-Sorrell & R. A. Hawkins (Eds.), *Advanced nursing practice* (pp. 131–135). Pittsburgh: Oncology Nursing Society.

McGavin, C. R., Artvinli, M., & Naoe, H. (1978). Dyspnea, disability and distance walked: Comparison of estimates of exercise performance in respiratory disease. *British Medical Journal, 2*(6132), 241–243.

Moody, L. E., & McMillan, S. (2003). Dyspnea and quality of life indicators in hospice patients and their caregivers. *Health and Quality of Life Outcomes, 1*(1), 9.

Moore, S., Corner, J., Haviland, J., Wells, M., Salmon, E., Normand, C., et al. (2002). Nurse led follow-up and conventional medical follow-up of patients with lung cancer: Randomized trial. *British Medical Journal, 325*(7373), 1145–1151.

Morel, D. R., Forster, A., Bachman, M., & Suter, P. M. (1984). Effect of intravenous midazolam on breathing pattern and chest wall mechanics in humans. *Journal of Applied Physiology, 57*(4), 1104–1110.

Nathan, P., Corey, H., & Lim, L. (2004). *Panic stations! Coping with panic attacks.* Perth, Australia: Centre for Clinical Interventions.

O'Donnell, D. E., McGuire, L., Semis, L., & Webb, K. A. (1995). The impact of exercise reconditioning on breathlessness in severe chronic airflow limitation. *American Journal of Respiratory Critical Care Medicine, 152*(6), 2005–2013.

O'Driscoll, M., Corner, J., & Bailey, C. (1999). The experience of breathlessness in lung cancer. *European Journal of Cancer Care, 8*(1), 37–43.

O'Neill, E. S. (2002). Illness representations and coping of women with chronic obstructive pulmonary disease: A pilot study. *Heart and Lung, 31*(4), 295–301.

Paintal, A. S. (1983). Lung and airway receptors. In D. J. Pallot (Ed.), *Control of respiration* (p. 78). London: Croom Helm.

Philip, J., Gold, M., Milner, A., Di Iulio, J., Miller, B., & Spruyt, O. (2006). A randomized double-blind, crossover trial on the effect of oxygen on dyspnea in patients with advanced cancer. *Journal of Pain and Symptom Management, 32*(6), 541–550.

Portenoy, R. K., Thaler, H. T., Kornblith, A. B., Lepore, J. M., Friedlander-Klar, H., Coyle, N., et al. (1994). Symptom prevalence, characteristics and distress in a cancer population. *Quality of Life Research, 3*(3), 183–189.

Prommer E. E., & Casciato, D. A. (2004). Supportive care. In D. A. Casciato (Ed.), *Manual of Clinical Oncology.* (pp. 102–130). Philadelphia: Lippincott Williams & Wilkins.

Qaseem, A., Snow, V., Shekelle, P., Casey, D., Cross, T. J., & Owens, D. K. (2008). Evidence-based interventions to improve palliative care of pain, dyspnea, and depression at the end of life: A clinical practice guideline from the American College of Physicians. *Annals of Internal Medicine, 148*(2), 141–149.

Quinn, S. (1999). Lung cancer: The role of the nurse in treatment and prevention. *Nursing Standards, 13*(41), 49–54.

Reis, A., Kaplan, R., Limberg, T., & Prewitt, L. (1995). Effects of pulmonary rehabilitation on physiologic and psychosocial outcomes in patients with chronic obstructive pulmonary disease. *Annals of Internal Medicine, 122*(11), 823–832.

Ripamonti, C., & Bruera, E. (1997). Dyspnea: Pathophysiology and assessment. *Journal of Pain and Symptom Management, 13*(4), 220–232.

Rousseau, P. (1996). Non-pain symptom management in terminal care. *Clinics in Geriatric Medicine, 12*(2), 313–327.

Sarna, L., & Brecht, M. L. (1997). Dimensions of symptom distress in women with advanced lung cancer: A factor analysis. *Heart and Lung, 26*(1), 23–30.

Sarna, L., Brown, J. K., Cooley, M. E., Williams, R. D., Chernecky, C., Padilla, G., et al. (2005). Quality of life and meaning of illness of women with lung cancer. *Oncology Nursing Forum, 32*(1), 9–19.

Sarna, L., Evangelista, L., Tashkin, D., Padilla, G., Holmes, M., Brecht, M. L., et al. (2004). Impact of respiratory symptoms on quality of life of long-term survivors of non-small cell lung cancer. *Chest, 125*(2), 439–450.

Simon, P. M., Basner, R. C, Weinberger, S. E., Fenci, V., Weiss, J. W., & Schartzstein, R. M. (1991). Oral mucosa stimulation modulates intensity of breathlessness induced in normal subjects. *American Review of Respiratory Disease, 144*(2), 419–422.

Skaug, K., Eide, G. E., & Gulsvik, A. (2007). Prevalence and predictors of symptoms in the terminal stage of lung cancer: A community study. *American College of Chest Physicians, 131*(2), 389–394.

Smoller, J. W., Polack, M. H., Otto, M. W., Rosenbaum, J. F., & Kradin, R. L. (1996). State of the art: Panic anxiety, dyspnea and respiratory disease. *American Journal of Respiratory Critical Care Medicine, 154*(1), 6–17.

Spruit, M. A., Janssen, P. P., Willemsen, S. C. P., Hochstenbag, M. H., & Wouters, E. F. M. (2006). Exercise capacity before and after an 8-week multi-disciplinary inpatient rehabilitation program in lung cancer patients: A pilot study. *Lung Cancer, 52*(2), 257–260.

Stover, D. E., & Kaner, R. J. (2001). Pulmonary toxicity. In V. T. Devita, S. H. Hellman, & S. A. Rosenberg (Eds.), *Cancer: Principles and practice of oncology* (6th ed., pp. 2894–2904). Philadelphia: Lippincott Williams & Wilkins.

Tanaka, K., Akechi, T., Okuyama, T., Nishiwaki, Y., & Uchitomi, Y. (2002). Factors correlated with dyspnea in advanced lung cancer patients: Organic causes and what else? *Journal of Pain and Symptom Management, 23*(6), 490–500.

Tarzian, A. J. (2000). Caring for dying patients who have air hunger. *Journal of Nursing Scholarship, 32*(2), 137–143.

Teel, C. S., Meek, P., McNamara, A. M., & Watson, L. (1997). Perspectives unifying symptom interpretation. *Image, 29*(2), 175–181.

Thoman, R. L., Stoker, G. L., & Ross, J. C. (1966). The efficacy of pursed-lips breathing in patients with chronic obstructive pulmonary disease. *American Review of Respiratory Disease, 93*(1), 100–106.

Thomas, J., & von Gunten, C. F. (2003). Management of dyspnea. *The Journal of Supportive Oncology, 1*(1), 23–33.

Thompson, E., Sola, I., & Subirana, M. (2005). Non-invasive interventions for improving well-being and quality of life in patients with lung cancer: A systematic review of the evidence. *Lung Cancer, 50*(2), 163–176.

Thorne, S. E. (1999). The science of meaning in chronic illness. *International Journal of Nursing Studies, 36*(5), 397–404.

Tishelman, C., Degner, L. F., & Mueller, B. (2000). Measuring symptom distress in patients with lung cancer: A pilot study of experienced intensity and importance of symptoms. *Cancer Nursing, 23*(3), 82–90.

Travers, J., Dudgeon, D. J., Amjadi, K., McBride, I., Dillon, K., Laveneziana, P., et al. (2007). Mechanisms of exertional dyspnea in patients with cancer. *Journal of Applied Physiology, 104*(1), 57–66.

Turk, D. C., & Okifuji, A. (2001). Psychological factors in chronic pain: Evolution and revolution. *Journal of Consulting Clinical Psychology, 70*(3), 678–690.

Viola, R., Kitely, C., Lloyd, N. S., Mackay, J. A., Wilson, J., & Wong, R. K. (2008). The management of dyspnea in cancer patients: A systematic review. *Supportive Care in Cancer, 16*(4), 329–337.

von Leupoldt, A., Mertz, C., Kegat, S., Burmester, S., & Dahme, B. (2006). The impact of emotions on the sensory and affective dimension of perceived dyspnea. *Psychophysiology, 43*(4), 382–386.

Wenger, A. F. Z. (1993). Cultural meaning of symptoms. *Holistic Nurse Practitioner, 7*(2), 22–35.

Whipp, B. J. (1987). *The control of breathing in man.* Manchester, UK: Manchester University Press.

Wickham, R. S. (1996). Managing dypsnea in cancer patients. *Development in Supportive Cancer Care, 2*(2), 33–40.

Woo, K. (2000). A pilot study to examine the relationships of dyspnea, physical activity, and fatigue in patients with chronic obstructive pulmonary disease. *Journal of Clinical Nursing, 9*(4), 526–533.

Zebraski, S. E., Kochenash, S. M., & Raffa, R. B. (2000). Lung opioid receptors: Pharmacology and possible targets for nebulized morphine in dyspnea. *Life Sciences, 66*(23), 2221–2231.

Zigmond, A. S., & Snaith, R. P. (1983). The Hospital Anxiety and Depression Scale. *Acta Psychiatrica Scandinavica, 67*(6), 361–370.

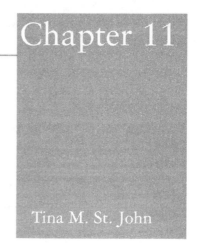

Chapter 11

Environmental Risk: Indoor Radon Exposure

Tina M. St. John

Introduction

Radon is a carcinogenic radioactive gas produced by the spontaneous decay of naturally occurring uranium in rock and soil. Radon is colorless, odorless, and tasteless. Unlike carbon monoxide and many other home pollutants, radon's adverse health effects are not immediate. Radon exposure can take place for many years without people suspecting its presence.

Radon emits alpha particles and produces several solid radioactive products called radon progeny (daughters). Radon-producing elements are virtually ubiquitous in the environment. Particularly high radon levels occur in regions where the soil or rock is rich in uranium deposits, including areas with large deposits of granite, limestone, shale, sandstone, and a variety of clays.

The National Research Council's Sixth Committee on Health Risks of Exposure to Radon (BEIR VI, 1999a) estimated that 15,400 to 21,800 lung cancer deaths in the United States in 1995 were attributable to indoor residential radon exposure. This study ranks indoor radon as the second leading cause of lung cancer, second only to cigarette smoking. The U.S. Environmental Protection Agency (EPA) states that exposure to indoor radon gas poses a significant risk of lung cancer (Office of Radiation and Indoor Air, 2003), and the Harvard Center for Risk Analysis ranked the inhalation of radon as the most important potentially fatal hazard in the home (DeAscentis & Graham, 1998).

The dangers of indoor radon are illustrated by the now infamous case of Mr. Stanley Watras. In 1984, Watras was an employee of the Limerick Nuclear Generating Station in Pennsylvania. As an electrical engineer, he did not work in an area of the plant where he could have encountered radioactive materials. However, Watras consistently triggered the plant's radioactive contamination alarms when leaving work each day. Watras speculated that the contamination was not occurring at the plant. He tested his theory by walking through the contamination sensors when he first arrived at work. As expected, Watras triggered the alarms, indicating that he was picking up the radioactive contamination *before* arriving at the power plant.

Plant and Pennsylvania state officials examined the Watras home and identified radon decay products throughout his property. The Watras family left the home during decontamination; radon mitigation devices were simultaneously installed.

After the radon concentration was reduced to acceptable levels, the family returned to their home.

Radon Effects on Health: Past to Present

Documentation of the detrimental occupational effects of mining on health dates back to the 15th century when citizens near mining towns in present-day Germany and Czechoslovakia described a "mountain sickness" that was believed to be caused by "subterranean dwarfs" (Lewis, 2006). The link between residential radon exposure and disease has heightened over recent years. In 1980, President Jimmy Carter ordered the establishment of the Radiation Policy Council (1980), arguably the first US governmental body to address the possible effects of indoor radon exposure. Nonetheless, the Watras case was a significant turning point in modern research on the negative health effects of indoor radon exposure.

Prior to the mid-1980s, the radon-lung cancer connection was researched primarily in the context of underground miners who were exposed to high concentrations of radon over prolonged periods. The confined area and long-term nature of the exposure were determined to be contributing factors to miners' high lung cancer rates (Samet, 1989; Harley, et al., 1986; Edling & Axelson, 1983). The Watras case focused attention on the presence of radon in homes in concentrations previously thought to occur only in underground mines.

Indoor Radon Exposure

Radon gas enters buildings as a result of the differential pressure gradient between the environment inside and the ambient air pressure outside. The gas moves up through the ground into the building through cracks and other holes in the foundation where it becomes trapped inside. Any building can become contaminated with indoor radon, including homes, schools, and business establishments. Homes are particularly susceptible because they are often less well ventilated than public structures. Radon can also be found in well water and is released into the air whenever the water is used, contributing to the total concentration of radon in the indoor air (National Research Council, 1999b).

Because uranium deposits occur throughout the earth's crust, radon gas can exist in the soil in diverse geographic areas. The EPA has created a Radon Zone map of the United States, which indicates the relative risk for elevated indoor radon levels by county (see Figure 11–1). The zones range from 1 to 3, in descending order of relative risk. The map was developed using five factors to determine radon risk potential: indoor radon measurements, geology, aerial radioactivity, soil permeability, and foundation type.

Zone 1 counties have the highest risk potential, with a predicted average indoor radon screening level greater than 4 pCi/L (pico curies per liter). Zone 2 and 3 counties have a predicted average indoor radon screening level between 2 and 4 pCi/L and < 2 pCi/L, respectively. However, the interpretation of these zones must be undertaken with caution. Even when armed with extensive geological information for a given area, predicting radon levels in individual homes is virtually impossible (Tanner, 1988). Local geology, home style, construction details, and usage patterns have been found to affect indoor radon levels (Henschel & Scott, 1986). Hence, there are many homes in zone 3 areas with dangerously high levels of radon, and conversely, many homes in zone 1 areas have safe radon readings.

The EPA estimates that nearly 1 out of every 15 homes in the United States has an elevated radon level (United States EPA, 2008). The EPA recommends immediate remedial action if test-

Figure 11–1 EPA Radon Risk Potential Zone Map.

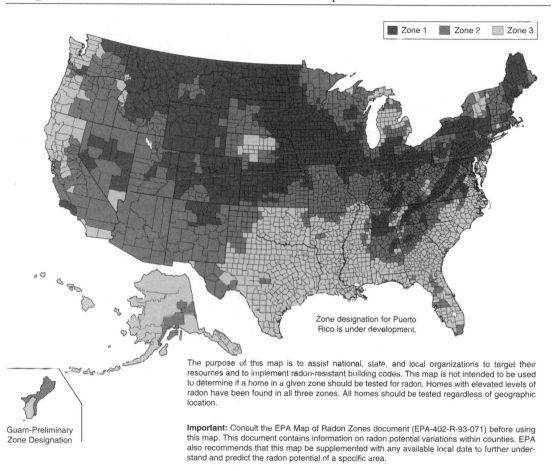

Zone designation for Puerto Rico is under development.

Guam-Preliminary Zone Designation

The purpose of this map is to assist national, state, and local organizations to target their resources and to implement radon-resistant building codes. This map is not intended to be used to determine if a home in a given zone should be tested for radon. Homes with elevated levels of radon have been found in all three zones. All homes should be tested regardless of geographic location.

Important: Consult the EPA Map of Radon Zones document (EPA-402-R-93-071) before using this map. This document contains information on radon potential variations within counties. EPA also recommends that this map be supplemented with any available local data to further understand and predict the radon potential of a specific area.

Source: http://www.epa.gov/radon/zonemap.html. Accessed June 25, 2008.

ing shows a level of ≥ 4 pCi/L. The EPA further states, "Radon levels less than 4 pCi/L still pose a risk, and in many cases may be reduced."

The Radon-Lung Cancer Connection

The carcinogenic effects of radon are caused by its decay into radioactive elements. Radon orig-

inates from uranium-238, which occurs naturally in most types of granite and soil in varying degrees. Radon-222 is the decay product of concern; as a gas, it seeps out of the rock or soil into the surrounding air (Figure 11–2). Radon progeny (formerly known as radon daughters) are fine, solid particles that result from the radioactive decay of radon gas. These particles are inhaled and accumulate in the lungs, where they cause

Figure 11–2 Radon production by radioactive decay of Uranium-238.

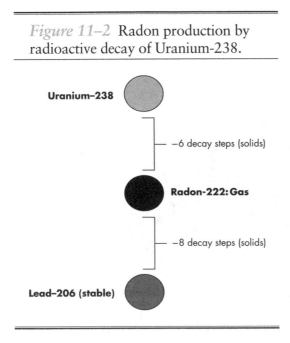

cellular damage by emitting ionizing alpha radiation. Although alpha radiation does not penetrate deeply into tissues, it can cause major genomic changes, including mutation and transformation in the cells that line the airways.

The causal relationship between atmospheric radon and lung cancer is well established. Both the International Agency for Research on Cancer and the United States National Toxicology Program list radon and its decay products as known human carcinogens with respect to pulmonary cancers. Analyses indicate that atmospheric radon does not pose a material risk of nonlung cancers (Darby, et al., 1995).

As reported in BEIR VI, the most important information concerning the health risks from radon comes from the epidemiologic studies of underground miners. In these cohort studies, lung cancer mortality is monitored over time in a group of miners and correlated with the miners' estimated past radon exposure. The BEIR

VI committee analyzed results from 11 separate miner cohorts, each of which shows a statistically significant elevation in lung cancer mortality with increasing radon exposure (Table 11–1) (National Research Council, 1999a; Office of Radiation and Indoor Air, 2003).

Extrapolating and applying the data from the underground miner studies to the risk of lung cancer attributable to the much lower level of indoor exposures in homes and public buildings initially proved to be challenging. However, in recent years, the risk predicted by the mathematical models of the BEIR VI committee have been borne out in indoor radon study data (Lubin, et al., 2004; Krewski, et al., 2005; Krewski, et al., 2006; Samet, 2006).

Today, the general consensus of the peer-reviewed literature is that long-term exposure to high levels of radon is associated with a significantly increased risk of lung cancer. The risk is substantially increased for smokers, because the effects of radon and tobacco smoke are synergistically cocarcinogenic.

Radon Information Resources

Radon-induced lung cancer is an important priority for many governmental and nongovernmental organizations. Radon has been classified as a known human carcinogen by the US Department of Health and Human Services (2005), the National Research Council (2005), the International Agency for Research on Cancer (1988), the National Environmental Health Association, the US Environmental Protection Agency, and the National Institutes of Health (NIH). These organizations' position on radon indicates official concern and support for radon mitigation programs. The U.S. Surgeon General and the EPA recommend that *all* homes be tested for radon.

Table 11–1 Miner Cohorts, Number Exposed, Person-Years of Epidemiologic Follow-Up, and Lung Cancer Deaths

Study	Type of Mine	No. of Workers	No. of Person-Years	No. of Lung Cancers
China	tin	13,649	134,842	936
Czechoslovakia	uranium	4,320	102,650	701
Colorado Plateau	uranium	3,347	79,536	334
Ontario	uranium	21,346	300,608	285
Newfoundland	fluorspar	1,751	33,795	112
Sweden	iron	1,294	32,452	79
New Mexico	uranium	3,457	46,800	68
Beaverlodge (Canada)	uranium	6,895	67,080	56
Port Radium (Canada)	uranium	1,420	31,454	39
Radium Hill (Australia)	uranium	1,457	24,138	31
France	uranium	1,769	39,172	45
TOTAL		60,606	888,906	2,674

Source: Health Effects of Exposure to Radon: BEIR VI. Committee on Health Risks of Exposure to Radon, Board on Radiation Effects Research, Commission on Life Sciences, National Research Council. National Academy Press, National Academy of Sciences, 1999; EPA Assessment of Risks from Radon in Homes. June 2003. Office of Radiation and Indoor Air, United States Environmental Protection Agency, Washington, DC.

Table 11–2 lists information and service resources for healthcare providers and patients.

January is observed as National Radon Action Month each year. Efforts are coordinated primarily by the EPA but also include activities by other federal and state agencies and non-governmental organizations. In January 2008, local groups conducted more than 700 National Radon Action Month activities and events across the country. Organizations from 39 states, three territories, and three tribal nations joined together to increase radon awareness and help save lives from radon-induced lung cancer.

Obstacles to Radon Testing, Exposure Prevention, and Mitigation

While testing for radon saves lives, there are obstacles that prevent individuals from surviving this deadly exposure. These include cost, lack of awareness, misperceptions, and lack of research studies. Each is described below.

Cost

The EPA estimates that the average cost for professional radon mitigation/correction is approximately $1,200, although it can range from $800 to $2,500. The cost is much less if a passive system was installed during home construction.

The public is often unaware that there are relatively inexpensive and simple methods they can use themselves to reduce radon levels in their homes, saving professional labor costs. These techniques include installing plastic piping systems outside the home that link to heating or cooling systems to circulate air from outside the home into the structure and increase ventilation. There are also concrete sealers formulated to block radon that homeowners can apply themselves. The New York State Department of

Table 11–2 Radon Information Resources

Agency/Organization	Contact Information	Products/Services
US EPA	URL: www.epa.gov/radon	EPA map of radon zones Indoor environments media campaigns Fact sheets Radon FAQs Health risks State/regional indoor environmental contacts
National Safety Council	URL: www.nsc.org Phone: 1-800-767-RADON (1-800-767-7236); recorded message Phone: 1-800-55-RADON (1-800-557-2366); speak with an information specialist	Information about radon exposure and mitigation
Spanish Radon Hotline	1-866-528-3187	Spanish-speaking information specialists
National Service Center for Environmental Publications	URL: www.epa.gov/nscep Phone: 1-800-490-9198 Fax: 301-604-3408 E-mail: nscep@bps-lmit.com	Publications from the EPA on radon topics
Indoor Air Quality Information Hotline	Phone: 1-800-438-4318 E-mail: iaqinfo@aol.com	This is a call-back service to answer questions regarding indoor air quality. The hotline also provides referrals to appropriate government agencies, research, public interest, and industry representatives.
The International Radon Project of the World Health Organization	URL: www.who.int/ionizing_radiation/env/radon/en/index.html	Launched in 2005, the working groups of the IRP collect and analyze information on radon risk, radon policies, radon mitigation and prevention, as well as risk communication.
Agency for Toxic Substances and Disease Registry (ATSDR)	URL: www.atsdr.cdc.gov/tfacts145.html	Toxicology and patient information; materials also available in Spanish.

Table 11–2 Radon Information Resources (continued)

Agency/Organization	Contact Information	Products/Services
	Phone: 1-888-42-ATSDR (1-888-422-8737) E-mail: ATSDRIC@cdc.gov	
National Radon Action Month (January)	URL: www.epa.gov/radon/nram/index.html	Activities, event planning kits, informational materials, poster contents information, etc.

Health conducted a survey that concluded that increasing awareness of radon's health risk along with introduction of cheaper methods for reducing radon might help in the public's willingness to voluntarily apply radon mitigation techniques (Wang, Ju, Stark, & Teresi, 1999).

A good resource to consult for information about radon testing and mitigation techniques is the EPA's "Consumer's Guide to Radon Reduction," which is available online (see Table 11–2) or from your state radon office.

Lack of Public Perceptions of Health Risk

Identifying public perceptions of radon as a health risk is an important component of radon mitigation programs. As all nurses and other healthcare providers well know, risk communication and the translation of risk perception to action are complex and multifactorial processes.

Overall, it appears that public media campaigns have been effective in making people aware of indoor radon. However, awareness and perception of personal risk are two very different things. For example, one telephone survey of 685 adults (in a radon zone 1 area) found that 92% of those who had heard of radon believed it to be a health risk, but only 4% believed they were at risk due to current exposure to high levels of radon (Mainous & Hagen, 1993). In this survey, younger and less educated individuals were more likely to perceive radon as a health risk. A northern Illinois study found that a significant number of the research subjects underestimated the seriousness of long-term radon exposure compared to the positions held by leading health organizations (Duckworth, Frank-Stromborg, Oleckno, Duffy, & Burns, 2002). Another study reported that proximity is an important factor in effective radon risk communications. The study found that people who live in high radon zones are more concerned about the risk of indoor radon than they are about other environmental risks that they do not perceive as having proximity (Poortinga, Cox, & Pidgeon, 2008). A report from the EPA's radon program suggests that "major gains in public health protection could be achieved through communication that effectively persuades people to accept personal responsibility for preventing voluntary risks, such as radon, and a more informed dialogue between the scientific community and the public concerning national priorities for environmental health protection" (Page, 1994).

This perception of radon as being less hazardous than hypothesized is consistent with the Risk Perception Model posited by Sandman (1987). One explanation for this perception could be that because radon is a natural product and its effects are not generally observable, little outrage is generated (Oleckno, 1995). In the northern Illinois study, almost 80% of the respondents indicated that they had not tested for radon. Even in a study of US women physicians (a group one would expect to understand the health risks of radon), 82% reported not having conducted radon testing in their homes (Baldwin, Frank, & Fielding, 1998). These findings are consistent with those of several other researchers (Ford & Eheman, 1997; Field, Kross, & Vust, 1993; Weinstein, Sandman, & Roberts, 1991).

False Health Beliefs

Using data from the 1990 National Health Interview Survey, an analysis was conducted to explore the links between demographic characteristics of the respondents and radon knowledge, perception of radon as a health hazard, and mitigation behavior. Less than one-third of the 28,000 respondents correctly identified lung cancer as a radon health effect and headaches (a false effect) as being caused by radon (Halpern & Warner, 1994). This study suggests that while there may be a general comprehension of the carcinogenic effects of radon, there may also be equally incorrect perceptions. There was a significant relationship between having accurate radon information and willingness to employ radon mitigation techniques when the perception of personal risk was high due to elevated radon measurements in the home. Similar results showing the public's misconceptions about the health effects of radon have been reported by other researchers (Duckworth, et al., 2002;

Ferng & Lawson, 1996; Weinstein, Klotz, & Sandman, 1988; Witte, et al., 1998) with a notable lack of knowledge regarding the synergistic effects of radon exposure and smoking (Hampson, Andrews, Lee, Lichtenstein, & Barckley, 2000; Lee, Lichtenstein, Andrews, Glasgow, & Hampson, 1999).

Paucity of Coordinated Radon Measurement Data

The need for research programs that collect radon measurement data is significant. Radon measurement programs have been largely piecemeal and without a large-scale coordination effort, though progress has been made in recent years in isolated pockets around the world (Krewski, et al., 2005; Darby, et al., 2005; Field, et al., 2001; Sandler, et al., 2006; Chen, Jiang, Tracy, & Zielinski, 2008; Cortina, Duran, & Lierena, 2008; Singh, Singh, Singh, & Bajwa, 2008; Celik, Cevik, Celik, & Kucukomeroglu, 2008; Gruber, Baumgartner, Seidel, & Maringer, 2008; Appleton, Miles, Green, & Larmour, 2008; Celik, Poffjin, Cevik, & Schepens, 2008; Al-Azmi, Abu-Shady, Sayed, & Al-Zayed, 2008). With increasing coordination among state radon offices and the new World Health Organization International Radon Project, there is an opportunity to validate the EPA's zone ratings of radon risk potential and to collect global data.

In the United States, the EPA has classified every county in the nation according to what it estimates to be the potential level of indoor radon (see Figure 11–1). Actual measurements in residences need to be taken in each county to validate the EPA radon map zoning. Measurements in a DeKalb, Illinois, study confirmed the EPA's zoning estimate for the county (Brookins, 1990). The EPA rates many states as zone 1, including the New England states and continuing south along the Appalachian Mountains. All the Midwestern states contain high radon potential zones, as well as states as far south as New Mexico and as far west as Washington. It is important to note that the EPA map is only an estimate of radon risk potential. All homes, regardless of where they fall on the EPA's classification of radon zones, should be tested because radon concentrations can vary greatly from one home to another and from one region to another.

Legal Concerns

Radon testing is a sensitive issue for homeowners. Many believe that test results are subject to disclosure to government agencies and could result in forced compliance with federal, state, or local regulations. For example, in the northern Illinois study (Duckworth, et al., 2002), many respondents questioned the confidentiality of the program and expressed reluctance to test for fear of reducing the salability of the home if high radon levels were identified.

Status of Indoor Radon Control Measures in the United States

In 1988, the federal Indoor Radon Abatement Act (IRAA) was enacted. The IRAA established the long-term goal that indoor air be as free from radon as the ambient air outside buildings. The law authorized funds for radon-related activities at the state and federal levels:

- Establishing state programs and providing technical assistance
- Conducting radon surveys of schools and federal buildings
- Establishing training centers and a proficiency program for firms that offer radon services

- Developing a citizen's guide to radon
- Developing model construction standards

In June 2008, 20 years after the enactment of IRAA, the Office of the Inspector General issued a report (2008) evaluating the effectiveness of the EPA's radon programs to date. The summary statements of the report are as follows:

Nearly two decades after passage of the 1988 Indoor Radon Abatement Act (IRAA), exposure to indoor radon continues to grow. Efforts to reduce exposure through mitigation or building with radon-resistant new construction have not kept pace. Of 6.7 million new single family detached homes built nationwide between 2001 and 2005, only about 469,000 incorporated radon-resistant features. Of 76.1 million existing single family homes in the United States in 2005, only about 2.1 million had radon-reducing features in place.

The IRAA established the goal that indoor air should be as free of radon as outdoor air. Since 1988, EPA has administered a voluntary program to reduce exposure to indoor radon by promoting awareness, testing, installation of radon mitigation systems in existing homes, and use of radon-resistant new construction techniques. Still, building codes in some areas do not require new homes to be built with radon-resistant new construction. Much of the progress made in reducing exposure has occurred as a result of real estate transactions. In those cases, a buyer, seller, mortgage lender, and/or real estate agent requested that a home be tested. Some States and localities do not require testing or the disclosure of test results during real estate transactions.

The radon program is not achieving greater results for several reasons. EPA's ability to achieve results with a voluntary program is limited. Potential loss of a sale represents a disincentive for real estate agents and sellers to conduct radon tests during real estate transactions. Added expense represents a disincentive for builders to use radon-resistant new construction. Opportunities exist within the federal community to substantially increase the number of homes tested and mitigated for radon. EPA has not decided how to use all the authorities or tools available to it to achieve the Act's goals. Also, EPA has not been reporting program results in relation to homes at risk in its performance reporting.

As noted in the Office of the Inspector General's (OIG) report, radon-related codes and regulations vary widely and are inconsistent. The EPA does not maintain current data of areas where builders are required to use radon-resistant new construction or which states require radon service providers to be certified, making it impossible to quantify the coverage or utilization of such measures. To date, the EPA has relied on the voluntary actions of key stakeholders, such as real estate agents, home buyers and sellers, home builders, and home inspectors to reduce the public's exposure to indoor radon. According to the EPA, > 85% of the radon testing/mitigation activity in the United States is real estate-driven (Office of the Inspector General, 2008).

The OIG 2008 report recommends that EPA "develop a strategy for achieving the long-term goal of the IRAA by considering using the authorities authorized by Congress under Section 310 of that Act, or explain its alternative strategy." This section of the Act authorizes the EPA to issue regulations as may be necessary to carry out the provisions of the Act. In its comments to the 2008 OIG report, the EPA agreed to develop a strategy as recommended by the OIG in

the context of EPA's available approaches, authorities, and resources. The strategy will need to balance the potential augmentation of disincentives for key stakeholders against the public health benefits of the long-term goal of IRAA.

Implications for Nursing Research

While there is extensive environmental health literature regarding the carcinogenic effects of radon exposure, there has been remarkably sparse nursing research in this arena. A search of the PubMed database limited to articles in nursing journals from 1960 through June 2008 produced only 25 citations, of which only 3 were research papers. Remarkably, 7 of the 25 citations addressed the purported therapeutic use of radon waters.

Although it is still a relatively new topic in oncology, radon's carcinogenic potential must be monitored. Exploration of the radon-lung cancer connection and research into radon-attributable lung cancer among high-risk communities is an important field for future research in cancer nursing. Nurses should take the opportunity of this emerging health issue to become leaders among healthcare professionals in researching radon and its health effects.

Implications for Nursing Practice

Indoor radon gas emissions should be a concern for nurses of all disciplines, particularly oncology nurses. Nurses need to determine their community's EPA radon potential rating. Based on the radon risk potential, nurses can establish community education programs regarding such indoor cancer risks. Health education programs need to include information on the serious health effects of chronic radon exposure as well as efforts to counter widespread misconceptions.

Following education campaigns to inform their communities, nurses can promote radon testing programs to determine actual radon levels in local homes. It is important that education programs be accompanied by information on actual radon levels in the community as well as efforts to promote testing and mitigation behavior. Awareness of radon as a health hazard and of its general presence in the community is less significant than the perception of personal risk from radon in promoting radon testing and mitigation behaviors.

All nurses must play a leading role in educating the public about the potential effects of radon exposure. Nurses are already important sources of information for the public on cancer prevention and early detection (Howell, Nelson-Marten, Krebs, Kaszyk, & Wold, 1998; Mahon, 1998; Hacihasanoglu & Gozum, 2008; Graham, 2005; Bailey, 2005). Radon awareness can be a component of nurses' discussions of cancer risks with their patients. Radon education can be incorporated into health awareness counseling sessions on cancer risks as one of several indoor environmental health hazards, such as smoking. This is especially important because radon exposure and cigarette smoking have been shown to be synergistically cocarcinogenic.

Nurses are in a unique position to disseminate radon risk information because of the nature of their contact with the public, and they should take advantage of this access to educate their patients and communities about radon-associated health risks.

References

Al-Azmi, D., Abu-Shady, A. I., Sayed, A. M., & Al-Zayed, Y. (2008). Indoor radon in Kuwait. *Health Physics, 94*(1), 49–56.

Appleton, J. D., Miles, J. C., Green, B. M., & Larmour, R. (2008). Pilot study of the application of Tellus airborne radiometric and soil geochemical data for radon mapping. *Journal of Environmental Radioactivity, 99*(10), 1687–1697.

Bailey, K. (2005). The nurse's role in promoting breast awareness. *Nursing Standard, 14*(30), 34–36.

Baldwin, G., Frank, E., & Fielding, B. (1998). U.S. women physicians' residential radon testing practices. *American Journal of Preventive Medicine, 15*(1), 49–53.

Brookins, D. G. (1990). *The indoor radon problem.* New York: Columbia University Press.

Celik, N., Cevik, U., Celik, A., & Kucukomeroglu, B. (2008a). Determination of indoor radon and soil radioactivity levels in Giresun, Turkey. *Journal of Environmental Radioactivity, 99*(8), 1349–1354.

Celik, N., Poffijn, A., Cevik, U., & Schepens, L. (2008b). Indoor radon survey in dwellings of the Kars province, Turkey. *Radiation Protection Dosimetry, 128*(4), 432–436.

Chen, J., Jiang, H., Tracy, B. L., & Zielinski, J. M. (2008). A preliminary radon map for Canada according to health region. *Radiation Protection Dosimetry, 130*(1), 92–94.

Cortina, D., Duran, I., & Lierena, J. J. (2008). Measurements of indoor radon concentrations in the Santiago de Compostela area. *Journal of Environmental Radioactivity, 99*(10), 1583–1588.

Darby, S., Hill, D., Auvinen, A., Barros-Dios, J. M., Baysson, H., Bochicchio, F., et al. (2005). Radon in homes and risk of lung cancer: Collaborative analysis of individual data from 13 European case-control studies. *British Medical Journal, 330*(7485), 223–227.

Darby, S. C., Whitley, E., Howe, G. R., Hutchings, S. J., Kusiak, R. A., Lubin, J. H., et al. (1995). Radon and cancers other than lung cancer in underground miners: A collaborative analysis of 11 studies. *Journal of the National Cancer Institute, 87*(5), 378–384.

DeAscentis, J. L., & Graham, J. D. (1998). Risk in perspective. Ranking risks in the home. *Harvard Center for Risk Analysis, 6*(4), 377–394.

Duckworth, L. T., Frank-Stromborg, M., Oleckno, W. A., Duffy, P., & Burns, K. (2002). Relationship of perception of radon as a health risk and willingness to engage in radon testing and mitigation. *Oncology Nursing Forum, 29*(7), 1099–1107.

Edling, C., & Axelson, O. (1983). Quantitative aspects of radon daughter exposure and lung cancer in underground miners. *British Journal of Industrial Medicine, 40*(2), 182–187.

Ferng, S., & Lawson, J. K. (1996). Residents in a high radon potential geographic area: Their risk perception and attitude toward testing and mitigation. *Journal of Environmental Health, 58*(6), 13–17.

Field, R. W., Kross, B. C., & Vust, L. J. (1993). Radon testing behavior in a sample of individuals with high home radon screening measurements. *Risk Analysis, 13*(4), 441–447.

Field, R. W., Steck, D. J., Smith, B. J., Brus, C. P., Fisher, E. F., Neuberger, J. S., et al. (2001). The Iowa radon lung cancer study—phase I: Residential radon gas exposure and lung cancer. *The Science of the Total Environment, 272*(1–3), 67–72.

Ford, E. S., & Eheman, C. R. (1997). Radon retesting and mitigation behavior among the U.S. population. *Health Physics, 72*(4), 611–614.

Graham, H. (2005). The nurse's role in promoting breast awareness to women. *Nursing Times, 101*(41), 23–24.

Gruber, V., Baumgartner, A., Seidel, C., & Maringer, F. J. (2008). Radon risk in alpine regions in Austria: Risk assessment as a settlement planning strategy. *Radiation Protection Dosimetry, 130*(1), 88–91.

Hacihasanoglu, R., & Gozum, S. (2008). Effect of training on the knowledge levels and beliefs regarding breast self-examination on women attending a public education centre. *European Journal of Oncology Nursing, 12*(1), 58–64.

Halpern, M. T., & Warner, K. E. (1994). Radon risk perception and testing: Sociodemographic correlates. *Journal of Environmental Health, 56*(7), 31–35.

Hampson, S. E., Andrews, J. A., Lee, M. E., Lichtenstein, E., & Barckley, M. (2000). Radon and cigarette smoking: Perceptions of this synergistic health risk. *Health Psychology, 19*(3), 247–252.

Harley, N., Samet, J. M., Cross, F. T., Hess, T., Muller, J., & Thomas, D. (1986). Contribution of radon and radon daughters to respiratory cancer. *Environmental Health Perspectives, 70*, 17–21.

Henschel, D. B., & Scott, A. G. (1986). The EPA program to demonstrate mitigation measures for indoor radon: Initial results. In *Indoor radon* (pp. 110–121). Pittsburgh, PA: Air Pollution Control Association.

Howell, S. L., Nelson-Marten, P., Krebs, L. U., Kaszyk, L., & Wold, R. (1998). Promoting nurses' positive attitudes toward cancer prevention/screening. *Journal of Cancer Education, 13*(2), 76–84.

International Agency for Research on Cancer (IARC). (1988). *Summaries & evaluations, 43,* 173. Retrieved June 21, 2008, from http://www.inchem.org/documents/iarc/vol43/43-02.html

Krewski, D., Lubin, J. H., Zielinski, J. M., Alavanja, M., Catalan, V. S., Field, R. W., et al. (2005). Residential radon and risk of lung cancer: A combined analysis of 7 North American case-control studies. *Epidemiology, 16*(2), 137–145.

Krewski, D., Lubin, J. H., Zielinski, J. M., Alavanja, M., Catalan, V. S., Field, R. W., et al. (2006). A combined analysis of North American case-control studies of residential radon and lung cancer. *Journal of Toxicology and Environmental Health, Part A, 69*(7), 533–597.

Lee, M. E., Lichtenstein, E., Andrews, J. A., Glasgow, R. E., & Hampson, S. E. (1999). Radon-smoking synergy: A population-based behavioral risk reduction approach. *Preventive Medicine, 29*(3), 222–227.

Lewis, R. K. (2006). *A History of radon: 1470 to 1984.* Pennsylvania Department of Environmental Protection, Bureau of Radiation Protection, Radon Division. Presented at the 2006 National Radon Meeting. Retrieved June 20, 2008, from http://www.google.com/search?q=cache:b5bObpo3toAJ:www.crcpd.org/radon/HistoryOfRadon.rtf+history+of+radon&hl=en&ct=clnk&cd=3&gl=us&client=firefox-a

Lubin, J. H., Wang, Z. Y., Boice, J. D., Jr., Xu, Z. Y., Blot, W. J., De Wang, L., et al. (2004). Risk of lung cancer and residential radon in China: Pooled results of two studies. *International Journal of Cancer, 109*(1), 132–137.

Mahon, S. M. (1998). Cancer risk assessment: Conceptual considerations for clinical practice. *Oncology Nursing Forum, 25*(9), 1535–1547.

Mainous, A. G., III, & Hagen, M. D. (1993). Public perceptions of radon risk. *The Family Practice Research Journal, 13*(1), 63–69.

National Research Council. (1999a). *Health effects of exposure to radon: BEIR VI.* Committee on Health Risks of Exposure to Radon, Board on Radiation Effects Research, Commission on Life Sciences. Washington, DC: National Academy Press.

National Research Council. (1999b). *Risk assessment of radon in drinking water.* Committee on Risk Assessment of Exposure to Radon in Drinking Water, Board on

Radiation Effects Research, Commission on Life Sciences. Washington, DC: National Academy Press.

National Research Council. (2005, June). *Health risks from exposure to low levels of ionizing radiation.* BEIR VII Committee, Nuclear and Radiation Studies Board. Washington, DC: National Academy Press.

Office of Radiation and Indoor Air. (2003, June). *EPA assessment of risks from radon in homes.* Washington, DC: United States Environmental Protection Agency.

Office of the Inspector General of the United States Environmental Protection Agency. (2008, June 3). *More action needed to protect public from indoor radon risks* (Report No. 08-P-0174). Retrieved December 3, 2008, from www.epa. gov/oig/reports/2008/ 20080603-08-P-0174.pdf

Oleckno, W. W. (1995). Guidelines for improving risk communication in environmental health. *Journal of Environmental Health, 58*(1), 20–23.

Page, S. D. (1994). Indoor radon: A case study in risk communication. *American Journal of Preventive Medicine, 10*(Suppl. 3), 15–18.

Poortinga, W., Cox, P., & Pidgeon, N. F. (2008). The perceived health risks of indoor radon gas and overhead powerlines: A comparative multilevel approach. *Risk Analysis, 28*(1), 235–248.

President Jimmy Carter. (1980, February 21). Executive Order 12194. Radiation Policy Council.

Samet, J. (2006). Residential radon and lung cancer: End of the story? *Journal of Toxicology and Environmental Health, Part A, 69*(7), 527–531.

Samet, J. M. (1989). Radon and lung cancer. *Journal of the National Cancer Institute, 81*(10), 745–758.

Sandler, D. P., Weinberg, C. R., Shore, D. L., Archer, V. E., Stone, M. B., Lyon, J. L., et al. (2006). Indoor radon and lung cancer risk in Connecticut and Utah. *Journal of Toxicology and Environmental Health, Part A, 69*(7), 633–654.

Sandman, P. M. (1987). Risk communication: Facing public outrage. *EPA Journal, 13*, 21–22.

Singh, H., Singh, J., Singh, S., & Bajwa, B. S. (2008, February 2). Regional variations pattern of indoor radon levels in some areas of Punjab and Haryana. *Radiation Protection Dosimetry.*

Tanner, A. B. (1988, March 30–31). The source of radon in homes. In N. H. Harley (Ed.), *Proceedings of the 24th Annual Meeting of the National Council on Radiation Protection and Measurements, Radon 10, Washington DC* (pp. 159–169). Bethesda, MD: NCRPM.

US Department of Health and Human Services, Public Health Service, National Toxicology Program. (2005). *Report on carcinogens* (11th ed.). Washington, DC: Author.

United States Environmental Protection Agency. (2008). *A citizen's guide to radon: The guide to protecting yourself and your family from radon.* Retrieved June 20, 2008, from http:// www.epa.gov/radon/pubs/citguide.html#results

Wang, Y., Ju, C., Stark, A. D., & Teresi, N. (1999). Radon mitigation survey among New York state residents living in high radon homes. *Health Physics, 77*(4), 403–409.

Weinstein, N. D., Klotz, M. L., & Sandman, P. M. (1988). Optimistic biases in public perceptions of the risk from radon. *American Journal of Public Health, 78*(7), 796–800.

Weinstein, N. D., Sandman, P. M., & Roberts, N. E. (1991). Perceived susceptibility and self-protective behavior: A field experiment to encourage home radon testing. *Health Psychology, 10*(1), 25–33.

Witte, K., Berkowitz, J. M., Lillie, J. M., Cameron, K. A., Lapinski, M. K., & Liu, W. Y. (1998). Radon awareness and reduction campaigns for African Americans: A theoretically based evaluation. *Health Education and Behavior, 25*(3), 284–303.

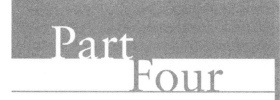

Part Four

Psychosocial Issues of Individuals with Lung Cancer

Chapter 12

Living with Hope: Lung Cancer

Katherine Katen Moore

"Hope: Expectation of something desired; desire combined with expectation."

Oxford English Dictionary, 1971, p. 1329

Introduction

People, including healthcare workers, use the term "hope" freely in discussions about cancer. It is used as though it were a life force, "he needs to have hope or he won't make it," and it is used as a rationale for futile treatment that may likely increase suffering: "I know this treatment won't do anything except make her weaker, but it gives her hope" (Arnold & Quill, 2003; Eliott & Olver, 2007). But what are we saying when we refer to hope? Why is it so important for the oncology nurse to assess, engender, and support hope in patients who are coping with lung cancer? Interestingly, despite the frequent and free use of "hope" in oncology practices and the literature about caring for cancer patients, Rustøen et al. (1998) and Clayton et al. (2005) found the term itself rarely defined, described, measured, and often not addressed in quality of life studies.

People might assume that hope can exist only as long as the possibility for cure exists; however, cancer patients frequently do not necessarily de-

scribe hope this way (Ballard, Green, McCaa, & Logsdon, 1997; Sand, Strang, & Milberg, 2008). Hope is not a static concept, but it is changeable depending on the person's realistic expectation of the future (Rustøen & Wiklund, 2000; Rustøen, et al., 1998; Arnold & Quill, 2003; Felder, 2004; Clayton, et al., 2005). Hope cannot be assumed to be present or absent without a discussion with the patient. The meaning of hope for that patient can and will change over the course of his or her life with lung cancer.

Uncertainty is not hopelessness. Uncertainty has a direct effect on the presence or absence of hope. Lung cancer is a disease group fraught with uncertainty, starting with its insidious growth before discovery in an advanced state (Chapple, Ziebland, & McPherson, 2004). It is a cancer in which a chemotherapy that provides two more months of life (perhaps just breathing in a bed) is something to be excited about. Uncertainty means that any remission is a potential threat to the patient's hope because remission puts the patient into a holding pattern. Uncertainty is also, however, frequently the result of lack of open discussion between patient and clinician because the patient has not been warned of the possible threat (The, Hak, Koeter,

& van Der Wal, 2000; Rustøen, et al., 1998; Clayton, et al., 2005; Griffin, et al., 2003). Uncertainty is also related to questions that the patient has but does not ask or patient's need for information that is not elicited by the providers, including the oncology nurse. Oncology nurses are in a position to address the threat of uncertainty through compassionate and therapeutic assessments and empathetic listening (Felder, 2004; Vellone, Rega, Galletti, & Cohen, 2006). Oncology nurses also have a duty to provide accurate and clear information that the patient can understand and assimilate (Wonghongkul, Moore, Musil, Schneider, & Deimling, 2000).

The antithesis of hope, hopelessness is commonly associated with lung cancer. Hopelessness, however, is a potentially pathological state (Rodin, et al., 2007; Sand, et al., 2008). Approximately 90% of all lung cancer cases that are now diagnosed in the United States are considered to be due to smoking (CDC, 2005). Lung cancer patients potentially experience hopelessness due to shame and guilt. These feelings are related to the tendency to perceive lung cancer as retribution for a "self-imposed" disease related to smoking behaviors. This peculiar characteristic of lung cancer may be the inadvertent result of vigorous public antismoking campaigns. The nihilistic attitude is further complicated by clinicians who do not recommend more than the best supportive care in nonsurgical lung cancer candidates despite clinical evidence that the newer treatment regimens may actually lessen suffering and prolong meaningful life (Hoffman, Mauer, & Vokes, 2000). Although it may be difficult, it is important to assure the patient that the oncology nurse is not the patient's judge. The endeavor of cancer nursing is to care and create a "therapeutic ambi-

ence" that will further the growth of both patient and oncology nurse (Chauhan & Long, 2000a).

This chapter will discuss the importance of hope at all times during the cancer trajectory. Hope, as has already been discussed, is what the patient says it is. However, supporting hope needs accurate and sensitive information to provide comfort to the patient. A case presentation of a woman with acute onset of what will be stage IV lung cancer will be discussed. Suggestions for nursing actions will be presented, although as of this writing there continue to be very few studies of hope interventions (Lin & Bauer-Wu, 2003). Most studies continue to focus on the description and measure of hope and its correlation to quality of life issues. It is for this reason that many of the articles cited in this chapter are older references.

Hope Interventions

Herth (2001) developed and evaluated a Hope Intervention Program (HIP) based on the Hope Process Framework (HPF) of Farran, Wilken, and Popovich. This framework describes common elements of a definition of hope in four attributes: (1) experiential, (2) spiritual or transcendent, (3) rational thought, and (4) relational processes. Herth found that by using HIP, oncology nurses could engender hope in their patients through direct intervention. HIP consists of eight weekly 2-hour group sessions. Each session explores a theme that expresses one of four domains of the HPF and uses various group and individual exercises to develop that theme. The themes that were used included building a community, searching for hope, connecting to others, expanding the boundaries, building a hopeful veneer, and, finally, reflecting back on the experience of the other seven sessions.

The participants were recruited from two outpatient oncology clinics. The entry criteria required that they be first-time recurrent cancer patients undergoing treatment. Although there was no control group, all study participants found the intervention useful and reported enhanced feelings of hope at the end of the intervention. Nine months after completing the 8-week program, the feelings continued to be reported.

Rustøen et al. (1998) used an experimental design to evaluate a nursing intervention's effect on cancer patients' hope and quality of life in a large study of newly diagnosed Norwegian cancer patients. The researchers used the Nowotny Hope Scale, which is based on Nowotny's definition of hope. This definition consists of six dimensions: (1) hope is dynamic; (2) it is future oriented and possible; (3) it comes from within; (4) it is fluid and actively engaged by the person; (5) it has a relationship to others or a higher being; and (6) it gives outcomes meaning.

The participants were randomized to three support groups, which met for eight 2-hour sessions, similar to the HIP intervention. All groups had an introductory and evaluation meeting. The first group received the intervention to increase hope. The intervention was a discussion based on each of the six attributes of the Nowotny definition. The themes were belief in one's self and one's own ability; emotional reactions after a cancer diagnosis; relationships with family, friends, and colleagues; active involvement; spiritual beliefs and values; and acknowledgment that there is a future. The second group had an intervention called "Learning to Live with Cancer," similar to the American Cancer Society's "I Can Cope" program.

The last group—the control group—was a traditional cancer support group.

The researchers found that the nursing intervention group reported increased feelings of hope immediately after the intervention was completed but not at six months. The researchers questioned the design of the intervention, suggesting that it needed more direct input from the participants about different aspects of hope that could be discussed other than the ones the researchers had determined.

It is not possible and likely not reasonable to initiate an 8-week program that will engender hope for every lung cancer patient, but the ideas in each intervention can be used for other intervention designs. Designed to effect long-term change, HIP allows the group to guide the exact focus of each discussion to work in more depth. Research is needed to learn if either design could be translated for use over a much shorter period of time with a patient who may not have eight weeks. Although the Norwegian study used very similar themes, it appears to have been more didactic and conversational than the HIP approach, which included exercises designed to illustrate and encourage nonverbal expression. For more acutely ill patients, as illustrated in the case presented here, the themes in these interventions will need to be concentrated and perhaps less exploratory.

The importance of the oncology nurse's role in influencing the support and maintenance of hope in the lung cancer patient is presented in the case that follows. The intention here is to remind the reader that hope is always present and can be supported by the oncology nurse at any point in the illness continuum. The essential role of an oncology nurse in influencing the level of hope in a patient involves time, care, and empathy.

Case Presentation

An inpatient oncology nurse is about to enter the hospital room of a new patient who was recently admitted for complications related to a newly diagnosed lung cancer. This woman's cancer history is typical of lung cancer patients. Over the past two to three months she recalled having been more fatigued than usual. She credited her fatigue to her full schedule of teaching graduate students and a persistent cough. She was treated with three courses of antibiotics for a suspected respiratory infection. When her cough never resolved, her primary care clinician finally ordered a chest X-ray. On the X-ray film, a large mediastinal mass was visualized. A CT guided needle biopsy was scheduled for the following week. However, the next day, the patient experienced severe dyspnea and upper-body swelling. Frightened by her sudden severe breathlessness and change of appearance, she called her primary care clinician. The clinician advised the woman to go directly to emergency department of the hospital.

In the emergency department, the woman was tachycardic and hypotensive. Her EKG was abnormal with occasional preventricular contractions. A routine pulse oximetry reading revealed 86% oxygen saturation on room air. A diagnostic chest CT showed the very large centralized mass involving her aorta, bilateral pleural effusions, and the possibility of a cardiac effusion. She was immediately put on oxygen via face mask and bed rest. The suspected diagnosis was superior vena cava syndrome, and she was admitted directly to the oncology unit.

After she was admitted, the woman's symptoms continued to worsen, and she became more anxious and fearful. The attending physician had the resident evaluate her, and the decision was made to insert a left-side chest tube

in the larger of the effusions and allow the fluid to drain. The woman's respiratory and cardiac status rapidly declined, and she became more unstable. She was moved to the cardiac ICU for a planned insertion of a chest tube and possible intubation. Aspiration of the pleural fluid showed malignant cells that would later be confirmed as adenocarcinoma of the lung.

The oncology nurse reviewed the chart and found that the patient's prior medical history was unremarkable. She is 58 years old, divorced, and has two adult children aged 28 and 21 years. She lives alone. She has no other concurrent health problems and is not on any medication. She had smoked inconsistently for over 40 years, approximately three cigarettes a week. She has no other risk factors for lung cancer. The oncology consult revealed that the woman's prognosis with the current presentation was very poor and that chemotherapy would be discussed as soon as her medical condition stabilized.

The sequence of events from the chest X-ray to her admission to the ICU all transpired in less than 24 hours of learning that her chest X-ray had a suspicious chest mass. This patient was clearly gravely ill from complications of her lung cancer, yet she was in no condition to undergo treatment. Getting to treatment, however, is only one of the goals in her care plan. At this moment, the primary goal for this patient is twofold: to stabilize her medically and at the same time to assess and support her through the enormous transitions she has just undergone and will continue to experience. The oncology nurse recognizes that this patient has been transformed from an independent adult with an X-ray showing a suspicious mass in her lung to an overwhelmed, dependent, medically unstable patient in the cardiac ICU.

Before the oncology nurse introduced herself, the patient looked up at her and said haltingly, "I can't eat, I can't sleep, I can't breathe. I don't know how long I can do this." A powerful silence follows. How the oncology nurse responds will determine whether this patient will be presented with the possibility of an alliance with the oncology nurse to help her reclaim her hope or if she will be left alone, with a sense of hopelessness.

Mental Health and Spiritual Counseling

Cancer patients are at higher risk for threats to psychological and spiritual well-being than the general population. However, they may not always be encouraged to seek help and get the referrals they need (Moore & Schmais, 2001). Feelings of hopelessness, grief, sadness, anger, and denial are expected reactions to any cancer diagnosis. It is helpful to reassure patients that these feelings are normal. On the other hand, anxiety and depression correlate with fears that are not elicited in discussions with healthcare workers.

Sometimes it may be enough to simply reassure the patient to prevent any progression to a pathological response. The oncology nurse can provide support and empathy by allowing the patient to express these feelings without any other intervention. The oncology nurse can also recognize the need to share silence as a commitment to the patient's well-being (Friedrichson, Strang, & Carlsson, 2000; Chauhan & Long, 2000a).

If the patient reports feelings that are overwhelming and/or more than the oncology nurse could appropriately assist with, the oncology nurse can suggest a referral to a mental health counselor. A referral is correct to give the patient access to clinical expertise in counseling, not because the oncology nurse is unwilling to provide empathy. The patient may need only a few sessions to get through the initial diagnosis period (Schofield, et al., 2001). Professional support groups for lung cancer patients may be available after the initial diagnosis and should be encouraged at the time of diagnosis.

A diagnosis of cancer may also trigger spiritual crises for a patient. Spiritual well-being and hope are intertwined. An interesting pastoral care study (Easterling, Gamino, Sewell, & Stirman, 2000) looked at the differences in bereavement between those who described their spirituality as regularly attending church with those who reported internalized spiritual experiences (regardless of church attendance). Their research found that there was a strong correlation with internalized spirituality and better grief adjustment. The researchers concluded that study participants with internalized spirituality found that it provided a readily available personal support mechanism. It was also a source of comfort and provided a contextual framework that gave meaning to crisis.

Pulchaski (1999) designed a quick and effective tool for the assessment of spiritual well-being: Faith or beliefs, Importance and influence, Community, and Address (FICA) (Ferrell, 2007). Conducting a spiritual assessment encourages and fosters open communication, compassion, and a sense of hope between the oncology nurse and the patient. The patient should be encouraged to include a spiritual counselor on the healthcare team. If one is not available, a referral can be made to the institution's pastoral care department (Pulchaski & Romer, 2000).

Communication and Uncertainty

An effective therapeutic relationship between the lung cancer patient and the oncology nurse depends on time, empathy, open communication, and individualized disclosure (Girgis & Sanson-Fisher, 1995; Chauhan & Long, 2000a, 2000b; Felder, 2004). Open communication consists of listening carefully to the patient's story and responding clearly and honestly to questions and concerns. Individualized disclosure recognizes and assesses the unique needs of the patient. The provided information is tailored to that patient (Girgis & Sanson-Fisher, 1995). The therapeutic relationship helps decrease a patient's uncertainty and feelings of threat (Wonghongkul, et al., 2000).

Let's review the case example again. Many oncology nurses have seen similar patients sitting upright in bed, gasping between each word, and visibly suffering. At that moment, the immediate intervention was to minimize the physical symptoms and to prevent the patient from perceiving them as hopelessly intractable. The oncology nurse must also ask other questions: Would explaining the symptom and why it is occurring be helpful? This tactic can help allay the patient's perception of uncertainty, especially with the presentation or persistence of symptoms that are not responsive, or responsive enough, to the intervention (Felder, 2004).

The patient in this case reported physiological symptoms that she identified as potentially intolerable by stating, "I don't know how long I can do this." This communication was a tenuous moment in the oncology nurse/patient relationship (Lin & Bauer-Wu, 2003; Sand, et al., 2008). It was not entirely clear what the patient was saying to the oncology nurse. Was she referring to her disease prognosis or her ability to tolerate her symptoms? Was she asking what she can expect if things get worse or better? Was she warning the oncology nurse that she feels that her fears, questions, and concerns are not being heard over the rush to medically stabilize

her? To know what the patient needs, the oncology nurse must be sure to ask the patient gentle, open-ended questions and allow the patient to speak at her own pace (Lin & Bauer-Wu, 2003; Sand, et al., 2008).

If the patient was asking about her prognosis, the oncology nurse must be truthful with her response. However, in the patient's current state of discomfort, a routine discussion outlining the risks and benefits of treatment would likely not be recommended or appropriate as an immediate intervention. A brief discussion of the patient's diagnosis and the complications she is experiencing, as well as the nurse's willingness to answer the patient's questions, is recommended. All of this discussion should occur simultaneously with effective interventions directed at relieving the patient's physical symptoms. Research has shown that patients prefer that their clinicians discuss prognosis openly and meaningfully. Patients also prefer that they receive clear information about the dying process when treatment is no longer helpful (Ambuel & Mazzone, 2001; Girgis & Sanson-Fisher, 1995; Grassi, et al., 2000; Parker, et al., 2001; The, et al., 2000; Felder, 2004; Griffin, Koch, Nelson, & Cooley, 2007; Clayton, et al., 2005; Lin & Bauer-Wu, 2003; Sand, et al., 2008).

Difficult information should be delivered after warning shots that bad news is to come. Warning shots are statements such as, "I am sorry to tell you news that may be difficult for you to hear," or, "I wish things were different than they are now." The point of the warning shot is not to deliver the bad news specifically but to give the patient time to process what will be coming and to stop further communication if that is what he or she needs to do. (There will be further discussion of this topic in the next section.)

The oncology nurse's empathy opens lines of communication and helps the patient to understand that hope still exists for comfort and compassionate care. These interventions allow the oncology nurse to practice "caring" and the patient to feel "cared for" (Chauhan & Long, 2000a). The patient is the source from which the oncology nurse gathers information. This patient data should be used when advocating for the patient during discussions with the healthcare team (Jurkovich, Pierce, Pananen, & Rivara, 2000; Chauhan & Long, 2000b). The oncology nurse influences the patient's feelings of hope by explaining symptoms and their meaning in relationship to his or her state of health (Wonghongkul, et al., 2000). By listening to the patient's feelings and fears and responding with empathy, the therapeutic relationship reduces the patient's risk of isolation (Felder, 2004). Soliciting the patient's own words validates the patient's experience of symptoms and disease (Baile, et al., 2000; Nail, 2001).

Warning Shots and Bad News

As the diagnostic process continues and the list of differential diagnoses gets shorter with each test, the patient can be given warning signs—statements by the clinician that clearly give voice to concern about possible negative outcomes of tests. This is to alert the patient that the diagnosis is likely to be worse than previously expected. Examples of warning signs would be to tell the patient, "I am afraid I have bad news to share with you," or, "I am very sorry to tell you that your tests have confirmed that the mass is cancer." Calling attention to these warning signs allows the patient to prepare for the possibilities and assimilate the news. It is also very important that the language used be accurate, common language and not medical jar-

gon, such as "unfortunate," "tests are not turning out as I would have wanted," or "malignant mass" to describe a cancer tumor. Following the warning shots, the discussion between the oncology nurse and the patient can also include modified expectations based on what the news could mean in terms of the individual patient (Girgis & Sanson-Fisher, 1995; Boyd, 2001; Chauhan & Long, 2000a; Baile, et al., 2000). In the case presented here, an example of a warning shot would be for the nurse to change the focus of the discussion from the patient's respiratory issues to her severely compromised cardiac status. Does the patient understand the physiological implications of the tumor mass involving her aorta?

Receiving the diagnosis of cancer falls into the category of bad news—knowledge that changes a person's usual lifestyle. This information limits the choices that the person assumed he or she already had. Bad news is a direct threat to the notion of future. The task of breaking bad news is stressful to both the oncology nurse and the patient. However, as stated earlier in the discussion of uncertainty, patients do want to be told the news clearly yet sensitively. The oncology nurse who delivers this news should prepare what will be said before presenting it to the patient and should anticipate the intense reaction of the patient to such life-changing news (Dosanjh, Barnes, & Bhandari, 2001; Boyd, 2001; Girgis & Sanson-Fisher, 1995; Parker, et al., 2001; Ptacek & Eberhardt, 1996; Ambuel & Mazzone, 2001; Schofield, et al., 2001; Baile, et al., 2000; Jurkovich, et al., 2000).

The oncology nurse should be aware that the patient's perspective regarding the news may not be that the news is entirely bad. It can be that hearing the diagnosis of lung cancer is a relief after the patient had experienced the uncertainty of symptoms and the unclear results of tests. Being allowed to ask questions and receiving clear answers serves to diminish uncertainty (Griffin, et al., 2003). If warning signs had been provided to this patient during the diagnostic process (for example, being forthright with the patient that there was suspicion of cancer before the test was done), the answer then either confirms the suspicion or puts it to rest (Ptacek & Eberhardt, 1996; The, et al., 2000; Rustøen, et al., 1998; Clayton, et al., 2005; Griffin, et al., 2003).

Respecting the Patient's Experience of Lung Cancer

The oncology nurse cannot honestly promise a patient that there will or will not be suffering during treatment. The oncology nurse can only promise that the patient's healthcare team will do their best to discuss and address the possibilities of relief and provide sufficient time to answer any questions or concerns of the patient. The patient's experience of lung cancer is unique to that patient no matter what the oncology nurse's previous experience was with other patients with similar conditions. If the oncology nurse dismisses a new problem or symptom, he or she has effectively shut the open communication with the patient (Nail, 2001). This type of response will increase the isolation and uncertainty of the patient. Interventions will be less effective because there is no open communication by which to assess effectiveness. On the same point, Baile and colleagues (2000) recommend that the patient never be told that "there is nothing more than can be done." There is always an intervention of caring that can be made to provide comfort and/or relief.

In a small study to improve antismoking interventions, conducted in the United Kingdom, Chapple et al. (2004) learned that patients report feeling stigmatized and ashamed to be smokers even before a lung cancer diagnosis. When the diagnosis of lung cancer was added, the patients felt responsible for their illnesses because of partaking in a controllable behavior. Indeed, the suffering of a former smoker with lung cancer is often used as a deterring image directed at young potential smokers. Sensitivity to the feelings of those with lung cancer is likely not considered in these campaigns. Oncology nurses must remain alert and sensitive to their own personal bias about smoking and not let them affect the care of their patients with lung cancer who either still smoke or formerly smoked.

Supporting Hope During Dying and Death

More than half of the patients who are treated for lung cancer die of their disease. The possibility of dying from lung cancer itself or complications from the disease exists simultaneously. When and if the patient asks about his or her prognosis, it is always important to be honest yet sensitive when discussing the grim realities of a lung cancer diagnosis. Hope can be communicated in the compassionate delivery of information and empathetic responses to the patient's concerns (Ptacek & Eberhardt, 1996).

The and her colleagues (2000) found an interesting dynamic they called "false optimism" in their small, yet thought-provoking, study of non-small cell lung cancer patients in the Netherlands. According to the study, observations of false optimism were the result of patients who were reluctant to question the meaning of worsening symptoms and of physicians who advocated adherence to a treatment plan despite worsening symptoms. Quirt et al. (1997) also found in their study of Canadian lung cancer patients undergoing therapy that physicians did not correct or clarify misconceptions regarding the goal of the patient's treatment. Both groups of researchers conclude that this lack of communication of accurate information denied the patients' autonomy in making treatment decisions and in preparing for end of life.

Uncertainty is a result of not knowing. It is reasonable to share an uncertain prognosis with the patient because some events may truly be unpredictable. However, it is deceitful to withhold information from a patient when the patient expresses concern about a symptom that is life threatening or means progression of the disease (Chauhan & Long, 2000a, 2000b). The patient trusts and desires that questions will be answered (Sand, et al., 2008). Contrary to what many may believe or fear, research does not support that accurate information, even if unfavorable, is harmful to the patient (Baile, et al., 2000).

Warning a patient that the treatment is no longer effective and that the disease is progressing can be done in a compassionate and caring manner (Friedrichson, et al., 2000). On the other hand, predicting the life expectancy of an individual patient is usually not a helpful discussion. Numerous studies have shown that prognostication is correct only in about 20% of the cases where this information is provided to patients (Griffin, et al., 2003). There are many factors that enter into prognostication accuracy, not least of which is the extent of the clinician's experience with the disease. More experienced clinicians have been found to be more accurate than less experienced clinicians. However, there is also a direct correlation between a clinician knowing the patient well and "overpredicting" life expectancy (Christakis & Lamont, 2000). When a patient asks the oncology nurse, "How long do I have?" it is reasonable to respond that the answer is not known. However, it is also reasonable to add that most patients with similar symptoms and similar disease have been known to survive a range of time (Field & Cassel, 1997).

Conclusion

Patients know how serious the diagnosis of lung cancer is before they receive the official report. It is up to the oncology nurse to be ready to help that patient with the physical symptoms of the disease and its treatment, including the psychosocial aspects, such as hope. In fact, physical symptoms may not be separated from the patient's perception of them. The patient's responses are influenced by all aspects of his or her experience of the disease.

Hope is a very personal, individualized concept that is worthwhile for the oncology nurse to explore with the patient throughout that patient's care. Hope changes according to the information provided and the patient's needs. What the patient calls hope can only be known by being willing to be an empathic listener and provide accurate information compassionately.

Hope is ephemeral, but it exists. The oncology nurse has a clear role to assess and support the lung cancer patient's hope. Listening to the patient's story and asking simple, caring questions validates the patient's experience of lung cancer and reinforces the therapeutic relationship between patient and oncology nurse. Answering the patient's questions clearly, accurately, and appropriately will diminish the patient's experience of uncertainty and its threat to hope. Warning the patient that there could be bad news or that treatment adherence may not be in the patient's best interest can help the patient to prepare and modify expectations and goals. Hope is possible at any point in the lung cancer continuum, and it means what the patient tells the oncology nurse it means.

There does not have to be hopelessness if an oncology nurse recognizes the profound influence of caring and empathy.

References

Ambuel, B., & Mazzone, M. (2001). Breaking bad news and discussing death. *Primary Care: Clinics in Office Practice, Palliative Care, 28*(2), 249–267.

Arnold R., & Quill, T. (2003). Hope for the best, and prepare for the worst. *Annals of Internal Medicine, 138*(5), 439–444.

Baile, W., Buckman, R., Lenzi, R., Glober, G., Beale, E., & Kudelka, A. (2000). SPIKES—a six-step protocol for delivering bad news: Application to the patient with cancer. *Oncologist, 5*(4), 302–311.

Ballard, A., Green, T., McCaa, A., & Logsdon, M. (1997). A comparison of the level of hope in patients with newly diagnosed and recurrent cancer. *Oncology Nursing Forum, 24*(5), 899–904.

Boyd, J. R. (2001). A process for delivering bad news: Supporting families when a child is diagnosed. *Journal of Neuroscience Nursing, 33*(1), 14–20.

Centers for Disease Control and Prevention. (2005). Annual smoking-attributable mortality, years of potential life lost, and productivity losses—United States, 1997–2001. *Morbidity and Mortality Weekly Report, 54*(25), 625–628.

Chapple, A., Ziebland, S., & McPherson, A. (2004). Stigma, shame and blame experienced by patients with lung cancer: Qualitative study. *British Medical Journal, 328*(7454), 1470.

Chauhan, G., & Long, A. (2000a). Communication is the essence of nursing care 1: Breaking bad news. *British Journal of Nursing, 9*(14), 931–938.

Chauhan, G., & Long, A. (2000b). Communication is the essence of nursing care 2: Ethical foundations. *British Journal of Nursing, 9*(15), 979–984.

Christakis, N., & Lamont, E. (2000). Extent and determinants of error in doctors' prognoses in terminally ill patients: Prospective cohort study. *British Medical Journal, 320*(7233), 469–473.

Clayton, J., Butow, P., Arnold, R., & Tattersall, M. (2005). Fostering coping and nurturing hope when discussing the future with terminally ill cancer patients and their caregivers. *American Cancer Society, 103*(9), 1965–1975. Retrieved on October 23, 2008, from http://www3.interscience.wiley.com/cgi-bin/fulltext/110432962/mail.html,ftx_abs

Dosanjh, S., Barnes, J., & Bhandari, M. (2001). Barriers to breaking bad news among medical and surgical residents. *Medical Education, 35*(3), 197–205.

Easterling, L., Gamino, L., Sewell, K., & Stirman, L. (2000). Spiritual experience, church attendance, and bereavement. *Journal of Pastoral Care, 54*(3), 263–275.

Eliott, J., & Olver, I. (2007). Hope and hoping in the talk of dying cancer patients. *Social Science and Medicine, 64*(1), 138–149.

Felder, B. (2004). Hope and coping in patients with cancer diagnoses. *Cancer Nursing, 27*(4), 320–324.

Ferrell, B. (2007). Meeting spiritual needs: What is an oncologist to do? [Editorial]. *Journal of Clinical Oncology, 25*(5), 467–468. Retrieved December 4, 2008, from http://jco.ascopubs.org/cgi/content/full/25/5/467

Field, M., & Cassel, C. (Eds.). (1997). *Approaching death: Improving care at the end of life.* Washington, DC: National Academy Press.

Friedrichson, M., Strang, P., & Carlsson, M. (2000). Breaking bad news in the transition from curative to palliative cancer care—Patient's view of the doctor giving the information. *Supportive Care in Cancer, 8*(6), 472–478.

Girgis, A., & Sanson-Fisher, R. W. (1995). Breaking bad news: Consensus guidelines for medical practitioners. *Journal of Clinical Oncology, 13*(9), 2449–2456.

Grassi, L., Giraldi, T., Messina, E., Magnani, K., Valle, E., & Cartei, G. (2000). Physicians' attitudes to and problems with truth-telling to cancer patients. *Supportive Care in Cancer, 8*(1), 40–45.

Griffin, J., Koch, K., Nelson, J., & Cooley, M. (2007). Palliative care consultation, quality-of-life measurements, and bereavement for end-of-life care in patients with lung cancer: ACCP evidence-based clinical practice guidelines (2nd ed.). *Chest, 132*(Suppl. 3), 404–422.

Griffin, J., Nelson, J., Koch, K., Niell, H., Ackerman, T., Thompson, M., et al. (2003). End-of-life care in patients with lung cancer. *Chest, 123*(Suppl. 1), 312–331.

Herth, K. (2001). Development and implementation of a hope intervention program. *Oncology Nursing Forum, 28*(6), 1009–1017.

Hoffman, P., Mauer, A., & Vokes, E. (2000). Lung cancer. *The Lancet, 355*(9202), 479–485.

Jurkovich, G., Pierce, B., Pananen, L., & Rivara, R. (2000). Giving bad news: The family perspective. *The Journal of Trauma: Injury, Infection, and Critical Care, 48*(5), 865–873.

Lin, H., & Bauer-Wu, S. (2003). Psycho-spiritual well-being in patients with advanced cancer: An integrative review of the literature. *Journal of Advanced Nursing, 1*(44), 69–80.

Moore, K., & Schmais, L. (2001). *Living well with cancer: A nurse tells you everything you need to know about managing the side effects of your treatment.* New York: Putnam.

Nail, L. (2001). I'm coping as fast as I can: Psychosocial adjustment to cancer and cancer treatment. *Oncology Nursing Forum, 28*(6), 967–970.

Parker, P., Baile, W., deMoor, C., Lenzi, R., Kudelka, A., & Cohen, L. (2001). Breaking bad news about cancer: Patients' preferences for communication. *Journal of Clinical Oncology, 19*(7), 2049–2056.

Ptacek, J., & Eberhardt, T. (1996). Breaking bad news: A review of the literature. *Journal of the American Medical Association, 276*(6), 496–502.

Pulchaski, C. (1999). A spiritual history. *Supportive Voice, 6*(5), 12–13.

Pulchaski, C., & Romer, A. (2000). Taking a spiritual history allows clinicians to understand patients more fully. *Journal of Palliative Medicine, 3*(1), 129–137.

Quirt, C., Mackillop, W., Ginsburg, A., Sheldon, L., Brundage, M., Dixon, P., et al. (1997). Do doctors know when their patients don't? A survey of doctor-patient communication in lung cancer. *Lung Cancer, 18*(1), 1–20.

Rodin, G., Zimmermann, C., Rydall, A., Jones, J., Shepherd, F., Moore, M., et al. (2007). The desire for hastened death in patients with metastatic cancer. *Journal of Pain and Symptom Management, 6*(33), 661–675.

Rustøen, T., & Wiklund, I. (2000). Hope in newly diagnosed patients with cancer. *Cancer Nursing, 23*(1), 214–219.

Rustøen, T., Wiklund, I., Hanestad, B., & Moum, T. (1998). Nursing intervention to increase hope and quality of life in newly diagnosed cancer patients. *Cancer Nursing, 21*(4), 235–245.

Sand, L., Strang, P., & Milberg, A. (2008). Dying cancer patients' experiences of powerlessness and helplessness. *Supportive Care in Cancer, 16*(7), 853–862.

Schofield, P., Beeney, L., Thompson, J., Butow, P., Tattersall, M., & Dunn, S. (2001). Hearing the bad news of a cancer diagnosis: The Australian melanoma patient's perspective. *Annals of Oncology, 12*(3), 365–371.

The, A-M., Hak, T., Koeter, G., & van Der Wal, G. (2000). Collusion in doctor-patient communication about imminent death: An ethnographic study. *British Medical Journal, 321*(7273), 1376–1381.

Vellone, E., Rega, M., Galletti, C., & Cohen, M. (2006). Hope and related variables in Italian cancer patients. *Cancer Nursing, 29*(5), 356–366.

Wonghongkul, T., Moore, S., Musil, C., Schneider, S., & Deimling, G. (2000). The influence of uncertainty in illness, stress appraisal, and hope on coping in survivors of breast cancer. *Cancer Nursing, 23*(6), 422–429.

Chapter 13

Meaning of Illness in Cancer

Pamela M. Calarese

Life has to be in the moment,
Spontaneous, and vulnerable.
There isn't any winning or losing.
Life itself is . . . The reward
And isn't always fun or easy . . .
The issue of happiness is irrelevant.
The relevant quest is the expansion of
consciousness.

Richard Moss, *The I That is We*

Background

Providing care for individuals and their families during their diagnosis and treatment of lung cancer provides an opportunity to initiate discussions that encompass an array of feelings such as hope, fear, anger, and utter disbelief. Providers commonly recognize that lung cancer is stressful. The expectation of many oncologists and nurse practitioners is that patients will eventually come to terms with their diagnosis and "fight" with the medical team to achieve as much of a cancer kill as possible (Keorner & Bunkers, 1994; Lazarus & Folkman, 1984).

Working in a comprehensive cancer center, specifically in thoracic oncology, a large percentage of patients present with stage III to stage IV non-small cell lung cancer (NSCLC) or extensive stage small cell lung cancer (SCLC) (NCCN, 2008; ACS 2008; Sequist, 2008). Most NSCLC patients present with advanced disease at the time of diagnosis, and 21% of patients have distant metastasis in the brain, bone, liver, or adrenal glands (De Petris, et al., 2006). Many individuals are referred by their primary healthcare provider for advice about the best approach to treatment. Because this disease is often diagnosed in later stages, it places the healthcare provider in a position of having to address potential end-of-life issues in conjunction with the stressors associated with lung cancer.

Most patients are quite up to date on the latest statistics and have done exhaustive research on the Internet for the best treatments and research studies. With that in mind, it is important to note that the overall statistics are not overwhelmingly optimistic. To highlight the devastation of lung cancer, it may be helpful to review the survival rates. If untreated, the median survival rate of NSCLC is 9 months for stage IB–IIIA and 13 months for patients who are diagnosed at stage IA (Raz, et al., 2007). The median survival is four to nine months for stages IIIB and IV. The median survival for SCLC, if untreated, is five to 12 weeks (Detterbeck, Rivera, Socinski, & Rosenman, 2001).

The overall 5-year survival in patients who are treated for lung cancer is only 14–20% (ACS, 2008). Each year approximately 165,000 people, male and female, will be diagnosed with lung cancer. Of those, 86% will die within five years of their diagnosis. The overall survival rate is 14%, which has increased over the last 30 years due to smoking cessation efforts. It is important to note that 10–15% of patients (17,000 to 26,000) are diagnosed with lung cancer who have either never smoked or smoked less than 100 cigarettes in their lifetime (Jemal, et al., 2008). Lung cancers that occur in never-smokers are four to five times more frequent in women compared to men (Jänne, 2007). Since 1987, deaths from lung cancer in women have surpassed deaths from breast cancer. While lung cancer in men has declined in recent years, a similar level of decline has not been achieved in women (Jemal, et al., 2008). It is worthwhile to report that lung cancer is currently the leading cause of cancer-related death in women, outnumbering deaths from cervical, uterine, breast, and ovarian cancers combined (ACS, 2008; Jemal, et al., 2008).

I experienced a powerful and unforgettable analogy of what it feels like to be given the diagnosis of lung cancer during the 2001 bombings of the World Trade Center in New York City. While watching the horror unfold on television, I was treating a patient with lung cancer in a bustling clinic. She looked up and asked me how it felt to be watching all of this unfold. My reaction was that of a surreal feeling. I could visualize the horror on the television screen and yet could not seem to assimilate the idea that this was actually happening. The patient said, "That, my dear, is how it feels to be told you

have lung cancer. You notice the day going on without you. You find yourself sort of stuck in a time warp. You feel like screaming but know that nobody will hear you."

As individuals with lung cancer digest the wealth of information related to their diagnosis and treatment, commonly asked questions are, "How long do I have?" "How will the end be?" and "How many people are cured from this?" While it is easy to recite statistics, oftentimes these numbers will relieve the individual and their family of any hope. It is vitally important to begin a dialog with patients that allow for the trajectory of diagnosis to death. Emphasis must be placed on maintaining hope throughout this entire journey (Groopman, 2004; Nail, 2001; Rhoden & McDaniel, 1996).

Oscar Breathnach, MD, had the most interesting approach to discussing the continuum of cancer, which encompassed diagnosis to death (McCray, 1994; Weisman & Worden, 1976). He received his oncology training in Ireland, where his education spanned the entire extent of the disease. He was quite respectful of the hospice system while being very aggressive in his approach to treating cancer. He began his discussion with all of his lung cancer patients in this manner. There are three phases of treatment in lung cancer. The first phase is the workup to determine the extent of disease. He would stress that this phase is the point of deciding which treatment modality would offer the most effective approach to kill cancer. He also acknowledged the emotional impact of the disease on the individual and family. He further reinforced that changes in lifestyles would occur as individuals begin to cope with the diagnosis of their disease (Breathnach, personal communication, 2001).

The second phase of treatment, as outlined by Dr. Breathnach, is the active treatment phase.

During this phase a multimodality approach is implemented, which encompasses surgery, chemotherapy, and radiation. During this phase of treatment, patients experience the emotional and physical ramifications of the treatment they receive. As a result, coping styles are modified and deepened as the overall experience of cancer is again changed and refocused (Groopman, 2004; Koerner, & Bunkers, 1994; Newman, 1994; Peteet, 2000). In the second phase of treatment, patients will most likely undergo a number of treatments aimed at decreasing or stabilizing the disease. When the cancer begins to progress, however, treatment approaches are reevaluated and changed. Patients and their families undergo a new active treatment cycle, with multiple clinic visits and a new set of potential side effects. This second phase can last for many months, and if there is a successful regression and stabilization, it can be longer than a year (Sequist, 2008; Groopman, 2004). It is during this phase of treatment that healthcare providers focus on "living with cancer."

The third and final phase of treatment occurs when the individual and/or the oncologist feel that the patient can no longer safely undergo aggressive treatment. This is when the focus is shifted from cure/stabilization to managing the symptoms associated with the cancer and ultimately maintaining comfort and dignity (Pantilat & Markowitz, 2001; Wilkes, Ingwersen, & Barton-Burke, 2000; Zhulhorsky, Abdullah, Richardson, & Walsh, 2000).

Theoretical Frameworks

There are many theoretical perspectives that discuss coping and physical illness. The works of Johnson et al. (1997), Leventhal and Nerenz (1982), and Lazarus and Folkman (1984) recognize the individual response to and the perception of disease. This response allows for individuals to perceive a situation and begin the process of setting up coping mechanisms that are as unique as the person who is diagnosed with cancer (Johnson, et al., 1997).

The Roy Adaptation Model focuses on the individual as an adaptive biopsychosocial being who uses innate and acquired coping mechanisms to deal with the changing environment (Roy, 1980). The person's behavior is affected by stimuli that are categorized as focal, contextual, and residual. The goal is to promote adaptation by manipulating stimuli and/or broadening adaptation levels.

The work of Margaret Newman and her theory of Health as Expanding Consciousness allows for the acknowledgment of disease, but it goes on to promote a sense of health within the continuum of illness (Newman, 1994; Paukstis-Laje & Laje, 2000). This framework also allows for providers to be present for the individual and his or her family as they begin their journey. The provider enables those involved to acknowledge the disease in all of its enormity but, at the same time, there is a refocusing to the positive aspects of the situation, such as deepening of shared emotion and communication that otherwise would not occur. This refocusing, also known as "patterning," fosters an expansion of consciousness, thus the emergence of health within illness (Newman, 1994; Paukstis-Laje & Laje, 2000). This theory allows for the meaning of illness to be an individual experience while providing a guide to assist the patient to achieve as much of a life response as possible (Koerner & Bunkers, 1994; Newman, 1994).

The Synergy Model for Patient Care is the nursing conceptual framework that guides patient and family care at Dana-Farber Cancer Institute. This framework views patients and family members as active participants in the patients' treatment (Curley, 2004). It seeks to match the healthcare provider's strengths to patients' and families' needs, recognizing that patients and family members may have different needs and that these needs will fluctuate at different points within the phases of treatment. Because lung cancer is usually diagnosed at a late stage, patients and family members have limited time to progress through the continuum of disease acceptance to the emergence of health within the illness. This condensed process makes the needs of lung cancer patients more complex than patients with other cancers. An interdisciplinary team approach that aligns patients' and family members' needs with the healthcare provider's strengths helps overcome some of the complexities in treating lung cancer patients.

The Diagnosis and the Individual Response

The diagnosis of lung cancer brings about a tremendous sense of living with uncertainty. Many lung lesions are found on routine physical exam. Of the approximate 165,000 new cases of lung cancer, a large number, 2–15%, of these will present asymptomatically (ACS, 2008; Kritz, 1997). The rate of lung cancer deaths in women has dramatically increased over the last decade, by approximately 160%. This is compared with a 20% rise in deaths for men within the same time period. There is a direct correlation between the use of tobacco and the rise in these figures (ACS, 2008; Minna, 2005; Sequist, 2008).

Along with the uncertainty of the diagnosis comes a sense of guilt over the chosen lifestyle of smoking. As a provider, it is vitally important to provide reassurance that smoking does not mean the individual deserves to have cancer. At the opposite end of that spectrum are individuals who develop lung cancer without ever smoking or being exposed to a known carcinogen. For this group, the sense that something is very wrong with their physical makeup is overwhelming because their bodies "have let them down" (ACS, 2008; Kritz, 1997; Zhulhorsky, et al., 2000).

The meaning of lung cancer and the manner in which people respond to the diagnosis will be a very individual response and will draw upon each person's response to past experiences that have required adaptation to stressful situations (Johnson, et. al., 1997; Lazarus & Folkman, 1984; Nail, 2001; Groopman, 2004). As individual as the person's response to cancer is, so too is the timing of diagnosis. For many, this seems to coincide with a family event, such as the birth of a child or grandchild, or an upcoming wedding (McCray, 1994; Nail, 2001; Peteet, 2000).

During the initial workup and staging of cancer, the individual may likely experience a variety of concerns that range from role and lifestyle changes to the likelihood that treatment may not effectively change the outcome. This is especially true in the younger population that is diagnosed with lung cancer (Spiegel, 1999).

To illustrate the impact of lung cancer on the patient, a case study is included, which will parallel the three stages of treatment (Detterbeck, et. al., 2001; Ginsberg, Kriss, & Armstrong, 1993).

Kathy, a 44-year-old lifelong nonsmoker, presented to her primary care physician with persistent low back pain. It began just after the

Thanksgiving holiday. She initially attributed her discomfort to jogging, carrying heavy bundles, and running after her two small children aged 4 and 6 years. Her primary care physician (PCP) prescribed nonsteroidal anti-inflammatory medication and physical therapy. These methods were successful for a few weeks, and then the discomfort turned into pain, radiating down her leg. She was evaluated again by her PCP, who ordered magnetic resonance imaging (MRI) of the lower spine to check for an abnormality in her lower back. The MRI revealed multiple lytic-looking areas in her entire lumbar thoracic spine, with no obvious spinal cord compression. She was then sent for further workup, which included a bone scan and computed tomography (CT) of the chest. The CT revealed a 1.5 cm spiculated mass in the left upper lobe of the lung and widely metastatic disease within the pelvis, hips, and ribs.

Kathy subsequently underwent biopsy of the hip bone, which revealed metastatic non-small cell lung cancer, adenocarcinoma in origin. She was then referred to a comprehensive cancer center for evaluation and initiation of treatment. Her staging at presentation was stage IV non-small cell lung cancer.

During her initial visit, Kathy was tearful and reserved. Her husband asked most of the questions, and Kathy seemed to listen but deferred any verbal interactions to her husband. They sat close together and held hands during the visit. At the end of the visit, Kathy was able to verbalize that her pain was oftentimes "so intense that it made it difficult for her to care for her children." She also made it very clear that she wanted to begin treatment as soon as possible to prevent further progression of disease.

A plan was made to incorporate a comprehensive pain regimen to enable Kathy to engage in some activities with her children. A return visit was arranged in an effort to allow Kathy the opportunity to digest all of the information she had been given within a very short period of time. Referrals to social services and a nutritionist were arranged to provide a comprehensive treatment plan and incorporate emotional support as well as provide her with the necessary tools to maintain adequate nutrition.

By the end of her first visit with her husband, Kathy was able to realistically articulate her hope that something could be done to allow her to live longer than she had read about online.

This example of one person's reaction to the diagnosis of lung cancer poignantly illustrates the dramatic life changes that ensue during this time of crisis (McDermott, 2000; Weisman & Worden, 1976). As a healthcare provider, it is vitally important to be present and listen to individuals as they process the information that is being related to them. Listening allows for the development of certain themes that arise from each individual's response to a situation, thus allowing for patterning and expansion of consciousness (Bramwell, 1984; Koerner & Bunkers, 1994; Newman, 1994; Rousseau, 2001). In this example the themes that stand out are:

- Independence
- Survival
- Spirituality and hope for a miracle
- Regression to an earlier stage of coping
- Loss of independence
- Bravery

Extracting these themes at the onset of developing a relationship is helpful in building a sound relationship with the patient and his or her family. This foundation fosters a sense of well-being and encourages the utmost in the continuum of health within illness (Newman, 1994). These same themes are deepened and patterned during the span of the disease, promoting emotional growth for all involved (Newman, 1994).

This assessment closely parallels "frequently worried about issues" that were identified and classified by Weisman and Worden (1976) as seven areas of predominant concern:

- Health concerns: A patient's level of worry is related to the individual's interpretation of disease spread and the significance of therapy-associated symptoms.
- Self-appraisal: Changes in physical appearance, along with changes in employment status, influence self-esteem and body image.
- Work and finance: Patients worry about their physical ability to continue working on a part-time basis or maintain full-time employment. Insurance issues and income concerns can be a tremendous source of emotional distress.
- Family and significant others: General mood swings, relationship issues, and sexual issues can strain relationships.
- Religion: Belief systems and attendance at church may allow some patients to feel comfort, while others feel abandonment.
- Friends and associates: The kindness of friends is cherished, but at the same time dependency is something with which the individual may not be comfortable.
- Existential concerns: Regardless of the diagnosis, individuals struggle with the finiteness of illness and the possibility of an early death (Weisman & Worden, 1976).

At this juncture, it is important to organize and implement a multidisciplinary team approach. The role of each of the healthcare providers is necessary to provide the standard in quality of care. Psychosocial issues can be identified by the healthcare provider but are best handled by social services, psychologists, and psychiatrists. Clergy and lay volunteers are wonderful resources for spiritual issues. Palliative care teams also provide input in pain and symptom management and act as liaisons to hospice. Navigators are new to the team. Navigators, who are trained as nurses or social workers, screen and help patients and their families move through the system to access the needed resources.

The Treatment Phase

Regardless of the number of combined treatments that are initially attempted, the treatment phase is a stressful period of time for patients and their families as they try to cope with the complexities of the treatment regimens. This is compounded by the need to navigate complex medical systems that traverse between chemotherapy, radiation, and surgery (John, 2000; Lazarus & Folkman, 1984). The patient may experience a sense of loss of control because of the extent of disease and also because of dependence upon others for transportation to and from large cancer centers that are far from home (Nail, 2001).

Along with the logistical aspects of treatment are the physical aspects. Lung cancer often presents with its own set of physical limitations.

Besides dyspnea, cough, and shortness of breath, pain is also an issue that individuals face. This symptom manifests as a result of the disease pressing on nerve groups or as a result of some of the diagnostic and therapeutic surgical interventions that the patient undergoes (Rhoden & McDaniel, 1996). The treatment regimen potentially causes nausea, vomiting, and dehydration. Alopecia is bothersome to both genders and in some cases, at the insistence of the patient, may result in the healthcare provider treating the patient with a different regimen to minimize this side effect. Taste alterations occur with both chemotherapy and radiation and can lead to a decrease in nutrition and ultimately in poor nutritional status (Rhoden & McDaniel, 1996).

Utilizing Newman's concept of Health as Expanding Consciousness is vital in attempting to prevent and minimize the side effects of treatment, such as nausea, vomiting, diarrhea, and dehydration, while at the same time being present for the individual to promote the health within illness (Levy, 1992; Rhoden & McDaniel, 1996). Promoting a sense of well-being will result in the highest level of quality of life, which, according to Campbell, is the ultimate in an individual's experience of life and may reflect his or her acceptance of the inability to meet a goal. As a healthcare provider, it is vital to allow individuals to achieve this level of quality within their cancer experience (McMillan & Weitzner, 2000; Rhoden & McDaniel, 1996). Returning to Kathy's situation, the case study continues.

Kathy's treatment was initiated with radiation therapy to the entire pelvic area. She obtained significant relief from the excruciating pain she had presented with and was able to be more involved in activities with her husband and children. However, she experienced myriad side effects, most notably diarrhea and resulting dehydration that required frequent IV infusions. She was taking high doses of narcotics for pain relief, which, along with the radiation, enabled her to continue activities with her family. A team approach that included social services, clergy, and patient peer support was also vital, allowing her to incorporate her disease into her daily life.

Kathy's initial chemotherapy was conventional carboplatin and paclitaxel, which resulted in stable disease after two cycles. However, after a short period of time she demonstrated progressive disease and required subsequent chemotherapies, which included multiple regimens of conventional chemotherapies as well as clinical trials aimed at interrupting the progress of the disease.

The cancer never regressed, but there were spans of time that afforded Kathy the opportunity to feel much better. At one point she was completely off her narcotic pain medications. Her clinic visits were part social and part therapeutic. She enjoyed sharing her stories of motherhood, shopping expeditions, and birthday planning with the staff. She was engaging and funny and spoke about the future with her husband and children.

However, consistent with what the lung cancer statistics illustrate, her cancer did ultimately grow to the point that she was no longer strong enough to tolerate chemotherapy. The focus of her treatment changed to palliation.

The same themes that were identified in the diagnostic phase are now more evolved and deepened in the treatment phase. The example presented reflects the theory of self-regulation as depicted by Johnson et al. (1997) and Leventhal and Nerenz (1982), which attempts to explain the mechanisms underlying the behavioral component of coping in response to a stressful event. Because the team of providers was present with Kathy during her treatment phase, she was truly able to pattern her experience and reach her own level of health within illness (Johnson, et al., 1997). Living with cancer requires that the individual and family adapt to the experience and the associated changes that occur over time. Both the occurrence of symptoms and the distress that each symptom presents requires readjustment and deepening of coping mechanisms (John, 2000; Roy, 1980).

End of Life: The Third Phase

The third phase of treatment brings with it the realization that the end of life is nearing. It is also the period of intense partnership between the patient, family, and healthcare providers. Care must be taken to fulfill the promises made at the outset of this journey to keep the individual as comfortable as possible. This means adequate pain control, nurturing for the patient and family, and decreasing the symptoms of end-stage lung cancer, such as increased cough and breathlessness (McDermott, 2000; Paukstis-Laje & Laje, 2000).

The benchmark of work that has been done on death and dying lies in the research of Kubler-Ross, which identifies the five stages of dying: denial, anger, bargaining, depression, and acceptance (Kubler-Ross, 1969). This work is furthered by Kavanaugh, who hypothesized that two tasks must be completed before an individual can die. The first task is for the dying person to receive permission from the important people

that he or she will leave behind. The second task is for the dying person to let go of all possessions and persons held dear (McCray, 1994). We continue Kathy's journey in the third and final phase.

As Kathy deteriorated and her disease began to grow; seemingly more rapidly, she openly discussed her fears and her sadness at leaving her two young children. She tried desperately to plan her daughter's birthday party and was adamant that she be involved. She was successful in doing so, but she participated from her hospital bed because she was too weak to be at home. The nursing staff supported her and provided a room full of balloons for her daughter for a family party in the hospital, with a "friends" party, which had been fully planned by Kathy, to take place the following day.

Kathy finally expressed a desire to just "let go." She was transferred to an inpatient hospice unit because she and her husband did not want to have her die at home with the kids. She did die with her husband by her side, and before she died she dictated letters to both children.

Ultimately, Kathy maintained her sense of control and ultimately died with the same grace and dignity that she exemplified during her short life.

Kathy's case is an individual review of the meaning of illness in lung cancer. She exemplified Weisman and Worden's seven areas of concern (1976, 1986). She also achieved health within illness as expressed by Newman's concept of Health as Expanding Consciousness (Newman, 1994).

Kathy's example of hope, bravery, and coping is humbling. Yet she mirrors the many heroes that also travel this path. Their journey is as unique and special as the individuals they are themselves.

References

American Cancer Society (ACS). (2008). *Cancer facts & figures*. Atlanta, GA: Author.

Bramwell, L. (1984). The use of life history in pattern identification and health promotion. *Advances in Nursing Science, 7*(1), 37–44.

Campbell, J., Cousineau, P., & Brown, S. (2003). *The hero's journey: Joseph Campbell on his life and work*. Novato, CA: New World Library.

Curley, M. A. (2004). The state of synergy. *Excellence in Nursing Knowledge*. Retrieved June 20, 2008, from http://www.nursingknowledge.org/

De Petris, L., Crino, L., Scagliotti, G. V., Gridelli, C., Galetta, D., Metro, G., et al. (2006). Treatment of advanced non-small cell lung cancer. *Annals of Oncology, 17*(Suppl. 2), ii36–ii41.

Detterbeck, F., Rivera, M., Socinski, M., & Rosenman, J. (2001). *Diagnosis and treatment of lung cancer: An evidence-based guide for the practicing clinician*. Philadelphia: W. B. Saunders.

Ginsberg, R., Kriss, M., & Armstrong, J. (1993). Cancer of the lung. In V. Devita, S. Hellman, & S. Rosenberg (Eds.), *Cancer principles and practice of oncology* (4th ed., Vol. 1). Philadelphia: Lippincott Williams & Wilkins.

Groopman, J. (2004). *The anatomy of hope: How people prevail in the face of illness*. New York: Random House.

Jänne, P. (2007). Non-small cell lung cancer in never smokers: A biologically and clinically distinct type of lung cancer. *American Society of Clinical Oncology 2007 Education Book* (pp. 401–405).

Jemal, A., Siegel, R., Ward, E., Hao, Y., Xu, J., Murray, T., et al. (2008). Cancer statistics, 2008. *CA: A Cancer Journal for Clinicians, 58*(2), 71–96. Retrieved May 20, 2008, from http://caonline.amcancersoc.org/cgi/content/full/58/2/71

John, L. (2001). Quality of life in patients receiving radiation therapy for non-small cell lung cancer. *Oncology Nursing Forum, 28*(5), 807–813.

Johnson, J. E., Fieler, V. K., Jones, L. S., Wlasowicz, G. S., & Mitchell, M. L. (1997). *Self regulation theory: Applying theory to your practice*. Pittsburgh, PA: Oncology Nursing Press.

Kavanaugh, R. (1976). Dealing naturally with the dying. *Nursing. 6*(10), 23–29.

Koerner, J. G., & Bunkers, S. S. (1994). The healing web: An expansion of consciousness. *Journal of Holistic Nursing, 12*(1), 51–63.

Kritz, F. L. (1997, January 1). Lung cancer risk is underestimated, especially by women. *Body and Soul: In the News*, p. 1.

Kubler-Ross, E. (1969). *On death and dying*. New York: Macmillan.

Lazarus, R. S., & Folkman, S. (1984). *Stress, appraisal and coping*. New York: Springer.

Leventhal, H., & Nerenz, D. R. (1982). A model for stress research and some implications for the control of stress disorders. In D. Meichenbaum & M. Jaremko (Eds.), *Stress prevention and management: A cognitive behavioral approach* (pp. 5–38). New York: Plenum Press.

Levy, M. (1992). Constipation and diarrhea in cancer patients. *Cancer Bulletin, 43*, 412–422.

McCray, N. (1994). Psychosocial issues. In S. Otto (Ed.), *Oncology nursing* (2nd ed.). Pittsburgh, PA: Oncology Nursing Press.

McDermott, M. (2000). Cough. In D. Camp-Sorrell & R. Hawkins (Eds.), *Clinical manual for the oncology advanced practice nurse*. Pittsburgh, PA: Oncology Nursing Press.

McMillan, S. C., & Weitzner, M. (2000). How problematic are various aspects of quality of life in patient's cancer at the end of life. *Oncology Nursing Forum, 27*(5), 817–823.

Minna, J. D. (2005). Neoplasms of the lung. In T. R. Harrison, et al. (Eds.), *Harrison's principles of internal medicine* (16th ed., pp. 552–568). New York: McGraw-Hill.

Nail, L. (2001). I'm coping as fast as I can: Psychosocial adjustment to cancer and cancer treatment. *Oncology Nursing Forum, 28*(6), 967–970.

National Comprehensive Cancer Network (NCCN). (2008). *Practice guidelines in oncology: Non-small cell lung cancer. V.2.2008*. Retrieved May 20, 2008, from http://www.nccn.org

Newman, M. (1994). *Health as expanding consciousness* (2nd ed.). New York: NLN Press.

Pantilat, S. Z., & Markowitz, A. J. (2001). Initiating end-of-life discussions with seriously ill patients. *Journal of the American Medical Association, 285*(22), 2906.

Paukstis-Laje, R., & Laje, G. (2000). Quality at the end of life. *Journal of the American Medical Association, 284*(12), 1513–1515.

Peteet, J. (2000). Cancer and the meaning of work. *General Hospital Psychiatry, 22*(3), 200–205.

Raz, D., Zell, J., Ignatius Ou, S., Gandara, D., Hoda, A.-C., & Jablons, D. (2007). Natural history of stage I non-small cell lung cancer: Implications for early detection. *Chest, 132*(1), 193–199. Retrieved May 27, 2008, from http://www.medscape.com/viewarticle/560050

Rhoden, V., & McDaniel, R. (1996). The symptom experience: Impact on quality of life. In S. Groenwald, M. H. Frogge, M. Goodman, & C. Yarbro (Eds.), *Cancer symptom management* (pp. 3–19). Sudbury, MA: Jones and Bartlett.

Rousseau, P. (2001). Kindness at the end of life. *Western Journal of Medicine, 174*(4), 292.

Roy, C. (1980). The Roy Adaptation Model. In J. P. Riehl & C. Roy (Eds.), *Conceptual models for nursing practice* (2nd ed., pp. 179–188). New York: Appleton-Century-Crofts.

Sequist, L. (2008). Non small cell lung cancer. In B. Chabner, D. Longo, & T. Lynch (Eds.), *Manual of oncology* (pp. 455–466). New York: McGraw-Hill.

Spiegel, D. (1999). A 43-year-old woman coping with cancer. *Journal of the American Medical Association, 282*(4), 371–378.

Weisman, A. D., & Worden, W. J. (1976). The existential plight of cancer: Significance of the first 100 days. *International Journal of Psychiatric Medicine, 7*(1), 1–15.

Weisman, A. D., & Worden, W. J. (1986). The emotional impact of recurrent cancer. *Journal of Psychosocial Oncology, 3*(4), 5–16.

Wilkes, G., Ingwersen, K., & Barton-Burke, M. (2000). *2000 Oncology nursing drug handbook*. Sudbury, MA: Jones and Bartlett.

Zhulhorsky, D., Abdullah, O., Richardson, M., & Walsh, D. (2000). Clinical evaluation in advanced cancer. *Seminars in Oncology, 27*(1), 24–33.

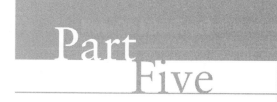

Part Five

*Assistance and
Resources for
Individuals Facing
Lung Cancer*

Chapter 14

Navigators Helping During the Cancer Journey

Amy Kuhns Roberts
Angelina Esparza

It is expected that about 2.5 million people in the United States will be newly diagnosed with cancer in 2008 (American Cancer Society, 2008). In addition, it is estimated that there are 10 million survivors living with the aftereffects of cancer. It is clear that diagnosis, treatment, and care for these individuals is a significant undertaking for the healthcare system and has a significant impact on the country. Those who are diagnosed with cancer are often confronted with a number of diverse challenges in accessing, utilizing, and navigating the healthcare system. The current healthcare system can present many barriers to the newly diagnosed and leave many to face a system that is often fragmented and disempowering. The American Cancer Society Patient Navigator (PN) program is designed to help meet these challenges and improve patients' access to resources to assist in their fight with the disease. Some patient navigator programs choose to focus on a subgroup of patients (i.e., lung cancer population), while other programs are more generalized, assisting any patient who has been diagnosed with cancer.

Numerous barriers to health care have been cited as the primary reason for the failure of many Americans to obtain quality care (Adler,

Boyce, Chesney, Folkmann, & Syme, 1993; Larson, Nelson, Gustafson, & Batalden, 1996; Yabroff, et al., 2004). Additive to the barriers that many face are the compounding factors associated with health and healthcare disparities among subpopulations of Americans (Bach, et al., 2002; Bacon & Kawachi, 2002; Nelson, 2003). Unnecessary suffering and death have been attributed to an inability to access the healthcare system and resources. Even when a person is able to access care, multiple factors are associated with failure to access appropriate resources needed prior to and through the treatment and recovery. These factors include: race (Chu, et al., 2001), gender (Landis, Murray, Bolden, & Wingo, 1999), age (Landis, et al., 1999), culture (Grossfeld, et al., 2002), education, functional and health literacy (Bennet, et al., 1998; Bilodeau & Degner, 1996; Kim, et al., 2001; Lannin, et al., 1998), transportation (Weinrich, Greiner, Reis-Starr, Yoon, & Weinrich, 1998), finances (Polednak, 1997), insurance (Penson, et al., 2001), interpersonal communications (Capirci, et al., 2005), and belief systems (Chavez, Hubbell, Mishra, & Valdez, 1997; Lambert, Fearing, Bell, & Newton, 2002; Nelson, Geiger, & Mangione, 2002). Cancer care, timely diagnosis, and treatment require the integration of efforts among multiple providers. Patient navigation is a means to fill the discovery–delivery gap by removing barriers to appropriate and timely health care. This chapter will describe how patient navigation has been proposed as a means to create assistance to cancer patients and describe the role of the navigator as the liaison between the healthcare system and the patient.

Patient Navigation and Health Disparities

The concept of patient navigation was conceived by Dr. Harold Freeman in the 1990s. Patient navigation originated following the American Cancer Society's "Report to the Nation; Cancer in the Poor" (1989) under the leadership of the then President Freeman. Dr. Freeman held hearings around the country to understand the needs and challenges faced by those within the lowest of socioeconomic levels when diagnosed with cancer. The report revealed that low-income persons frequently face financial and nonfinancial barriers when attempting to seek cancer diagnostics tests and treatment and often do not seek proper and/or timely care because of these barriers. Due to late stage cancer diagnosis and/or incomplete cancer treatment, the poor disproportionately experience pain, suffering, and death. Furthermore, the poor describe higher levels of fatalism, which often prevents them from seeking care.

Freeman and colleagues were the first to identify an association between low socioeconomic status and racial differences in cancer survival (Freeman, 2004). Based on the needs articulated by those who experienced barriers to care and his personal experience as a surgical on-

cologist in Harlem, Freeman created the first program that he termed "patient navigator." The program was started at the Harlem Hospital and was supported by a grant from the American Cancer Society. As a physician for that community, he often watched as women finally sought care at the latest stages of the disease, often incurable, leading to high mortality and morbidity for this population. The program focused on delivering services to women who had an abnormal screening result from initial mammography screening. It was the job of the patient navigator to assure that these women were able to receive timely diagnosis, treatment, and resolution.

The results of the program were dramatic. The project showed that 85.7% of patients that received navigation after initial suspicious finding upon screening received a recommendation for breast biopsy versus only 56.6% of nonnavigated patients. In addition, there was a significant shift in 5-year survival rate from 39% to 70% with the implementation of navigation. Dr. Freeman's landmark work showed that the concept of patient navigation showed promise in addressing barriers to care and follow-up that often contributed to health disparities in the Harlem population. The improvements shown by Dr. Freeman's program ignited a movement to implement patient navigators as a way to address health disparities. While many programs exist and differ in their approach, it is important to understand that addressing health disparities is not an easy task. Multiple factors are believed to play a role in discrepancies in health among populations, and patient navigation can only address some factors. However, understanding the impact and complexity of health disparities is helpful in assessing the need for these types of programs in the current complex, and often inequitable, health system that exists.

In 1999, the Institute of Medicine (IOM) (Haynes & Smedley, 1999) published a report that started many discussions on health disparities. The report, entitled, "The Unequal Burden of Cancer," was commissioned by the US Congress to review many of the institutes of the National Institutes of Health (NIH), including the National Cancer Institute. This section of the report evaluated the spending on cancer research relative to minorities and the medically underserved, examined the communication of existing research findings on the topic to affect prevention and treatment programs, and examined the adequacy of NIH procedures to assure the inclusion of women and minorities in clinical trials. After much research and investigation of trends and outcomes, the report concluded that, "Despite scientific gains, not all segments of the US population have benefited to the fullest extent from advances in the understanding of cancer" (p. 10).

Health disparities and cancer are as variable as the disease itself, and many proposed root causes have been discussed: socioeconomics, health belief systems, insurance coverage, access to care, cultural barriers, and biological differences (Haynes & Smedley, 1999).

Gansler, et al. (2005) investigated the role of health literacy and decision making related to breast cancer screening. The authors discussed sociodemographic variables, health literacy, attitudes, and beliefs as well as the effect that knowledge and utilization of screening may have on suboptimal health decisions about disease prevention, early detection, and treatment, which may contribute to health disparities (Boulware, Cooper, Ratner, LaVeist, & Powe, 2003; Nielsen-Bohlman, Panzer, & Kindig, 2004). The study was designed to interview a varied sample to ascertain knowledge about cancer and the likelihood of having misconceptions about cancer. The authors found that subjects with higher education and income were more likely to be more knowledgeable about cancer and less likely to have misconceptions. Subpopulations including nonwhites (African Americans and Hispanics), subjects greater than 65 years of age, and those from the South reported not being informed about cancer and had the highest misconception scores.

The literature has documented disparities in lung cancer and identified factors from myths about disease and treatment to practitioner bias. Margolis, et al. (2003) conducted a survey among lung cancer patients in five pulmonary thoracic surgery outpatient clinics in the United States. A misbelief that lung cancer is spread by exposure to the air at the time of surgery was more prominently discussed by African-American patients (19%) than by white patients (5%). What was most notable was the influence of this belief on treatment. Fourteen percent of the African-American respondents and 5% of the white respondents expressed opposition to lung cancer surgery on the basis of this belief, and furthermore they would reject the advice of the physician to have surgery as a course of treatment (Margolis, et al., 2003). Clearly, there are different beliefs among subpopulations, and understanding the origins of these beliefs is complex.

In part, the historical discrimination and disenfranchisement of populations may add to a level of distrust among communities against the healthcare system as a whole. It is in these instances that the use of a patient navigator, a person outside of the clinical team, may help to bridge the patients' gap of concerns and provide information to assist the patients in making the best choices for their treatment and care. A patient navigator who is the broker between patients, the patient support system, and the medical team may help to elucidate the need for improved communication and assist the patients in understanding how to discuss these concerns with their healthcare providers.

Patient navigation has also been used to increase screening and address delays in follow-up after the discovery of a suspicious finding, particularly in cancer with reliable screening tests. Delays in follow-up cancer screening have been associated with health disparities in cancer outcomes, particularly among racial and ethnic minority populations. Battaglia et al. (2007) conducted a study to examine the role of patient navigation and follow-up care. After an adjusted analysis, the authors found that women who received navigation had 39% greater odds of having timely follow-up after initial screening. Timely follow-up was defined as 120 days or less. The investigators also found that some patient characteristics showed a stronger relationship to the intervention (patient navigation) success. These characteristics include women over 65 years of age, those with private insurance, those referred to a hospital-based practice, and those who have an abnormal mammogram.

Follow-up to screening requires a number of steps to be completed. First the results have to be communicated to both the healthcare provider and the patient, then the appropriate diagnostic follow-up must be determined and explained, the provider and site for follow-up care must be determined, and the patient must make and keep the appointment. Within these many steps exist challenges for the patients and may prove to be overwhelming for some. While this sequence outlines follow-up care, a similar set of activities and tasks is associated with treatment. This is where the patient navigator has shown to be most helpful in the coordination and assistance of completing each of these steps and addressing and eliminating barriers as they arise.

Socioeconomic status (SES) factors have long been associated with the differences in screening rates; however, most studies have shown that SES alone does not account for the differences in utilization. Even when universal access is present, there are still differences in screening rates (Farley & Flannery, 1989). Cultural factors, including beliefs, attitudes, and knowledge about cancer, have been suggested as possible contributing factors. It is accepted that it is most likely the combination of cultural barriers in combination with limited access to care, either through limited insurance coverage, physical access, limited physicians, and other structural barriers, that may help to elucidate possible reasons for the lower screening rates and thus lower survival rates and increased morbidity (Chu, Charisse, & Freeman, 2003).

Unequal treatment may also pose a problem that is a difficult subject for many to discuss because inherent in the discussion is the idea of deep-seated racial bias and social injustice. In the "Unequal Treatment" report (Smedley, Stith, & Nelson, 2003), the IOM discussed the influence of unequal treatment through three main sources: healthcare system, patient level, and disparities arising from clinical encounters. Examples cited of healthcare system barriers include linguistic and cultural barriers, lack of a stable relationship between the patient and provider, financial limitation, and the fragmentation of the system. Racial and ethnic minority patients are more likely than white patients to refuse treatment, but differences in refusal rates are generally small, and minority patient refusal does not fully explain healthcare disparities (Smedley, et al., 2003).

These differences in treatment selection have been noted in the treatment of lung cancer. Although little difference has been noted in survival for those in late-stage disease, the most important discrepancies relate to early stage resectable disease. Greenwald, et al. (1998) found in three diverse treatment sites that of individuals with stage I non-small cell lung cancer who were diagnosed between 1980 and 1992, African Americans were 20% less likely to undergo surgery and 31% less likely to survive 5 years. A similar study conducted by Bach et al. (2002), with a sample of elderly patients in 10 US sites, reported 13% lower rate of surgery and 8% lower survival rate among African Americans (Greenwald, et al., 1998).

Types of Navigation Services

The National Cancer Institute has provided the following definition of navigation: "Assistance offered to healthcare consumers to help them access and chart a course through the healthcare system and overcome barriers to care."

While this definition provides a solid framework to describe patient navigation in general, variations on this theme are exhibited in the multiple types of current navigation programs. Although there are variations in the structure of the program, ultimately the core principles of the program are the same and reflect the previous definition. Program delivery can differ by services, characteristics of the patient navigator, time at which services are offered, and location of program delivery, to name a few (Dohan & Schrag, 2005).

The use of lay navigators is common, and this was the original model used by Dr. Freeman. Lay navigators, sometimes referred to as lay health advisors, have not received professional training related to a healthcare field. These navigators are juxtaposed to navigators who are associated with a professional degree or title, such as nurses (sometimes referred to as nurse navigators) or social workers who function in the role of patient navigators. This distinction does not take into account any formal education that the patient navigator may have received or any additional experience in a healthcare field. There is no data to suggest that a professional title or education attainment has any influence or advantage as one functions in the position. In some cases there may be a preference for a skill set that aligns most closely with the overall goals of a particular program. Within the American Cancer Society Patient Navigator (PN) program, which will be discussed at length, there is no professional requirement, and success has been noted by using patient navigators of diverse educational backgrounds and experiences.

Navigation can begin at any point of entry along the cancer continuum and varies among programs depending on the goals and structure of the navigation program. Some programs, as in the case with Harlem Hospital, begin with assisting individuals through screening and resolution. Because many who have a suspicious finding on initial screening resolve without a cancer diagnosis, only a percentage of cases are then navigated as cancer patients. Most of the research to date has focused on this type of navigation service.

Other programs focus on the time after a patient is diagnosed and offer peer support, for example, cancer survivors as guides or patient navigators through the system. The American Cancer Society PN program begins navigation at the point of a definitive diagnosis and partners with cancer treatment facilities. The patient navigator is actually placed within the treatment facility to provide one-on-one services and guidance to the patient, caregiver, and loved ones. The patient is assisted throughout the treatment process as barriers arise during and following treatment. This continuous contact with a patient allows for the full use of programs and services offered by the American Cancer Society that are appropriate to address the changing information and service needs of the patient throughout the cancer continuum.

The location of the patient navigator, either in a healthcare setting or community based, can present its own challenges. The use of navigation in a community setting may be selected based on the purpose of the program. In some cases, the use of navigation in a community setting assists in encouraging utilization of screening or other health promotion activities. This may also include assistance in navigation through a healthcare facility, even though the patient navigator is not physically located in the treatment center. As previously mentioned, some programs, such as the American Cancer Society PN program, are located within the healthcare facility, which provides direct access to the patient and healthcare providers. The location of the patient navigator within the healthcare setting may also create a sense of integration of the navigator into the services offered to the patient. It is important to note that both of these approaches are important to the overall care of the patient and the need to address concerns and barriers. Each environment, the community and treatment facility, provides its own types of challenges to overcome. The patient navigator can be a successful part of addressing the needs of the individual within and across these environments as he or she moves from screening to diagnosis, treatment, and aftercare. In a site-specific navigation program, such as a patient navigator whose focus is lung cancer, the navigator may work directly with the cardiothoracic surgeon, often contacting pa-

tients by phone prior to a definitive diagnosis and just after a suspicious scan or finding. The navigator may help to provide encouragement and resources in an effort to secure a timely result so that if the person does have cancer, treatment delays are minimized. The surgeon will appreciate the added attention that a navigator can provide and will include navigation services even before a diagnosis is made.

Services of programs may vary, and a combination of services may be offered through one program. A limited list of the combination of services that are offered most often are: provision of information about disease prevention, site-specific and treatment options, practical advice on dealing with the disease, psychosocial support (professional), patient advocacy, peer support, financial assistance and guidance, referral to multiple resources, and one-on-one assistance. While this is not an exhaustive list, it does represent the most common types of services. These services may be provided in person or using a telephone-based call center or Web site. Programs may also focus on one type of cancer, such as lung cancer, or a particular population or geographic area.

The American Cancer Society provides navigation in a variety of mechanisms. Navigation can include the use of the Society's Web site (www.cancer.org), calls to the National Cancer Information Center (1-800-227(ACS)-2345), and the use of community offices and services throughout the country. The presence of the American Cancer Society throughout many communities allows the organization to be able to support constituents where they work and live. However, each of these mechanisms requires constituents to reach out to the Society and retrieve information. The American Cancer Society PN program is an attempt to reach out to patients in healthcare facilities as a way to proactively promote the awareness and utilization of the Society's programs and services. In addition, the PN program helps to identify hospital-, national-, and community-based resources, assist the patient in accessing these services, and coordinate the resources to address the patient's barriers and needs.

Patient Navigation in Action

The most compelling information about patient navigation can be shared through case examples. A description of a patient navigation program located in a semiurban setting is discussed in this section. To protect patients' and families' confidentiality, some general demographic information may be omitted or slightly altered. The navigation program that is discussed serves patients and families with any cancer diagnosis (with the top two sites consisting of breast and lung cancers) and is utilized in an outpatient clinic setting; however, the navigator occasionally meets with patients and families in the acute hospital setting. When considering the examples that do not specify the type of cancer, one can interject that persons who are facing a lung cancer diagnosis will likely encounter the same barriers with similar solutions.

When a person hears the word "cancer" for the first time, he or she ultimately does not hear much else after that surreal moment. Many people have difficulty making sense of all this information following the shocking diagnosis of cancer. If you ask a patient or family who has just received a cancer diagnosis if they have any questions, you might hear something like, "I don't know what I need," or, "I am not sure

what I am supposed to be asking. You tell me, is there something I am missing?" Many times people feel exhausted after spending 45 minutes listening to the physician explain chemotherapy, surgery, and radiation. Some people feel better prepared, but often people wonder if they can or will comprehend what they have just heard and how much new information they can absorb at one time. Often patients and families haven't slept in the last few days or weeks worrying over the unknown result of a pathology report.

Often healthcare systems are overwhelming and foreign to people. Barriers limit people's ability to access services that already exist. Navigators step in just after a diagnosis. They listen to what a patient and their family needs. If a patient is too overwhelmed, the navigator can begin to direct him or her each step of the way. Navigators help to highlight the special skills, training, and knowledge of the myriad professionals who can be available to patients and help patients know what services to request during their cancer journey. A navigator serves as a liaison to these incredibly valuable resources and helps people learn to access these resources at a time when they are feeling numb and in shock. A navigator is not meant to replace desperately needed hospital staff that is so crucial in helping patients and families during their care. Many times patients and families just aren't sure who to ask, where to turn, or that a resource even exists that could meet their needs.

Fostering Communication and Informed Decisions

Navigators foster communication and help promote understanding during the cancer experience. They do this by assisting people with cancer and their support system (family members, caregivers, etc.) in gaining an understanding of the healthcare system while also working to help the healthcare system understand the cultural, economic, and psychosocial perspectives of individuals. Navigators work with individuals to help them communicate with their medical team for health care that respects and complements the individual's needs. One effective way to accomplish this is having the navigator work as a part of a multidisciplinary team that respects the unique talents, training, and gifts of each team member. In this way, the navigator can utilize the wealth of knowledge and resources that are available at the hospital level. Navigators can direct patients and families to people who give tremendous insight and guidance through a terribly overwhelming and confusing matrix of medical demands. Patients or families are often unaware of resources and professionals at the hospital level and what exactly each can provide. This collaboration, networking, and partnerships are what allow navigators to accomplish their goals of eliminating barriers to care, alleviating stress, and providing support. A case example of a Hispanic female (Mrs. N), who speaks primarily Spanish, is presented to show how a navigator may help to foster communication and understanding within a medical setting.

> *Mrs. N is often tearful during her care, and it is understood that she is in quite a bit of pain from her cancer and her treatments. The navigator is able to place a consultation for pastoral care to sit with her and an interpreter to visit so that they may talk. The navigator learns that in addition to the physical pain Mrs. N is experiencing, she also misses her mother, who is in Mexico, terribly and that her mother's health*

> *is not well. In addition to this increased spiritual support and understanding, Mrs. N was also linked to a support group for people who have similar diagnoses and treatments. At the group the presenter speaks both English and Spanish, and Mrs. N learns about other supportive programs, such as physical therapy services.*

Another way to foster communication and understanding is with education by linking patients and families to information about their cancer, treatments, clinical trials, health care, and support programs. Many patients and families have never faced this before and don't know what to expect. Being informed about the disease and treatments may help them feel more in control and allow them to begin to comprehend what is happening. A navigator helps in this orientation to cancer by providing patients and their families with reliable information about their diagnosis and treatment in easy-to-understand terminology. Navigators may also serve as coordinators in many ways by scheduling scans, consultations, and appointments for people who may not be able to manage this aspect of their care. In this setting a survivor's guidebook can be created to help orient patients and families to the healthcare system and to cancer. It could include maps to the various treatment centers, descriptions of the medical team members, a brief overview of the types of treatments available, blank calendars, sample questions for patients to discuss with their medical team, logs to record questions for physicians and nurses, and a list of local services that are most commonly needed during the cancer journey. In a lung cancer site-specific navigation program, this guidebook could be tailored to specifically include resources and treatments that relate to lung cancer. The guidebooks can be distributed to local physician offices, clinics, and treatment areas where people are most likely to learn of a new diagnosis. The book should include a description of the navigator program and how to get connected for services.

For many patients and families, barriers (fear, culture, anxiety, pain, health literacy, language, etc.) will influence the way education is provided to them. They may need the one-on-one guidance and encouragement of the navigator and healthcare team, interpreters to bridge language barriers, or a connection to a survivor who shares similar cultural, racial, or socioeconomic experiences. Linking patients to knowledge empowers them to actively participate in their medical plan, ask questions of their team members, and make well-informed decisions about their care. Patients are provided with the toll-free number to the American Cancer Society's Cancer Information Specialists, linked to healthcare team members, provided with a list of questions they may want to talk with their physician about, provided with easy-to-understand literature, and given encouragement for utilizing reliable, trusted Internet sites. The navigator, as well as the American Cancer Society Cancer Information Specialists, informs patients of resources specific to their diagnosis. For example, a person who is facing lung cancer may be provided with information about local lung cancer support groups; Caring Ambassadors Program (CAP) for Lung Cancer, which includes a Web page called Lung Cancer Ask a Doc, a publication entitled *With Every Breath: A Lung Cancer Guidebook*, and support; and the Lung Cancer Alliance (LCA) Survivors Support Community Phone Buddy Program. Navigators help guide patients through the process of finding information and show patients and families how to access these resources in the future.

Navigators Identify Patient and Family Needs

As mentioned earlier in the general outline of where navigation starts, it is imperative that navigators understand what barriers people face and listen to the individual perspectives of people who are considered to be at risk for falling through the cracks. It is critical to include the healthcare team members in the navigation process as a patient's needs become complicated and counseling is indicated for the patient and/or family members. In these cases a referral to appropriate healthcare providers and resources would be made by the navigator. The American Cancer Society (ACS) model of patient navigation encourages collaborative efforts with other disciplines.

While a navigator does not function in the role of a clinical social worker, the theoretical framework of "ecological perspective" or "person in environment," which has been a basic framework for the profession of social work since the mid-1970s, may help to illustrate not only the impact of the specific disease state but also the many aspects of the individual patient's needs and concerns (Hepworth, Rooney, & Larsen, 1997).

The Person in Environment Theory can be attributed to the work of Carel Bailey Germain. She first developed the concept of an ecological perspective while teaching at Columbia and later elaborated upon it in collaboration with a colleague, Alex Gitterman (Carel Bailey Germain, 1922–1998). The Person in Environment Theory, or the ecological perspective model, suggests that one cannot just consider one aspect of a person but needs to consider the relationship of how the environment and person are interconnected. For example, if a navigator only addresses the barrier of transportation but does not consider a person's fear and anxiety relating to medical costs, coordinating a ride could be ineffective. The individual may need to secure applications for health insurance funding and meet with a counselor to help the person cope with their lung cancer diagnosis.

A common barrier that patients and families cope with is living in poverty or with limited financial means. It might be helpful to consider the Person in Environment Theory when looking at poverty as a barrier to health care. Having a diagnosis of cancer may affect a person's physical and psychosocial components, including but not limited to: income, work, socialization/isolation, emotional well-being, physical well-being, mental health, transportation, relationships, spirituality, housing, food, utilities, etc. A second viewpoint could be that a diagnosis of poverty can affect overall health, cancer, and treatment outcomes. This is illustrated by the previously referenced "Cancer in the Poor" report, which shows that people in poverty, who are more likely to die from cancer and endure greater suffering, are less likely to seek care if they cannot afford it, and often have belief systems that mirror fatalism (American Cancer Society, 1989).

In the following case example, the initial response to the need may be strictly economic. However, upon closer exploration, challenges may lie in myriad factors, making it hard to distinguish the differing effects of poverty or disease on outcomes. The effects of poverty and some of the challenges it represents when coupled with a cancer diagnosis are reiterated by the following case example.

Ms. C is a single woman in her mid-40s who has recently been diagnosed with lung can-

cer. Due to her diagnosis, Ms. C was unable to work, so she decided to leave her residence and job, consequently losing her healthcare coverage in an effort to be in a more emotionally supportive environment. Ms. C now has no primary residence. The lack of income has affected her housing and her transportation, which means she "cannot make it to treatment until she finds somewhere to live." She admits to feeling depressed and feeling tired all the time. Her feelings of being tired have made her inactive and could possibly contribute to her depression. Her inability to work has isolated her socially. In this example, one can see how her diagnosis of cancer can affect other areas of her life as they become intertwined and interrelated.

The navigator talks with Ms. C about her plans for treatment. Ms. C is worried about the many expenses she needs to cover, not only related to care, but also to survival (rent, gas, utilities, medications, food). Despite efforts to offer assistance with housing and transportation, she is resistant to start treatments, stating that she "just wants to get a place to live first." After continued conversation with the patient navigator, Ms. C begins to share her personal beliefs, which include some aspects of fatalism related to the disease. She states, "I have lived a very rough life," and alludes to her cancer diagnosis as possibly a reasonable consequence or a reason to allow death to occur. The environment (multiaspects), her feelings of depression, and her personal belief system may contribute to her inability or desire to access treatment.

Using the information that Ms. C provided and understanding the larger context of the patient's financial situation, cultural beliefs, personal barriers, and family support system, the navigator is able to provide assistance to help mitigate the effects of these combined influences.

This example reminds one to look at the entire person in his or her environment and the importance of culture and belief systems when surviving with limited financial resources and facing cancer. Although a navigator may know how to secure transportation resources, contact the local housing authority agency, apply for medication assistance programs, and obtain Medicaid coverage (which is a significant and major aspect of patient navigation), if the navigator is not trained to look at the person in environment and deliver culturally competent care, all the resources at his or her disposal may not be utilized. It is important to start where the client is and have the person with cancer take part in establishing a treatment plan that is relevant to his or her environment, belief system, and culture.

Several other barriers are listed in Tables 14–1, 14–2, 14–3, and 14–4.

The following example illustrates how a person with cancer (one could interject lung cancer) who is coping with basic access to resources was assisted by the patient navigation program.

Mr. M is a 60-year-old gentleman who has been undergoing radiation treatment for a cancer diagnosis. He has worked his entire life doing construction but did not have health insurance coverage or any income during his treatments. The county he lives in has one of the highest mortality rates from cancer than other counties in this region. Mr. M was linked to financial assistance programs for medications and for the cost of gas during his treatments. Mr. M said, "I would not have been able to afford the medicines period, it is just that simple. {The navigator} has bent over backwards to help me."

Table 14–1 Healthcare Coverage and Associated Financial Challenges

Lack of health insurance.

Difficulty understanding, accessing, and fully implementing healthcare coverage provided by insurer.

Financial burden associated with copayments and deductibles.

Lack of income or healthcare coverage during the waiting process for federal- and state-based programs.

Dissolution of assets is required to be eligible for federal- and state-based programs.

Limited or no prescription coverage plans.

Loss of job, income, and/or healthcare coverage.

Ineligibility for government assistance because the person will not be out of work for a full year (mandated by Social Security Disability Insurance) and has no option for short-term or long-term disability income through his or her employer. The patient may be out of work for 6 months due to treatment but still not qualify for financial assistance services to maintain his or her basic needs.

Table 14–2 Health-Related Challenges

Mental illness (including but not limited to: alcoholism, addiction, dementia, depression, personality disorders, developmental delays, disorders of sleep, adjustment, mood, anxiety, etc.).

Emotional distress (including fear, anxiety, grief, adjustment difficulties relating to a new diagnosis).

Comorbidities including both preexisting and new onset (diabetes, heart disease, chronic obstructive pulmonary disease, home oxygen requirements, etc.).

Physical disabilities (including preexisting) and physical changes related to disease or treatment.

Pain that is uncontrolled or unrelieved.

Table 14–3 Resources and Environmental Challenges

Physical distance from treatment facilities, transportation.

Unavailable or nonexistent family, social, and/or spiritual support systems.

Increased cost of living.

Limited health (medical) literacy skills or limited knowledge about diagnosis and treatments.

Housing, substandard housing, homelessness, inability to maintain home during illness, no working telephone, water, etc.

Weather-related and other environmental challenges, such as ice, snow, and storms, specifically for those living on mountainous terrain where county disability transport systems cannot access the roads.

Table 14–4 Systems-Related Challenges

Systems may not be easily accessed or may not be user friendly for the general public.

Provider bias.

Fragmented systems and services.

Taking Action

When a navigator is able to establish what challenges or needs the patient and family face, taking into consideration culture and belief systems, he or she is now ready to begin to assist the entire family. Patients, their families, and healthcare providers are often unaware of all the services that exist and how to access them. Resources and support programs are available to people who are affected by cancer, but many times the patient and family do not access these resources. Patient navigators have listened to

survivors express frustration and anger when they felt that they hadn't been properly informed of these programs or been made aware of these resources.

Many times, knowing about a resource is not enough. Although patients may be encouraged to contact Medicaid, Social Security, and their employer about the Family and Medical Leave Act and short-term disability, often some patients are unable to follow through with these demands. A call for help may just seem like one more thing on an already overwhelming checklist of things to do. This is where the navigation program steps in to fill the gap that exists in many healthcare systems. Not everyone is able to make these phone calls or knows what to say when they do call. Not everyone can fill out the forms or keep up with the expectations of such complex treatment demands. The following example illustrates how a single woman in her 50s, with limited family support, may face challenges when accessing resources and how the patient navigation program assisted her. This case example could easily be the same story of a person who is coping with a lung cancer diagnosis and illustrates how accessing systems can be a challenge to some individuals.

Ms. N is a patient who needs services. The patient navigator made endless phone calls to help her keep heat in her home during the winter, help her with medical bills, and help give her hope that, despite all the barriers and fears, she could receive the recommended medical treatment. She often described that her "memory is no good." Her anxiety and fear inhibited her from making the calls herself. She even began to avoid answering the telephone, fearing potential calls from bill collectors. One day she told the navigator, "I could never do that." When asked, "Do what?" she stated, "That," She pointed at the phone, "calling all those people, thank you so much." She said that without the navigator she would have "gone cold" this winter and that she would not have been able to get her treatment.

By keeping the navigation role focused on accessing information and resources, and eliminating gaps or barriers, navigators have the time and ability to follow through that many specialized healthcare professionals may not have in today's demanding healthcare system. This is just one example of many people who have fallen into the category of being medically underserved due to limited health literacy, financial resources, or environmental factors. In addition to the medically underserved, a gap has been bridged for people who do not fit into these categories: people who have financial resources, people with supportive families, and people with some knowledge of medicine. Sometimes just pointing people in the right direction for guidance can be a lifeline. If you have never had cancer, you may not be aware of what is available.

This quote belongs to a young lady who knew how to use the Internet and a toll-free number and who had an intricate understanding of her disease because she had been living with cancer for many years.

The Patient Navigator has been a fabulous advocate and friend. She came to me, rather than being a resource-in-name only. Encouraging me with her knowledge of available resources, I've referred others, including my mother, to her, and she's had something to offer everyone. This office, and {navigator} in particular, fills an emotional, financial, and medical need that is part of what elevates the Hospital/ACS Navigator program to a truly life saving program. That's what anyone with cancer really

wants; to keep as much of their life as they can, for as long as they can. (A. Carpenter, Personal Communication, August 9, 2007)

Eliminating Gaps

An ACS Patient Navigator (PN) works in collaboration with healthcare professionals instead of personally eliminating every barrier that faces patients and their families. The PN's role is to identify gaps within communities and healthcare systems and raise awareness about those resource gaps. A PN's direct connection to patients' experiences and stories allow him or her to serve as an advocate and a direct link to other groups. PNs serve in work groups at hospitals, partner with ACS field staff, and actively network with community agencies. In this way, PNs can present the challenges people with cancer face and identify the gaps in the systems that provide services. The PN's input can help to develop solutions and programs that eliminate gaps in resources, not only for one patient and family, but for larger groups of individuals who are in need.

Networking, advocacy, and collaboration are all at the heart of being an effective navigator. Navigators must know the resources and how to access the many systems that patients encounter. Navigators serve as a vital link to financial counselors, pastoral care members, hospital social workers, and nurses. Many times navigators work side by side with oncology nurses and oncology social workers to assist patients. Nurses and physicians provide vital clinical assessments about patients' medical needs, care plans, and expected side effects, and they are excellent resources to help provide patients with further education about their disease and treatments. These assessments and close communication allow navigators to deliver services appropriately.

Nurses are also excellent resources for case management needs, for example, knowing whom to call in the medical setting and helping the navigator understand how all the pieces fit together. Oncology social workers are typically MSW-level clinicians who initiate clinical psychosocial assessments and have specialized training in assessment and intervention in the medical setting. Oncology social workers can provide brief counseling relating to adjustment to illness, grief, crisis intervention, and more. Their assessments of patients' needs are critical in appropriately interacting with patients and families and understanding family systems, culture, mental illness, and individual needs. Navigators collaborate with nurses, social workers, physicians, and many others on a daily basis to best meet patients needs.

Navigators connect patients and families to national nonprofit organizations that help with medical bills and copays, to community health departments and clinics that provide patient assistance programs for medications, and to local transportation programs, hospitality houses, homeless shelters, and Medicaid offices.

> **Tip: To help a person with no prescription coverage, visit the Web site www.needymeds.org. It provides a comprehensive list of every medication and provides a link to the pharmaceutical company's medication assistance program if there is one available. In many cases you can download the application directly from the site.**

Navigators often rely on local organizations, such as the council on aging, for services like respite care, Meals on Wheels, and other services for the elderly who are facing cancer. It seems to be impossible to describe a navigator's typical day because no day seems to be typical. The navigator fills out forms, talks with team members, calls agencies, informs people of resources, and helps to develop resources and services where gaps occur. Navigators spend time listening to caregivers, family members, and patients. One large reason the ACS Patient Navigator program is effective is that the PN's role is clearly defined and intentionally focused on resources that increase knowledge about cancer and treatment options and eliminates barriers to care. This clear focus and goal truly allow time to become an expert on the large amount of resources needed and to develop the resources or awareness where gaps exist. So many times, it is a comfort to know that there is a person who can help give patients and their families the hope and strength they need to move out of fear and shock and begin to face the path ahead of them. In summary, the final case example allows us to see firsthand how a navigator's help in managing the struggles of finances, health coverage, and resources can translate into hope and success for the person who is facing cancer. Ms. F is a very pleasant 70-year-old female who is facing cancer.

Ms. F has Medicare coverage and a supplemental plan, and at age 70, she was still working part time. She took a lot of pride in the fact that she worked her entire life. After being told she had cancer, she had to quit due to daily radiation therapy treatments. She later shared that she had paid incredible debts for the health care of a loved one in her past; she had sold her home to pay for medical care and never asked for a single penny in all her life. When she was told about her own cancer, she was ready to give up hope.

The navigator was able to link Ms. F to resources to change her supplemental insurance so that she could afford medications as well as assist her in applying for Medicaid to pick up the large copays she was responsible for. In addition to this, the navigator provided Ms. F with some gas vouchers to help with the costs of traveling 30 minutes each way for treatments. Ms. F shared, before meeting with the navigator, "I was very low, you helped me get emotionally stable, after getting the resources {in place.}"

Ms. F continued, "When you are sick and have all these bills piling up on you, you feel like there is no light at the end of the tunnel." "You {the navigator} helped with all of that, so that I could quit focusing on that and start to fight."

"The Navigator was such an encouragement." (Personal Communication, 2007)

All of the quotations and case examples provided in this chapter are testimonies of patients and families who were served by a patient navigator program. Some basic demographic information was altered slightly to protect patient confidentiality.

How Does the American Cancer Society Help?

The ACS Patient Navigator program is a 50/50 partnership between hospitals and the American Cancer Society. This partnership allows patients and caregivers to access two networks of resources and support, both from the hospital level and that of the American Cancer Society, all in a single interaction with an on-site navigator. Navigators function as full-time members of the hospital oncology team; they are trained by both ACS and the hospital staff and can network with both agencies to mobilize the wealth of expertise that the staff brings to patient care.

The primary goals of American Cancer Society Patient Navigators are to eliminate barriers to health care and increase quality of life for patients and their families. This is achieved in a variety of ways, with linkage to resources (easy-to-understand information, help with day-to-day needs, and emotional support) as the primary intervention. The Patient Navigator program is a proactive, rather than reactive, approach to helping cancer patients. Navigators reach cancer patients and their families early in the treatment decision-making process and, in many cases, immediately after diagnosis. Navigators support patients in need of assistance by providing one-on-one contact and helping them maneuver through healthcare systems, insurance systems, national resources, and local community programs.

ACS strives to promote informed decision making by providing easy-to-understand information to help patients make decisions about their care. Patients, families, and healthcare workers can access this information by telephone at 1-800-227-2345, by visiting www.cancer.org, or by e-mail when utilizing the ACS online service request intake form. The American Cancer Society provides reliable literature about treatment options, diagnosis, and support. ACS provides access 24 hours a day, 7 days a week to Cancer Information Specialists through the 1-800-227-2345 call center. The ACS National Call Center maintains the most up-to-date information about clinical trials. ACS also maintains a comprehensive resource database that can be accessed by an on-site navigator, online by patients, families, and healthcare workers, or by calling the National Call Center.

ACS offers help with the day-to-day barriers that patients and families are faced with by linking them to financial and insurance resources, help with transportation and prescription medications, and assistance with lodging. ACS provides emotional support for patients by providing one-on-one contact after diagnosis by a visit from the on-site Patient Navigator (where available); Reach to Recovery program; Look Good . . . Feel Better classes; a local Resource Room for wigs, bras, prosthetics, and information; access to a registered dietitian through the Dietitian on Call program; and linkage to a licensed clinical social worker for emotional support through the ACS Patient Advocate program. ACS provides support programs at hospitals and in communities. Please refer to Table 14–5 for a list of ACS support programs.

In addition to these programs, local field staff from each served community partners with the on-site Patient Navigator, hospital partners, and local churches and communities to identify gaps in service and develop and sustain community programs. Local field staff also ensure that the American Cancer Society Division Call Center, National Call Center, and Local Patient Navigator have the most up-to-date and comprehensive list of community-based resources, state resources, and national programs in the database. The navigator, in turn, ensures that the database has the most up-to-date and comprehensive information about the hospital's support programs.

For funding opportunities for a patient navigation program in your facility, you can contact the American Cancer Society at 1-800-227-2345 and ask about their Patient Navigation programs. Navigation funding opportunities may also be available through the federal government; contact the National Cancer Institute for additional information.

Table 14–5 ACS Support Programs

Look Good . . . Feel Better	Helps women overcome the appearance-related side effects of cancer treatment
Reach to Recovery	Peer support program for women with breast cancer
Road to Recovery	Volunteer driver transportation program
Online survivorship network	Online community of support
I Can Cope	Support group and educational program for people who are facing all types of cancer
Man to Man	Peer support and educational program for men who are dealing with prostate cancer
American Cancer Society Resource Room	Provides free wigs, hats, prostheses, and bras for uninsured/ underinsured women who are in treatment
Specific to the South Atlantic Division of ACS	Dietitian on Call program and Patient Advocate program are available by telephone

References

Adler, N., Boyce, W., Chesney, M., Folkmann, S., & Syme, S. (1993). Socioeconomic inequalities in health: No easy solution. *Journal of the American Medical Association, 269*(24), 3140–3145.

American Cancer Society. (1989). A summary of ACS report to the nation: Cancer in the poor. *CA: A Cancer Journal for Clinicians, 39*(5), 263–265 Retrieved on October 10, 2008, from http://caonline.amcancersoc.org/cgi/reprint/39/5/263?hits=10&FIRSTINDEX=0&FULLTEXT=report+to+the+nation%3B+cancer+in+the+poor&SEARCHID=1&gca=canjclin%3B39%2F5%2F263&

American Cancer Society. (2008). *Cancer facts & figures 2008*. Atlanta, GA: Author.

Bach, P. B., Schrag, D., Brawley, O. W., Galaznik, A., Yakren, S., & Begg, C. B. (2002). Survival of blacks and whites after cancer diagnosis. *Journal of the American Medical Association, 287*(16), 2106–2113.

Bacon, C. G., & Kawachi, I. (2002). Quality-of-life differences among various populations of localized prostate cancer: 2001. *Current Urology Reports, 3*(3), 239–243.

Battaglia, T. A., Roloff, K., Posner, M. A., & Freund, K. (2007). Improving follow-up to abnormal breast cancer screening in an urban population. *Cancer, 109* (Suppl. 2), 359–367.

Bennet, C. L., Ferreira, M. R., Davis, T. C., Kaplan, J., Weinberger, M., Kuzel, T., et al. (1998). Relation between literacy, race, and stage of presentation among low-income patients with prostate cancer. *Journal of Clinical Oncology, 16*(9), 3101–3104.

Bilodeau, B. A., & Degner, L. F. (1996). Information needs, sources of information, and decisional roles in women with breast cancer. *Oncology Nursing Forum, 23*(4), 691–696.

Boulware, L. E., Cooper, L. A., Ratner, L. E., LaVeist, T. A., & Powe, N. R. (2003). Race and trust in the healthcare system. *Public Health Report, 118*(4), 358–365.

Capirci, C., Feldman-Stewart, D., Mandoliti, G., Brundage, M., Belluco, G., & Magnani, K. (2005). Information priorities of Italian early-stage prostate cancer patients and their health-care professionals. *Patient Education and Counseling, 56*(2), 174–181.

Carel Bailey Germain Papers, Sophia Smith Collection, Smith College, Northampton, Mass. (1922–1998). Retrieved October 10, 2008, from http://asteria.fivecolleges.edu/findaids/sophiasmith/mnsss24_admin.html

Chavez, L. R., Hubbell, F. A., Mishra, S. I., & Valdez, R. B. (1997). The influence of fatalism on self-reported use of Papanicolaou smears. *American Journal of Preventive Medicine, 13*(6), 418–424.

Chu, K., Anderson, W. F., Fritz, A., Lynn, A. G., Ries, M. S., & Brawley, O. W. (2001). Frequency distributions of breast cancer characteristics classified by estrogen receptor and progesterone receptor status for eight racial/ethnic groups. *Cancer, 92*(1), L37–L45.

Chu, K. C., Charisse, L. A., & Freeman, H. P. (2003). Racial disparities in breast carcinoma survival rates, separating factors that affect diagnosis from factors that affect treatment. *Cancer, 97*(11), 2853–2860.

Dohan, D., & Schrag, D. (2005). Using navigators to improve care of underserved patients: Current practices and approaches. *Cancer, 104*(4), 848–855.

Farley, T. A., & Flannery, J. T. (1989). Late-stage diagnosis on breast cancer in women of lower socioeconomic status. *American Journal of Public Health, 79*(11), 1508–1512.

Freeman, H. P. (2004). A model patient navigation program. *Oncology Issues: Oncology Economic & Program Management, 19*(5), 44–46.

Gansler, T., Henley, J. S., Stein, K., Nehl, E. J., Smigal, C., & Slaughter, E. (2005). Sociodemographic determinants of cancer treatment health literacy. *Cancer, 104* (3), 653–660.

Greenwald, H. P., Polissar, N. L., Borgatta, E. F., McCorkle, R., & Goodman, G. (1998). Social factors, treatment, and survival in early stage non-small cell lung cancer. *American Journal of Public Health, 88*(11), 1681–1684.

Grossfeld, G. D., Latini, D. M., Downs, T., Lubeck, D. P., Mehta, S. S., & Carroll, P. R. (2002). Is ethnicity an independent predictor of prostate cancer recurrence after radical prostatectomy? *The Journal of Urology, 168*(6), 2510–2515.

Haynes, M. A., & Smedley, B. D. (1999). *The unequal burden of cancer; an assessment of the NIH research and programs for ethnic minorities and the medically underserved*. Washington, DC: National Academy Press.

Hepworth, D. H., Rooney, R. H., & Larsen, J. A. (1997). *Direct social work practice: Theory and skills* (5th ed.). Pacific Grove, CA: Brooks/Cole Publishing Company.

Kim, S. P., Knight, S. J., Tomori, C., Colella, K. M., Schoor, R. A., Shih, L., et al. (2001). Health literacy and shared decision making for prostate cancer patients with low socioeconomic status. *Cancer Investigation, 19*(7), 684–691.

Lambert, S., Fearing, A., Bell, D., & Newton, M. (2002). A comparative study of prostate screening health beliefs and practices between African American and Caucasian men. *The ABNF Journal, 13*(3), 61–63.

Landis, S. H., Murray, T., Bolden, S., & Wingo, P. A. (1999). Cancer statistics, 1999. *CA: A Cancer Journal for Clinicians, 49*(1), 9–31.

Lannin, D. R., Mathews, H. F., Mitchell, J., Swanson, M. S., Swanson, F. H., & Edwards, M. S. (1998). Influence of socioeconomic and cultural factors on racial differences in late-stage presentation of breast cancer. *Journal of the American Medical Association, 279*(22), 1801–1807.

Larson, C. O., Nelson, E. C., Gustafson, D., & Batalden, P. B. (1996). The relationship between meeting patients' information needs and their satisfaction with hospital care and general health status outcomes. *International Journal for Quality in Health Care, 8*(5), 447–456.

Margolis, M. L., Christie, J. D., Silvestri, G. A., Kaiser, L., Santiago, S., & Hansen-Flaschen, J. (2003). Racial differences pertaining to a belief about lung cancer surgery: Results from a multicenter survey. *Annals of Internal Medicine, 139*(7), 558–563.

Nelson, A. R. (2003). Committee on Understanding and Eliminating Racial and Ethnic Disparities in Health Care. Institute of Medicine. *Unequal treatment: Confronting racial and ethnic disparities in health care.* Washington, DC: National Academy Press.

Nelson, K., Geiger, A. M., & Mangione, C. M. (2002). Effect of health beliefs on delays in care for abnormal cervical cytology in a multi-ethnic population. *Journal of General Internal Medicine, 17*(9), 709–716.

Nielsen-Bohlman, L., Panzer, A. M., & Kindig, D. A. (Eds.). (2004). *Health literacy. A prescription to end confusion.* Washington, DC: National Academy Press.

Penson, D. F., Stoddard, M. I., Pasta, D. J., Lubeck, D. P., Flanders, S. C., & Litwin, M. S. (2001). The association between socioeconomic status, health insurance coverage, and quality of life in men with prostate cancer. *Journal of Clinical Epidemiology, 54*(4), 350–358.

Polednak, A. P. (1997). Stage at diagnosis of prostate cancer in Connecticut by poverty and race. *Ethnicity & Disease, 7*(3), 215–220.

Smedley, B. D., Stith, A. Y., & Nelson, A. R. (Eds.). (2003). *Unequal treatment: Confronting racial and ethnic disparities in health care.* Washington, DC: National Academy Press.

Weinrich, S. P., Greiner, E., Reis-Starr, C., Yoon, S., & Weinrich, M. (1998). Predictors of participation in prostate cancer screening at worksites. *Journal of Community Health Nursing, 15*(2), 113–129.

Yabroff, K. R., Breen, N., Vernon, S. W., Meissner, H. I., Freedman, A. N., & Ballard-Barbash, R. (2004). What factors are associated with diagnostic follow-up after abnormal mammograms? Findings from a U.S. national survey. *Cancer Epidemiology Biomarkers and Prevention, 13*(5), 723–732.

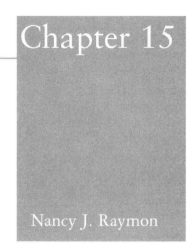

Chapter 15

Support Programs for Individuals with Lung Cancer

Nancy J. Raymon

Introduction

Over the past 30 years, cancer support groups have evolved as a common component of a comprehensive cancer support program. Early support groups were open to patients with any form of cancer. In recent years, the trend toward specialization in treatment of cancer has been paralleled by the development of an increasing number of support groups that are tailored to meet the needs of subgroups of cancer survivors with specific types of cancer. Advocacy groups that have arisen among patients with specific types of cancer have also contributed to the development of site-specific support groups. A literature search that was conducted in 2000, when planning for the lung cancer support group that is described later in this chapter, revealed numerous articles citing groups for breast cancer patients (Helgeson, Cohen, Yasko, & Schulz, 2000; Rice & Szopa, 1988; Cope, 1995; Geiger, Mullen, Sloman, Edgerton, & Petitti, 2000), young adults with cancer (Roberts, Piper, Denny, & Cuddeback, 1997), adolescents with cancer (Heiney, Wells, Coleman, Swygert, & Ruffin, 1990), prostate cancer patients (Chin-

A-Loy & Fernsler, 1998; Coreil & Behal, 1999), leukemia patients (McGrath, 1999; Moss, 2001), brain cancer patients (Leavitt, Lamb, & Voss, 1996), and ovarian cancer patients (Sivesind & Baile, 1997). Even though Zabora et al. (2001) have demonstrated that the prevalence of distress among lung cancer patients is the highest of any cancer type (35.1% for general cancer patients versus 43.4% among lung cancer patients), when the lung cancer support group that is described in this chapter was initiated, there were no references to support groups that were specifically designed for lung cancer patients (Zabora, et al., 2001).

As the support group movement has matured and broadened, meeting venues and formats have expanded from the traditional medical facility as a setting into getaway retreat sites (Rutledge & Raymon, 2001), patients' homes via radio (Van Scoy-Mosher & Schimmel, 1998), and the Internet (Fernsler & Manchester, 1997; Bliss, Allibone, Bontempo, Flynn, & Valvano, 1998; Finfgeld, 2000). Groups have also been developed to meet the specific needs of family members and the support system of the patient (McGee & Burkett, 1998; Heiney & Lesesne, 1996).

With 12.5 million health-related information searches per day, the Internet has become a powerful tool in the hands of patients seeking knowledge about a variety of diseases and treatments. The World Wide Web has created a new option in the world of cancer known as the electronic support group (ESG) (Eysenbach, 2003). While most in-person support groups routinely attract 10 to 12 attendees (Steinberg, 2004), ESGs conducted through e-mail lists can have hundreds or thousands of members (Nonnecke & Preece, 2000). Virtual communities can form when groups of participants participate in online discussions with sufficient duration and intensity of feeling "to form webs of personal relationships in cyberspace" (Wellman, 1997: 227).

Owen et al. (2005, 2007) studied support group use among 1844 cancer survivors and 4951 patients with noncancer chronic illnesses. They found that patients who attended cancer support groups were less likely to have a diagnosis of anxiety or depression than those who attended noncancer support groups. The authors concluded that this finding suggests that there are reasons besides emotional distress that drive cancer survivors to attend support groups. In addition to emotional support, benefits of support groups for cancer survivors include finding a community of those who share similar cancer experiences (Weis, 2003), obtaining information about cancer or its treatment (Ussher, Kirsten, Butow, & Sandoval, 2006, and learning how to cope with cancer sequelae (Stevens & Duttlinger, 1998). The emotional benefits of support group attendance include the opportunity to discuss fears related to disease recurrence or death (Spiegel & Classen, 2000) and a sense of camaraderie and giving back that is gained by providing support to others who are confronting similar issues (Owen, et al., 2005).

While organizations such as Susan G. Komen for the Cure (http://cms.komen.org/komen/index.htm) have been bringing attention to the issues of breast cancer survivors since 1982, the lung cancer patient population has been slower to form support or advocacy groups in spite of the desperate need. The first advocacy organization for lung cancer patients, Alliance for Lung Cancer Education Support and Advocacy (ALCASE; http://www.ALCASE.org), was formed in 1995. When choosing the design for a lung cancer support ribbon, ALCASE used clear plastic for a pin to symbolize "the invisible population of people with lung cancer." The experience of founder Mort Liebling is described as follows: "He began talking with other lung cancer survivors and their families and physicians and found out that there was a whole 'invisible' population out there who needed the same support and resources that he did."

In recent years, specific support for lung cancer patients has increased. ALCASE, now known as Lung Cancer Alliance (www.lungcanceralliance.org), lists 74 lung cancer support groups in 21 states, up from 43 groups in 20 states in 2003. In addition to in-person support group listings, the Lung Cancer Alliance Web site provides information about a number of online opportunities for group and one-on-one support for lung cancer patients as well as information about facilitated face-to-face groups run by hospitals, cancer centers, and community organizations. Another developing support system is offered by Caring Ambassadors Program (CAP; www.lungcancerguidebook.org), a site where patients can post questions for their medical director and view responses posted online.

A trend toward increased public awareness and understanding of lung cancer seems to have begun in 2005 with the death of respected news anchor Peter Jennings. Another celebrity, Dana Reeve, actress and wife of Christopher Reeve, brought additional attention to the disease when she publicly discussed her illness. Her death in 2006 shocked the world because she was young (aged 44 years), female, and a non-smoker. The fact that Ms. Reeve did not smoke increased public awareness that lung cancer can and does happen to people who do not smoke.

Development of Support Services in a Comprehensive Community Program

Beginning in August 2000, a lung cancer program was developed at a comprehensive community cancer program in Southern California where more than 2000 new cancer diagnoses are made annually, with over 200 new diagnoses of lung cancer each year. This cancer center has already developed successful site-specific programs for breast, brain, and prostate cancers, including support groups for each site. Lung cancer was targeted as the fourth site to be developed due to the high volume, complexity of care, necessity for an interdisciplinary approach, and the perception that the patient population had unmet needs for education and support. The Lung Cancer Support Group continually operates and is expanding each year. The following is a description of the program.

Focus Group Experience

Prior to initiating the support group, a focus group of lung cancer patients was convened in April 2000. The participants were asked to consider the needs for education and support, both at the time of diagnosis and on an ongoing basis. The needs assessment revealed the following:

- Meetings to be inclusive of those who have been treated for lung cancer and are surviving
- Forums to discuss the impact of having a lung cancer diagnosis, which was most likely caused by smoking, the related guilt and regret, as well as response of friends, family, and other cancer survivors
- Education about lung cancer in general, lung cancer staging, and treatment, with written materials for later reference
- Information about the specific long-term effects of treatment modalities, such as shortness of breath, incisional pain, and loss of libido, as well as more general effects, such as fatigue
- A discussion forum to open communication between patients and healthcare providers

Support Group Format

The Lung Cancer Support Group began as an evening group, meeting once a month in the cancer center with an oncology clinical nurse specialist and an oncology social worker as co-facilitators. Due to the fact that many patients in this group had diminished performance status from the time of diagnosis and the staff's belief that cancer affects the entire family, the group convened at 6:30 p.m. to accommodate family members' work schedules and to facilitate the patients' reliance on family members for transportation. The format included open discussion sessions alternating with educational presentations. Presentation topics were repeated because of the positive responses shown in Table 15–1.

Table 15–1 Educational Topics for Support Groups

- Overview of lung cancer treatment
- Ask the pulmonologist—questions and answers from the expert
- Radiation therapy—a treatment option
- Nutrition for the cancer patient
- Cancer and the law
- Coping with cancer at holiday time
- Imaging techniques for lung cancer
- Coping with fear
- Radio-frequency ablation for lung cancer
- Breathing and exercise rehabilitation for lung cancer patients
- Movement and wellness for lung cancer patients
- Sexuality and cancer treatment
- Advance care planning
- Understanding pathology reports
- Meditation for stress management

Description of First-Year Participants

Forty-five participants attended 21 support group sessions during the first year. A higher percentage was attended by females (76%) than males (24%). Over half of the participants were in their 60s and 70s, with 37% in their 50s and the rest in their 40s. Ranging from two to 11 participants per session, an average of six patients attended the meetings. Two support persons attended the meetings, with patients sometimes meeting on their own (range 0 to 5).

During the first few months, it became apparent that lung cancer patients had an acute need for accurate and understandable information regarding their disease and its treatment. Patients who attended the group had very little comprehension of how treatment was tailored to specific individuals, what the staging system meant and how it guided treatment, and how treatment modalities are combined. Approximately 70% of the patients in this support group were stage III or IV at the time of diagnosis and were already symptomatic, with less energy to focus on learning about cancer and its treatment than patients with some other types of cancer, such as breast and prostate cancer. Because there were limited courses of treatments prescribed, patients might have been less motivated initially to seek out information than if they were making a major decision between different treatment options.

Based on the patients' stated need for information about the complex treatment options they were facing, a 6-week educational series was developed for newly diagnosed patients. The content covered a general overview of lung cancer, types of lung cancer and staging, treatment modalities, the impact of a cancer diagnosis, coping with a cancer diagnosis, and resources (see Table 15–2). The first four sessions were taught by nurses, and the fifth and sixth sessions, covering psychosocial issues and resources, were taught by a nurse and a social worker. The series was presented three times over the first year. Because attendance over the summer months was lower than expected, the series was not offered again during the summer. The group of patients who attended the first educational series expressed interest in an ongoing group experience, but some patients were not able to attend at night. In response to this need, a daytime support group session was added. Over time, the 6-week educational series was discontinued, and educational presentations were incorporated into the support group schedule. The Lung Cancer Support Group is now

---

Table 15–2 Session Topics for Lung Cancer Educational Series

- Introduction to lung cancer
- Surgical treatment/minimally invasive surgery for lung cancer
- Chemotherapy for lung cancer
- Radiation therapy for lung cancer
- Meeting the demands of a lung cancer diagnosis
- Moving forward . . . putting this knowledge to use

---

held twice a month, one afternoon and one evening session, to accommodate differences in patients' schedules. Educational sessions alternate with facilitated open discussion.

Some patients have been group members since the Lung Cancer Support Group began in August 2000! These long-term survivors and group members are very helpful to newly diagnosed patients who benefit from their presence and their willingness to share their experiences. This group of long-term survivors provides a beacon of hope for patients who are newly diagnosed with a disease that is commonly perceived as an automatic death sentence. The long-term attendees state that their motivation for continued attendance is that they feel a strong sense of satisfaction from the experience of offering support and hope to those who are newly diagnosed with lung cancer. In addition, because cancer is a chronic disease, most of the long-term survivors have experienced either recurrence or a situation that they describe as "a scare" or a "bump in the road." They describe the ongoing support from members of the group and facilitators as a comfort and source of strength in times of stress and uncertainty.

Patient Recruitment

Patients were informed about the support group and educational series through various methods:

- Fliers were distributed to physicians' offices and additional sites throughout the cancer center.
- Direct referrals were made by physicians, nurses, and cancer center staff members.
- Invitations were sent to the facilitators of the group and the Lung Cancer Nurse Coordinator, who works with a high percentage of newly diagnosed lung cancer patients and is a cofacilitator of the group.
- Schedules were posted on the cancer center Web site (http://www.hoagcancercenter.org), including a description of the group and dates and times of the meetings. The Web site has been one of the most effective recruitment strategies for bringing in patients from outside the system.
- Although not originally posted, the group is now listed on the Lung Cancer Alliance Web site (www.lungcanceralliance.org).

Many lung cancer patients had diminished performance status at the time of diagnosis, and patients often were not well enough to attend the support group when they were first diagnosed. Therefore information about the group was offered not only at the time of diagnosis but also after the patient had time to recover from thoracotomy or adapt to their treatment routine. This ongoing flow of information about the support program was provided by the Lung Cancer Nurse Coordinator as well. Due to the prolonged recruitment process, patients often joined the group four to six months or longer after their diagnosis.

Discussion Themes

The following themes were common during open discussion sessions:

- Fear of recurrence and death
- Sharing of common experiences related to side effects of treatment
- Impact of negative responses from others to a diagnosis of lung cancer and the stigma of smoking
- Guilt related to smoking
- Issues related to communication with family and friends
- Concerns about effective communication with the treatment team
- Enthusiasm and support offered by longer-term survivors

Challenges

Working with the support group format as described can be challenging because there is no stratification of patients to subgroups of any type; patients bring unique perspectives from being newly diagnosed to having various stages and progression of the disease. The disparity in treatment options, prognosis, and physical status of attendees sometimes creates a situation where patients have little in common except the diagnosis of lung cancer.

Another challenge can be for the facilitator(s). Effective facilitation by a person who knows the long-term attendees can result in important insights for those in attendance. However, meeting the interests of all attendees can be challenging. Verbal comments and written feedback from evaluation forms have indicated that both the support groups and educational offerings for lung cancer patients were extremely well received by patients and family members alike. Patients report feeling more capable of understanding their disease and treatment plan, and they are comforted in the knowledge that there is a place to share their experiences with other lung cancer patients. Participants also report that a new sense of hope is conveyed to them through the experience of meeting long-term lung cancer survivors. While there are numerous challenges, this lung cancer support group is very rewarding for patients, caregivers, and moderators.

Lung Cancer Awareness Month Program

The lung cancer support group experience has led to an additional program component, which focuses on survivorship and new developments in the field of lung cancer treatment, in the form of a community symposium. Even though many of the participants were diagnosed years prior to the symposium and they have long since completed treatment, they still find the educational element to be enlightening and interesting. The first symposium was held in November 2006, and it was so well received that it has become an annual event. The program highlight is the announcement of the "Most Inspirational Lung Cancer Survivor" of the year. The nominees for this award come from members of the lung cancer support group, and the name of the award recipient is kept secret until the announcement during the program. This program component is particularly meaningful and poignant because lung cancer patients have such a strong sense of their own mortality and the aforementioned stigma of a lung cancer diagnosis. An additional component of the program is a survivor panel discussion in which panelists are asked to answer the question, "How have you been able to create meaning in your life related to your lung cancer diagnosis?" Panel members are chosen based on their unique experiences and known ability to express themselves in front of the support group. We have been successful in finding funding for these symposia through private donations and industry support.

Conclusion

Informed consumers in today's world are looking for specific information and services targeted to their medical needs. Lung cancer patients, with their specific set of physical and emotional requirements, are looking for programs that address their immediate and long-term needs. Nurses who work with lung cancer patients throughout the treatment trajectory have the opportunity to provide invaluable ongoing care and support to patients who are facing the challenges of this difficult disease. An important component of the nurse's role is to inform patients of available resources, including support groups, and to participate in organizing and facilitating these groups as appropriate, based on the level of his or her education and experience.

References

Bliss, J., Allibone, C., Bontempo, B., Flynn, T., & Valvano, N. E. (1998). Creating a web site for on-line social support. Melanocyte. *Computers in Nursing, 16*(4), 203–207.

Chin-A-Loy, S., & Fernsler, J. (1998). Self-transcendence in older men attending a prostate cancer support group. *Cancer Nursing, 21*(5), 358–363.

Cope, D. (1995). Functions of a breast cancer support as perceived by the participants: An ethnographic study. *Cancer Nursing, 18*(6), 472–478.

Coreil, J., & Behal, R. (1999). Man to man prostate cancer support groups. *Cancer Practice, 7*(3), 122–128.

Eysenbach, G. (2003). The impact of the Internet on cancer outcomes. *CA: A Cancer Journal for Clinicians, 53*(6), 356–371.

Fernsler, J., & Manchester, L. (1997). Evaluation of a computer-based cancer support network. *Cancer Practice, 5*(1), 46–51.

Finfgeld, D. (2000). Therapeutic groups online: The good, the bad, and the unknown. *Issues in Mental Health Nursing, 21*(3), 241–255.

Geiger, A., Mullen, E., Sloman, P., Edgerton, B., & Petitti, D. (2000). Evaluation of a breast cancer patient information and support program. *Effective Clinical Practice, 3*(4), 157–165.

Heiney, S., & Lesesne, C. (1996). Quest: An intervention program for children whose parent or grandparent has cancer. *Cancer Practice, 4*(6), 324–329.

Heiney, S., Wells, L., Coleman, B., Swygert, E., & Ruffin, J. (1990). Lasting impressions: A psychosocial support program for adolescents with cancer and their parents. *Cancer Nursing, 13*(1), 13–20.

Helgeson, V., Cohen, S., Yasko, J., & Schulz, R. (2000). Group support interventions for women with breast cancer. *Health Psychology, 19*(2), 107–114.

Leavitt, M. B., Lamb, S. A., & Voss, B. S. (1996). Brain tumor support group: Content themes and mechanisms of support. *Oncology Nursing Forum, 23*(8), 1247–1256.

McGee, S. J., & Burkett, K. W. (1998). Building a support group for parents of children with brain tumors. *Journal of Neuroscience Nursing, 30*(6), 345–349.

McGrath, P. (1999). Findings from an educational support course for patients with leukemia. *Cancer Practice, 7*(4), 198–204.

Moss, D. (2001). Leukemia support groups: How are they doing? *Cancer Control, 4*(5), 407–412.

Nonnecke, B., & Preece, J. (2000, April 1–6). Demographics: Counting the silent. *Proceedings of CHI 2000, Hague, The Netherlands.* Retrieved December 3, 2008, from www.Ifsm.umbc.edu/~preece/paper

Owen, J. E., Goldstein, M. S., Lee, H. J., Brent, J., & Rowland, J. H. (2007). Use of health-related and cancer-specific support groups among adult cancer survivors. *Cancer, 119*(12), 2580–2589.

Owen, J. E., Klapow, J. C., Roth, D. L., Shuster, J., Bellis, J., Meredith, R., et al. (2005). Randomized pilot of a self-guided Internet coping group for women with early-stage breast cancer. *Annals of Behavioral Medicine, 30*(1), 54–64.

Rice, M. A., & Szopa, T. J. (1988). Group intervention for reinforcing self-worth following mastectomy. *Oncology Nursing Forum, 15*(1), 33–37.

Roberts, C. S., Piper, L., Denny, J., & Cuddeback, G. (1997). A support group intervention to facilitate young adults' adjustment to cancer. *Health and Social Work, 22*(2), 133–141.

Rutledge, D., & Raymon, N. J. (2001). Changes in well-being of women cancer survivors following a survivor weekend experience. *Oncology Nursing Forum, 28*(1), 85–91.

Sivesind, D., & Baile, W. (1997). An ovarian cancer support group. *Cancer Practice, 5*(4), 247–251.

Spiegel, D., & Classen, C. (2000). *Group therapy for cancer patients.* New York: Basic Books.

Steinberg, D. M. (2004). *The mutual aid approach to working with groups: Helping people help one another* (2nd ed.). Binghamton, NY: Haworth Press.

Stevens, M. J., & Duttlinger, J. E. (1998). Correlates of participation in a breast cancer support group. *Journal of Psychosomatic Research, 45*(3), 263–275.

Ussher, J., Kirsten, L., Butow, P., & Sandoval, M. (2006). What do cancer support groups provide which other supportive relationships do not? The experience of peer support groups for people with cancer. *Social Science & Medicine, 62*(10), 2565–2576.

Van Scoy-Mosher, M., & Schimmel, S. (1998). The group room: A syndicated radio cancer support group. *The Oncologist, 3*(1), 61–63.

Weis, J. (2003). Support groups for cancer patients. *Support Care Cancer, 11*(12), 763–768.

Wellman, B. (1997). An electronic group is virtually a social network. In S. Kiesler (Ed.), *Culture of the Internet* (pp. 179–205). Mahwah, NJ: Lawrence Erlbaum.

Zabora, J., BrintzenhofeSzoc, K., Curbow, B., Hooker, C., & Piantadosi, S. (2001). The prevalence of psychological distress by cancer site. *Psychooncology, 10*(1), 18–28.

Understanding and Treating Tobacco Dependence in Adults with Lung Cancer

Mary Lou Heater

Introduction

The diagnosis of lung cancer provides a compelling reason to quit smoking. Simply put, cigarette smoking causes lung cancer (Dubey & Powell, 2008). In 2008, there will be an estimated 161,840 deaths from lung cancer (90,810 among men and 71,030 among women), and smoking is responsible for 87% of lung cancer deaths (Amos, 2008). Studies indicate, however, that up to 50% of people continue smoking after their diagnosis (Davison and Duffy, 1982; Dresler, Bailey, Roper, Patterson, & Cooper, 1996; Garces, et. al., 2004, Gritz, Nisenbaum, Elashoff, & Holmes, 1991, Schnoll, et al., 2003). Failure to quit smoking is attributable in large part to the addictive properties of nicotine (Benowitz, 1999). To provide assistance to those who are motivated to quit smoking, it is essential to understand nicotine dependence, the chronic nature of tobacco use disorders, and the range of interventions that are available to those who are ready to quit smoking. This chapter provides information about tobacco dependence, the role of addiction in promoting dependence, and the benefits of smoking cessation in adults with lung cancer.

Clinical interventions to promote smoking cessation are reviewed, and treatment issues specific to smokers with lung cancer are identified.

Tobacco Dependence

Progress has been made in understanding the nature of tobacco dependence. Now understood that tobacco dependence shows many features of a chronic disease (Fiore, 2004), it was the Surgeon General's report on nicotine addiction in 1988 that first provided conclusive evidence that cigarettes and other forms of tobacco are addicting in the same way as other drugs that determine addiction (US Department of Health and Human Services, 1988). Nicotine was identified as the dependence-producing substance in tobacco. In fact, nicotine was found to be just as addictive as heroin and cocaine (Fiore, et al., 2008; Henningfield, Cohen, & Slade, 1991). Furthermore, in 2000, nicotine dependence and withdrawal was included as a substance use disorder in the *Diagnostic and Statistical Manual of Mental Disorders,* Fourth Edition (*DSM-IV-R*).

Tobacco dependence is a chronic disorder evidenced by periods of remission and relapse. But what exactly is dependence? Although the

DSM-IV-R (American Psychiatric Association, 2000) cited that some of the generic dependence criteria do not apply to nicotine, tobacco use does cause physical dependence characterized by withdrawal symptoms. Individuals continue use despite a professed desire to quit and/or despite negative consequences, because nicotine has psychoactive and tolerance-producing effects (Fiore, 2004; Frank & Jaen, 1993). Tolerance develops rapidly and intensely; smoking even a few cigarettes may result in dependence (DiFranza, et al., 2000). Similar to other drug addictions, the number of cigarettes smoked gradually increases over several years. When an individual becomes dependent it is very difficult to quit smoking. The road to successful cessation is often long and arduous. The quitting process is characterized by repeated cycles of abstinence, relapse, and then recycling back to another quit attempt (Fiore, 2004; Ockene, et al., 2000). Most successful quitters average at least two to three attempts before being able to maintain long-term cessation. Tobacco dependence is a complex process that involves biological, psychological, social, and behavioral factors (Fisher, Lichtenstein, &

Haire-Joshu, 1993). Nicotine is the dependence-producing substance in tobacco products. It acts as a potent drug throughout the body and affects the reward center of the brain. After tobacco use, nicotine enters the brain and interacts with nicotinic receptors in the tissue. The number of receptors within the brain increases two- to threefold after exposure to nicotine. As the number of receptor sites increases, the ability of these receptors to function adequately decreases, thereby increasing tolerance to nicotine effects (Collins, Luo, Selvaag, & Marks, 1994).

Nicotinic receptor activation results in release of various neurotransmitters, including dopamine, norepinephrine, acetylcholine, beta-endorphin, and serotonin (Benowitz, 1999). These chemicals are responsible for many of the pleasurable and mood-altering side effects associated with nicotine (see Table 16–1).

Moreover, nicotine produces cardiovascular, neural, endocrine, and skeletal muscle effects resultant from the release of glutamate, growth hormone, prolactin, and ACTH. All effects are dependent on the dose of nicotine, rate of administration, tolerance level of the person, and rate of

Table 16–1 Neurotransmitter-Induced Effects of Nicotine

Neurotransmitter	Physiologic Effect
Acetylcholine	Increase stimulation
	Increase cognitive performance
Beta-endorphin	Decrease anxiety and tension
Dopamine	Increase pleasure
	Decrease appetite
Norepinephrine	Increase stimulation
	Increase alertness and vigilance
	Decrease appetite
Seratonin	Increase relaxation
	Decrease stress
	Decrease appetite

Source: Benowitz, 1999; Ferry, 1999.

elimination. Nicotine tolerance can be demonstrated by a decreased response to repeated doses and a subsequent increase in tobacco intake. Withdrawal symptoms occur in the face of abstinence in dependent smokers. Common withdrawal symptoms are irritability, sleep disturbance, anxiety, difficulty concentrating, restlessness, headache, weight gain, and drowsiness. Craving, an important part of the withdrawal process, may account for the difficulty that individuals have with achieving cessation.

Rustin (2000) grouped the criteria for all addictive substances into four categories that can be used to assess dependence on nicotine:

- Compulsion: The intensity with which the desire to use a chemical overwhelms thoughts, feelings, and judgments
- Control: The degree to which chemical use can or cannot be controlled after use is started
- Cutting down: The effects of use reduction; withdrawal symptoms
- Consequences: Denial or acceptance of the damage caused by the chemical

Tobacco smoke is comprised of more than 4,000 chemicals, at least 69 of which are known to cause cancer (Karam-Hage & Cinciripini, 2008). Evidence suggests that genetic variations increase lung cancer risk among smokers and ex-smokers. Not only have genes been identified that influence smoking behavior and the metabolism of nicotine (Lerman, et al., 1999; Lerman, et al., 2000; Rossing, 1998), but scientists recently identified two single nucleotide polymorphisms (SNPs) that are strongly associated with lung cancer in individuals who smoke (Amos, 2008). In addition, Landi and colleagues (2008) found that expression of specific genes strongly differentiates smokers from nonsmokers in lung tumors and early stage

tumor tissue, which is consistent with lung carcinogenesis induced by smoking. However, studies that examine genetic influences on smoking behaviors remain in their infancy (Kendler, 2001). Further research is needed to elucidate the role of specific genes, whether these genes are associated with certain subgroups of smokers, and whether certain subgroups of smokers (i.e., those with psychiatric disorders, alcoholics, and substance abusers) would benefit most from treatment with pharmacological cessation aids (Walton, Johnstone, Munafo, Neville, & Griffith, 2001). In addition, research continues to identify specific genes that are associated with nicotine dependence, response to treatment, and cancer susceptibility (Lerman & Berrettini, 2003; Hung, et al., 2008).

Psychological and social factors also play a significant role in tobacco use. Several studies have identified a high prevalence of smoking and increased difficulty quitting among persons with psychiatric disorders, including other substance use comorbidities (Anda, et al., 1990; Degenhardt & Hall, 2001; Niaura, et al., 2001; Ranney, Melvin, Lux, & McClain, 2006). Individuals with mental health disorders are more likely to be nicotine dependent than those without such diagnoses (Price, Jordan, Jeffrey, Stanley, & Price, 2008). Nicotine acts as a psychomotor stimulant but also has anxiolytic and antidepressant properties. The latter psychopharmacologic effects may enhance its addictive properties in individuals with underlying affective disorders and may promote self-medicating behaviors.

Social factors influence tobacco use. Smokers and ex-smokers are routinely exposed to stress, tobacco advertising campaigns, social groups with high smoking rates, social norms about smoking in recreational settings, and free or discounted products (DePue & Linnan, 2003). Although there has been a recent social movement to eliminate smoking from public and private venues, factors such as lower income, educational, and occupational levels and being male, unemployed, and single are associated with increased risk of smoking among all racial and ethnic groups (Cataldo, Cooley, & Giarelli, 2001). Social support seems to be an important protective factor, especially among women who are trying to quit smoking. Partner facilitation was a primary predictor of abstinence for women six to eight weeks after they quit smoking (Coppotelli & Orleans, 1985). Moreover, women who remained abstinent for eight weeks were more likely to have partners who were ex-smokers or partners who successfully quit smoking with them as compared to those who were not abstinent. In a recent longitudinal study (Pizacani, et al., 2008) that examined the affect of adopting a smoking ban in households with at least one smoker, it was found that those who adopted this supportive action had over three times the odds of quitting smoking for at least 3 months.

Conditioning is a major behavioral factor that increases the risk for relapse after a period of cessation. The tobacco user begins to associate specific moods and situations with the pleasurable side effects associated with nicotine. The association between such cues, the anticipated effects of nicotine, and the desire to smoke is a type of conditioning that occurs in cigarette smoking (Benowitz, 1999). Results of a recent study (Bradley, et al., 2007) suggest that a bias to maintain attention on smoking-related cues is primarily a function of the drug relevance of the cue. Multiple such cues exist within the smoker's environment. The sight of others smoking in person or in the media, the smell of cigarette smoke, and frequenting locations where smoking is commonplace (i.e., gambling casinos) are powerful triggers. Other common examples of cues are drinking coffee or alcohol, taking breaks at work, or facing stressful situations. Cues associated with smoking can elicit strong cravings and other withdrawal signs, making smoking abstinence difficult among individuals who are newly abstinent and even among those who have been abstinent for quite some time (Abrams, 1986; Hatsukami, Hughes, & Pickens, 1985).

Smoking Cessation in Adults with Cancer

Smoking cessation after the diagnosis of cancer is associated with improved response to treatment, decreased treatment complications, decreased number of second primary malignancies, and improved survival (Cinciripini, Gritz, Tsoh, & Skaar, 1998; McBride & Ostroff, 2003; Gritz, et al., 2005). Often called a "teachable moment," patients are more likely to comply with advice to quit smoking at the time of an acute illness (Gritz, et al., 2005; Schwartz, 1987; Taylor, et al., 2006). The diagnosis and treatment for cancer is a strong motivator for behavioral change. Several studies have documented an extremely high interest in smoking cessation interventions among smokers who have been diagnosed with cancer and a belief that quitting smoking would be beneficial to their health (Denmark-Wahnefried, Peterson, McBride, Lipkus, & Clipp, 2000; Pinto, Eakin, & Maruyama, 2000). In fact, studies have documented that more than 80% of smokers with lung or head and neck cancers attempt to quit smoking (Gritz, et al., 1991; Ostroff, et al., 1995). A sizable proportion of these patients, however, are unable to quit. Among those who continue to smoke, patients often remain motivated to quit and make multiple attempts to quit smoking. However, as Gritz and colleagues (2005) point out, very few smoking cessation interventions have been empirically tested with cancer patients or are readily accessible to those who are motivated to quit (Meert, Mayer, Milani, Beckers, & Razavi, 2006).

Most smokers (85%) who attempt to quit smoking prefer to make a self-initiated quit attempt using abrupt cessation, gradual reduction, or some other self-help approach to cessation (Fiore, Novotny, & Pierce, 1990). Similar to community-based samples, Ostroff and colleagues (1995) found that patients with head and neck cancer most often used self-initiated quit attempts (69%) in their cessation efforts, followed by listening to a physician's recommendation (39%), support from family and friends (35%), and use of nicotine replacement treatment (31%). Relapse rates among self-quitters are high and often occur in the early days and weeks after the quit attempt. Garvey and colleagues (1992) followed 235 adults for one year after self-initiated quit attempts and found that the majority of relapses occurred in the first few weeks after quitting: 13% relapsed within one day, 32% within three days, 49% within one week, and 62% after two weeks of the quit attempt. Schnoll et al. (2003) conducted a longitudinal study to examine the ability of patients to maintain abstinence after being newly diagnosed with lung or head and neck cancer. Data was accrued from 74 patients who were classified as smokers (39%) or recent quitters (61%). This study revealed at the 3-month follow-up that 45% were now classified as smokers and 55% as nonsmokers. It was found that patients who remained smokers or relapsed to smoking focused more on the disadvantages of quitting rather than the health benefits of abstinence.

Evidence suggests overall survival rates of nonsmokers are more favorable than those of former or current smokers. Bryant and Cerfolio (2007) found that the overall 5-year survival rate of stage I non-small cell lung cancer patients was greater in never-smokers (64%) than in smokers (56%). The 5-year survival rate was significantly lower in patients who had a smoking history of less than 20 pack years. A retrospective review (Videtic, et al., 2003) of 215 patients diagnosed with small cell lung cancer who received chemotherapy and radiotherapy found that those patients who continued to smoke had poorer survival rates than those who abstained throughout treatment. Additionally, in a review of 1,370 cases, Tsao and colleagues (2006) found that patients with advanced non-small cell lung cancer who never smoked had higher treatment response rates (19%), lower rates of progressive disease (49%), and higher overall survival rates than those who continued to smoke through treatment or were recent or remote quitters. Further, Ford et al. (2003) found that female breast cancer patients ($n = 280$) who underwent thoracic radiotherapy (XRT) and who continued to smoke or were former smokers had an increased risk of developing lung carcinoma. Overall, the odds ratio for smokers who received XRT, compared with smokers who did not receive XRT, was 9.0 (95% confidence interval). In other words, some continuing or former smokers increase their risk of developing lung cancer even after they survive breast cancer treatment.

One recent study of note (Knoke, Burns, & Thun, 2008) examined lung cancer risk modification by quitting smoking. Citing that the principal effect of smoking cessation on lung cancer risk is a change in the frequency with which normal cells turn malignant, the reduction in excess risk of death from lung cancer in former smokers is profound. Compared to smokers, individuals who quit smoking at age 30 years had a less than 3% chance of dying from lung cancer 20 years after smoking cessation, and individuals who quit smoking at age 50 years had a less than 8% chance after 20 years.

Treatment for Tobacco Dependence

Effective treatments for tobacco dependence are now available. Oncology nurses can play an important role in delivering smoking cessation interventions during a time when patients are motivated and willing to quit smoking (Andrews, Tingen, & Harper, 1999; Cooley, Sipples, Murphy, & Sarna, 2008). In a recent Cochrane review that included 42 studies of nursing interventions for smoking cessation, Rice and Stead (2008) found reasonable evidence that nursing intervention is effective. The challenge, they contend, is incorporating smoking cessation monitoring and interventions as part of standard practice. Mahon (2005) noted that nurses should not view tobacco cessation education and brief intervention as something to do if time permits but rather as a requirement of comprehensive nursing care.

The clinical practice guidelines for treatment of tobacco use and dependence have been updated (Fiore, et al., 2008). The guidelines recommend using the five A's—(1) Ask (screen for tobacco use); (2) Assess willingness to quit; (3) Advise patients to stop; (4) Assist with quitting; and (5) Arrange follow-up—as strategies for clinical interventions. The guidelines discuss each of these clinical interventions, and the roles of pharmacological cessation aids and behavioral counseling in tobacco dependence treatment are presented. Treatment issues specific to smokers with lung cancer are also discussed. In addition, the guideline provides a separate booklet for nurses to implement the five A's intervention. The implementation of a system that ensures tobacco use status is obtained and recorded at every patient contact, such as identifying tobacco use as the sixth vital sign in all nursing assessment documentation, is suggested.

Consistent identification and documentation of smokers is the first step in providing tobacco dependence treatment. Several simple methods exist to incorporate assessment into daily practice. Common examples include the use of a preprinted progress note that includes a place for tobacco assessment, the use of stickers applied to the chart to indicate that the patient is a smoker, or a vital sign stamp that has a place for tobacco assessment (Fiore, et al., 2008). Having information available about the smoking status of a patient acts as a prompt and increases the likelihood of clinical intervention. In fact, in settings where a systemwide approach to assess smoking behaviors is in place, clinicians are three times more likely to provide clinical intervention When a system is in place to identify tobacco users, an assessment should be done to determine the person's smoking and tobacco history, level of nicotine dependence, presence of any psychiatric comorbidities, and willingness to make a quit attempt. Obtaining information about the average number of cigarettes smoked per day and the time of the first cigarette helps identify those who are more likely to be highly dependent smokers. The Fagerstrom Test for Nicotine Dependence is a standard instrument that is used to assess the intensity of dependence (Heatherton, Kozlowski, Frecker, & Fagerstrom, 1991). The higher the score, the more dependent the individual. Light-level smokers usually smoke between 1 and 10 cigarettes per day, whereas moderate smokers smoke between 15 and 24 cigarettes, and heavy smokers smoke more than 25 cigarettes. Highly dependent smokers smoke even more cigarettes per day, smoke their first cigarette within 5 minutes after awakening in the morning, experience severe withdrawal reactions upon abstinence from tobacco, and have greater difficulty with quitting smoking (Killen, Fortmann, & Telch, 1988).

The prevalence rate of tobacco use among those with psychiatric disorders (i.e., chemical dependency, major depressive disorder, bipolar illness, and anxiety) is higher than the general population. Because the presence of these disorders is associated with an increased difficulty with quitting smoking, identification and treatment for these underlying disorders should be done prior to the quit attempt. When treatment for the underlying disorder is optimized, cessation efforts can be initiated. Ongoing assessment of any changes in mental health after reduction of nicotine is essential. Detection of underlying depression is an especially important issue in adults with lung cancer because de-

pression is common even among those with a good prognosis (Hopwood & Stephens, 2000; Uchitomi, et al., 2000). Therefore, screening for depressive symptoms should be a routine part of tobacco dependence assessment in adults with lung cancer. Determining the motivation and readiness of the smoker to quit is essential to decide upon the most appropriate clinical interventions. Increased motivation and confidence in the ability to quit smoking has been associated with increased abstinence. The Transtheoretical Model provides a framework to assess the smokers' readiness to quit smoking. This model postulates that there are five stages of change: (1) precontemplation, (2) contemplation, (3) preparation, (4) action, and (5) maintenance. The stage of change can be ascertained by asking a few questions (see Figure 16–1). Interventions

---

Figure 16–1 Stage of change (short form) questionnaire.

Are you currently a smoker?
- Yes, I currently smoke.
- No, I quit within the last 6 months. (Action Stage)
- No, I quit more than 6 months ago. (Maintenance Stage)
- No, I have never smoked. (Nonsmoker)

For smokers only:
In the last year, how many times have you quit smoking for at least 24 hours?
Are you seriously thinking of quitting smoking?
- Yes, within the next 30 days. (Preparation Stage if the person had one quit attempt in the past year; if no quit attempt, then Contemplation Stage)
- Yes, within the next 6 months. (Contemplation Stage)
- No, not thinking of quitting. (Precontemplation Stage)

Definitions for stage of change:
- Precontemplation: Not considering quitting in the next 6 months.
- Contemplation: Considering quitting in the next 6 months.
- Preparation: Ready to quit in the next month.
- Action: Taking steps toward cessation. Quit date set or has quit within the last 6 months.
- Maintenance: Has not smoked for more than 6 months.

Sources: Prochaska, Redding, & Evers, 1997; DiClemente, et al., 1991; Velicer, et al., 1995.

can be tailored to the patient's readiness to quit smoking (DiClemente, et al., 1991; Velicer, et al., 1995).

Every patient who uses tobacco should receive a strong message from his or her healthcare provider to quit smoking. For patients who are not yet ready to quit, providing personalized motivational messages built around the five R's shown in Table 16–2 may help move them forward in the stage sequence (Fiore, et al., 2008; Prokhorov, Hudman, & Gritz, 1997).

In the event that the patient is ready to quit smoking, a quit date should be determined, treatment with pharmacological cessation aids and behavioral counseling should be offered, and follow-up contacts should be arranged. The optimal time for follow-up is within one to two days after the quit date and at least one other contact within the first month. Contacts can be done either in person or by telephone. However, there is a strong dose-response relationship between the session length and successful outcome. If feasible, healthcare providers should strive to meet four or more times with individuals who are quitting tobacco use.

Tobacco Cessation Approved Pharmacotherapies

There are no published data on the efficacy of pharmacologic treatments for cancer patients who continue to smoke (Lerman, Patterson & Berrettini, 2005). However, medications have been found to double long-term smoking cessation rates in the general public. The most appropriate choice for medication is based on the patient's unique clinical factors (i.e., cancer treatment side effects), past experience with

Table 16–2 Providing Motivational Messages for the Patient Unwilling to Quit Smoking

The "5 R's" for Those Unwilling to Quit	
Relevance	• Provide information about quitting that is relevant to the patient's specific situation (i.e., disease status, having children in the home).
Risks	• Identify potential negative consequences or risks of tobacco use that are most relevant to patient (i.e., shortness of breath, cancer recurrence, impotence, infertility).
Rewards	• Identify potential benefits associated with quitting smoking (health improves, food will taste better, good example set for children).
Roadblocks	• Identify barriers or impediments to quitting and note elements of treatment (problem solving or pharmacotherapy) that could address barriers. • Find solutions for common barriers, which may include withdrawal symptoms, fear of failure, weight gain, depression, lack of support.
Repetition	• Repeat the motivational intervention when the unmotivated person visits the clinic setting. • Encourage tobacco users who have failed in previous quit attempts by telling them that most people make repeated quit attempts before they are successful.

Source: US Department of Health and Human Services, 2000.

pharmacological cessation aids, and preference for a specific agent. First-line medications for use in tobacco dependence are varenicline, bupropion, and nicotine replacement treatment (NRT) (see Table 16–3). These medications are generally safe, effective, and have been approved by the US Food and Drug Administration for tobacco-dependence treatment. Second-line medications include clonidine and nortriptyline.

Several forms of NRT are now available, including gum, patch, nasal spray, inhaler, and lozenge. Nicotine gum, patches, and lozenges can be purchased as over-the-counter products, whereas nicotine spray and inhalers are available through prescription. The relative efficacy of the various nicotine replacement products on smoking cessation rates has been described through meta-analysis. All of the current forms of NRT

Table 16–3 Tobacco Cessation Pharmacotherapy

Medication	Dosing	Contraindications	Common Side Effects	General Instructions
Varenicline	0.5 mg 1 mg	Renal failure	Nausea Vivid dreams Gas Constipation Headache	Take 0.5 mg PO daily × 3 days then BID × 4 days; on eighth day take 1 mg PO BID; take on full stomach and with full glass of water
Bupropion SR	150 mg	Seizures, heavy alcohol use, eating disorders	Insomnia Headaches Tremor Anxiety	Take 150 mg PO daily × 3 days and then BID
Nicotine patch	21 mg 14 mg 7 mg	Unstable angina	Skin irritation Sleep disturbance Palpitations	21 mg × 6 weeks 14 mg × 2 weeks 7 mg × 2 weeks
Nicotine gum	4 mg 2 mg	Unstable angina Mouth sores	Mouth irritation Sleep disturbance Palpitations	Chew and park up to 20 pieces/day Don't eat/drink during use
Nicotine lozenge	4 mg 2 mg	Unstable angina Mouth sores	Mouth irritation Sleep disturbance Palpitations	Dissolve over 20–30 minutes Don't eat/drink during use
Nicotine inhaler	10 mg	Unstable angina Mouth sores	Cough (if inhaled) Sleep disturbance Palpitations	Puff, do not inhale Don't eat/drink during use

are effective and should be considered for use in those who wish to quit smoking. Nicotine gum is available in 2 mg and 4 mg preparations. The 4 mg gum seems to be more effective for those who smoke 25 or more cigarettes per day. It is best to use one piece of gum every 1 to 2 hours for a maximum dose of 24 pieces per day of the 2 mg gum or 20 pieces of 4 mg gum (Thompson and Hunter, 1998). On average, most people find that between 10 and 15 pieces of gum per day provide relief from withdrawal symptoms. The recommended duration of therapy is approximately 6–14 weeks. Common side effects associated with use of the gum are mouth soreness, hiccups, dyspepsia, and jaw ache. Most of these side effects are transient and may be corrected by instruction about using the proper chewing technique. Gum should be chewed slowly until a peppery or mint taste emerges and then should be parked to facilitate nicotine absorption through the oral mucosa.

Nicotine lozenges are available in 2 mg and 4 mg dosing as well. It is recommended that patients initiate the 4 mg lozenge if they smoke their first cigarette of the day within 30 minutes of awakening. The usual duration is 6–12 weeks, and no more than 20 lozenges should be used per day. The lozenge is placed in the mouth and allowed to dissolve slowly (over 20–30 minutes) while moving the lozenge from one side of the mouth to the other until it is dissolved (Fiore, 2004).

Nicotine transdermal patches are available as either a 16- or 24-hour preparation. The 16-hour patch is followed by an 8-hour drug-free period. Potential advantages of this dosage schedule are that sleeping disturbances and tolerance to the effects of nicotine are lessened. The 24-hour preparation provides higher morning blood levels of nicotine and has the potential to lessen

early morning craving (Shiffman, et al., 2000). The usual duration is 6–14 weeks, although no optimal dosage or length of treatment for the patch has been identified. Treatment may be initiated on the quit day with a dose of 21 mg. Heavier smokers (10 or more cigarettes per day) usually receive treatment with 21 mg, whereas those who are light to moderate smokers receive treatment with the lower dose of nicotine (14 mg). Using a 10-week schedule, the patient would start with a 21 mg patch for 6 weeks, reduce to the 14 mg patch for 2 weeks, and end with the 7 mg patch for 2 weeks. Because the patches can be applied once a day, they provide a convenient way to deliver a steady dose of nicotine replacement. The most common adverse side effect associated with the patch is skin irritation at the patch site. Insomnia and vivid dreams are associated with use of the patch during the night.

Nicotine nasal spray was designed for rapid delivery and absorption of nicotine into the system. The initial starting dose is one spray (0.5 mg) to each nostril one to two times per hour on a regular basis. This dose may be supplemented by additional doses for a maximum daily dose of eight doses per hour or 40 doses per day. The recommended length of treatment is three months, followed by a gradual taper over the next three months. The most common side effects associated with the nasal spray are nasal and throat irritation, rhinitis, sneezing, coughing, and lacrimation during the first week of use. It is not recommended for use in those with severe reactive airway disease. The nicotine inhaler consists of a small capsule containing nicotine-impregnated cotton that is placed within a plastic cylinder. The patient puffs on the plastic cylinder for several minutes to release the nicotine. The vaporized nicotine is then delivered and absorbed through the buccal mucosa. The initial starting dose is approximately six capsules per day, not to exceed a maximum of 16 capsules per day. One advantage of using the inhaler is that it simulates the behavioral action of smoking. Common side effects are mouth and throat irritation. The recommended length of treatment is up to six months, followed by a gradual taper over the last six to 12 weeks of treatment.

Bupropion was the first nonnicotine agent to be approved for use in tobacco-dependence treatment. Although it is an atypical antidepressant medication, it does not appear to have greater efficacy in those with a history of major depression. One small study (Cullum, Wojciechowski, Pelletier, & Simpson, 2004) demonstrated that bupropion may reduce the fatigue that is experienced by cancer patients. In contrast to NRT, bupropion should be started one to two weeks prior to the quit date. The starting dose for treatment is 150 mg per day for three to seven days, followed by an increase to 150 mg twice a day. Treatment is continued for seven to 12 weeks. Recent evidence suggests that prolonged use may delay smoking relapse (Hays, et al., 2001). An added advantage is that bupropion results in less weight gain and may provide a benefit for those who are concerned about weight gain associated with smoking cessation (Hays, 2000). Common side effects associated with bupropion are dry mouth, sleep disturbance, and headache. Bupropion is contraindicated in individuals with a history of seizure disorder, a history of eating disorder, or who have used an MAO inhibitor in the past 14 days.

Combination NRT can be used if patients are unable to quit using a single type of treatment. The nicotine patch can be combined with a self-administered form of NRT (either gum or nasal spray) or bupropion. A meta-analysis of combination NRT demonstrated that the combination of a short-acting (gum or nasal spray) and long-acting (patch) NRT produced higher abstinence rates than did single-agent treatment. In particular, the use of nasal spray in combination with the patch seems to be promising in increasing long-term abstinence rates (Blondal, Gudmundsson, Olafsdottir, Gustavsson, & Westin, 1999). Bupropion alone or in combination with the nicotine patch resulted in higher abstinence rates as compared to the nicotine patch alone (Jorenby, et al., 1999; Jamerson, et al., 2001). Further research is needed to identify whether subgroups of smokers, such as those with higher levels of nicotine dependence, would benefit most from combined treatment.

Varenicline is the most recently released first-line pharmacotherapy for smoking cessation. Gaining FDA approval in 2006, this nonnicotine medication was specifically developed for smoking cessation. Varenicline is an alpha4beta2 nicotinic receptor partial agonist. By acting as a partial agonist, it inhibits the dopaminergic activation produced by smoking while simultaneously providing a moderate increase in mesolimbic dopamine, which may account for providing relief from the craving and withdrawal syndrome associated with tobacco cessation. The starting dose is 0.5 mg per day for the first three days, then twice a day for the following four days. On day eight, or the beginning of the second week, patients start taking 1 mg twice a day. The usual duration is three to six months. Unlike nicotine replacement therapy, varenicline treatment should begin treatment one to two weeks prior to the target quit date. It is available by prescription only and should be used with caution and dose reduction in patients with renal impairment. The most common side effects associated with varenicline are nausea, constipation, excess gas, headaches, sleep disturbance, and vivid dreams.

FDA added this warning in 2008: Some patients have reported changes in behavior, agitation, depressed mood, suicidal thoughts or actions when attempting to quit smoking while taking varenicline (Chantix) or after stopping varenicline. If agitation, depressed mood, or changes in behavior occur or if there is a development of suicidal thoughts or actions, stop taking the medication and call your healthcare provider right away. Also tell your healthcare provider about any history of depression or other mental health problems before taking varenicline, as these symptoms may worsen while taking this medication.

Many smokers with lung cancer have coexisting cardiovascular or pulmonary disease. Concerns may arise about the safety of pharmacological cessation aids among this subgroup of patients. The safety of NRT in patients with cardiovascular and pulmonary disease has been confirmed in several studies (Joseph, et al., 1996; Murray, et al., 1996). Moreover, neither bupropion nor varenicline has been associated with any significant cardiovascular side effects in any of the published drug studies. Caution should be exercised, however, in the use of NRT among patients who are within two weeks of postmyocardial infarction, those with serious arrhythmias, and those with serious or worsening angina pectoris. Otherwise, treatment can be individualized according to the patient's health status, his or her past experience with pharmacological cessation aids, and preference for a specific agent.

In reviewing pharmacotherapies for tobacco cessation, Karam-Hage and Cinciripini (2008) found that each of the medications have their place, often times in combination with other agents, in cancer patients who continue to smoke.

As noted, their initial experience with both varenicline and bupropion have been encouraging in the treatment of tobacco-dependent cancer patients, and future study is warranted in this population.

Behavioral Counseling

Pharmacological cessation aids and behavioral counseling each independently boost cessation success. Thus, behavioral counseling is an important and necessary component of tobacco-dependence treatment. Behavioral interventions that have been identified as effective include treatments involving person-to-person contact, such as individual meetings, group sessions, or telephone counseling. Person-to-person contact sessions usually include the provision of practical counseling and social support. Practical counseling sessions focus on helping the smoker to identify and anticipate potential triggers or cues associated with smoking and then to develop a list of coping strategies that may be used to delay the urge to smoke. Examples of potential strategies include deep breathing, leaving the situation, sucking on hard candy, or taking a walk. Social support during treatment consists of providing ongoing support and encouragement during the quit attempt. Smoking cessation advice as brief as three minutes is effective in increasing smoking abstinence rates and should be the minimal standard used with all smokers. Evidence suggests, however, that as the intensity of tobacco dependence counseling increases, so do smoking abstinence rates. A meta-analysis determined that the optimal smoking cessation treatment is four to seven person-to-person contact sessions during a period of at least eight weeks, with counseling sessions lasting at least ten minutes (Fiore, et al., 2008; Jorenby & Fiore, 1999).

The need exists to test new behavioral treatments targeted toward smoking cessation among adults with cancer (Brandon, 2001). For smokers who are highly nicotine dependent, such as those with lung cancer, the use of targeted intensive interventions may be particularly useful. Such an approach combines behavioral interventions with pharmacological cessation aids and is tailored to the needs of a specific group of smokers. Three studies have been conducted among smokers with lung cancer. Two of the studies used a minimal smoking cessation intervention among adults who were undergoing diagnostic testing or surgical procedures for their illness, while a third study used more intensive interventions, such as pharmacotherapy and behavioral counseling (Browning, Ahijevych, Ross, & Wewers, 2000; Griebal, Wewers, & Baker, 1998; Wewers, Jenkins, & Mignery, 1997). Further, there was one study (Clark, et al., 2004) that examined a self-help approach to improving cessation rates in patients who were being screened for lung cancer. At the one year follow-up, more patients in the intervention group (who were given handouts) reported an attempt to quit smoking than those in the control group. The results of these studies suggested that minimal smoking cessation interventions were of limited value in this group of patients. The efficacy of nurse-delivered intensive smoking cessation interventions seems promising, but further studies are needed.

Conclusion

Within the past 20 years, strides have been made in understanding and treating tobacco dependence. The 1988 surgeon general's report concluded that nicotine was the dependence-producing substance in tobacco and that it was just as addictive as heroin and cocaine. This knowledge provided the foundation for understanding that tobacco dependence is a chronic illness that requires assessment, intervention, and ongoing monitoring. Moreover, effective treatment is now available, but persistent efforts over repeated contacts are necessary to achieve long-term cessation. In fact, most successful quitters average at least three quit attempts before achieving long-term cessation. A growing body of evidence supports the conclusion that tobacco cessation is important for those with lung cancer. Oncology nurses can play an important role in delivering smoking cessation interventions during teachable moments when patients are willing and motivated to quit smoking. Knowledge of the available clinical interventions is critical to provide effective care. In particular, for smokers who are ready to make a quit attempt, the use of pharmacological cessation aids and behavioral counseling can double long-term quit rates. Further research is needed to identify the most effective treatment for tobacco dependence among adults with lung cancer.

References

Abrams, D. B. (1986). Roles of psychosocial stress, smoking cues, and coping in smoking relapse prevention. *Health Psychology, 5*(Suppl.), 91–92.

American Psychiatric Association. (2000). *Diagnostic and statistical manual of mental disorders* (4th ed.). Washington, DC: Author.

Amos, C., Wu, X., Broderick, P., Gorlove, I. P., Gu, J., Eisen, T., et al. (2008). Genome-wide association scan of tag SNPs identifies a susceptibility locus for lung cancer at 15q25.1. *Nature Genetics, 40*(5), 616–622.

Anda, R., Williamson, D., Esobedo, L., Mast, E., Giovino, G., & Remington, P. (1990). Depression and the dynamics of smoking. *Journal of the American Medical Association, 264*(12), 1541–1545.

Andrews, J. O., Tingen, M. S., & Harper, R. J. (1999). A model nurse practitioner-managed smoking cessation clinic. *Oncology Nursing Forum, 26*(10), 1603–1610.

Benowitz, N. L. (1999). Nicotine addiction. *Primary Care, 26*(3), 611–631.

Blondal, T., Gudmundsson, L. J., Olafsdottir, I., Gustavsson, G., & Westin, A. (1999). Nicotine nasal spray with nicotine patch for smoking cessation: Randomized trial with six-year follow-up. *British Medical Journal, 318*(7179), 285–289.

Bradley, B., Field, M., Healy, H., & Mogg, K. (2007). Do the affective properties of smoking-related cues influence attentional and approach biases in cigarette smokers? *Journal of Psychopharmacology, 22*(7), 737–745.

Brandon, T. H. (2001). Behavioral tobacco cessation treatments: Yesterday's news or tomorrow's headlines? *Journal of Clinical Oncology, 19*(Suppl. 18), 64S–84S.

Browning, K. K., Ahijevych, K. L., Ross, P. Jr., & Wewers, M. E. (2000). Implementing the Agency for Health Care Policy and Research's smoking cessation guideline in a lung cancer surgery clinic. *Oncology Nursing Forum, 27*(8), 1248–1254.

Bryant, A., & Cerfolio, J. (2007). Differences in epidemiology, histology, and survival between cigarette smokers and never-smokers who develop non-small cell lung cancer. *Chest, 132*(1), 185–192.

Cataldo, J., Cooley, M. E., & Giarelli, E. (2001). Smoking and cancer. In K. Jennings-Dozier & S. Mahon (Eds.), *Cancer prevention, detection and control: A nursing perspective* (pp. 101–156). Pittsburgh, PA: Oncology Nursing Press.

Cinciripini, P. M., Gritz, E. R., Tsoh, J. Y., & Skaar, K. L. (1998). Smoking cessation and cancer prevention. In J. C. Holland (Ed.), *Psycho-oncology* (pp. 27–45). New York: Oxford University Press.

Clark, M. M., Cox, L. S., Jett, J. R., Patten, C. A., Schroeder, D. R., Nirelli, L. M., et al. (2004). Effectiveness of smoking cessation self-help materials in a lung cancer screening population. *Lung Cancer, 44*(1), 13–21.

Collins, A. C., Luo, Y., Selvaag, S., & Marks, M. J. (1994). Sensitivity to nicotine and brain nicotinic receptors are altered by chronic nicotine and mecamylamine infusion. *Journal of Pharmacology and Experimental Therapeutics, 271*(1), 125–133.

Cooley, M. E., Sipples, R., Murphy, M., & Sarna, L. (2008). Smoking cessation and lung cancer: Oncology nurses can make a difference. *Seminars in Oncology Nursing, 24*(1), 16–26.

Coppotelli, H., & Orleans, C. (1985). Partner support and other determinants of smoking cessation maintenance among women. *Journal of Clinical Psychology, 53*(4), 455–460.

Cullum, J. L., Wojciechowski, A. E., Pelletier, G., & Simpson, J. S. (2004). Bupropion sustained release treatment reduces fatigue in cancer patients. *Canadian Journal of Psychiatry, 49*(2), 139–144.

Davison, A. G., & Duffy, M. (1982). Smoking habits of long-term survivors of surgery for lung cancer. *Thorax, 37*(5), 331–333.

Degenhardt, L., & Hall, W. (2001). The relationship between tobacco use, substance-use disorders, and mental health. Results from the National Survey of Mental Health and Well-being. *Nicotine and Tobacco Research, 3*(3), 225–234.

Denmark-Wahnefried, W., Peterson, B., McBride, C., Lipkus, I., & Clipp, E. (2000). Current health behaviors and readiness to pursue life-style changes among men and women diagnosed with early stage prostate and breast carcinomas. *Cancer, 88*(3), 674–684.

DePue, J. D., & Linnan, L. A. (2003). Contextual and systems factors that support treatment. In D. H. Barlow (Ed.), *The tobacco dependence treatment handbook* (pp. 249–276). New York: Guilford Press.

DiClemente, C. C., Prochaska, J. O., Fairhurst, S. K., Velicer, W. F., Velasquez, M. M., & Rossi, J. S. (1991). The process of smoking cessation: An analysis of precontemplation, contemplation, and preparation stages of change. *Journal of Consulting and Clinical Psychology, 59*(2), 295–304.

DiFranza, J. R., Rigotti, N. A., McNeill, A. D., Ockene, J. K., Savageau, J. A., St. Cyr, D., et al. (2000). Initial symptoms of nicotine dependence in adolescents. *Tobacco Control, 9*(3), 313–319.

Dresler, C. M., Bailey, M., Roper, C. M., Patterson, G. A., & Cooper, J. D. (1996). Smoking cessation and lung resection. *Chest, 110*(5), 1199–1202.

Dubey, S., & Powell, C. A. (2008). Update in lung cancer 2007. *American Journal of Respiratory and Critical Care Medicine, 177*(9), 941–946.

Fiore, M. C. (2004). *Treating tobacco use and dependence.* Retrieved May 27, 2008, from www.medscape.com/viewprogram/8840

Fiore, M. C., Jaen, C. R., Baker, T. B., Bailey, W. C., Benowitz, N. L., Curry, S. J., et al. (2008). *Treating tobacco use and dependence: 2008 update.* Clinical practice guideline. Rockville, MD: US Department of Health and Human Services.

Fiore, M. C., Jorenby, D. E., Schensky, A. E., Smith, S., Baue, R., & Baker, T. (1995). Smoking status as the new vital sign: Effect on assessment and intervention in patients who smoke. *Mayo Clinic Proceedings, 70*(3), 209–213.

Fiore, M. C., Novotny, T. E., Pierce, J. P., Giovino, G. A., Hatziandreu, E. J., Newcomb, P. A., et al. (1990). Methods used to quit smoking in the United States: Do cessation programs help? *Journal of the American Medical Association, 263*(20), 2760–2765.

Fisher, E. B., Lichtenstein, E., & Haire-Joshu, D. (1993). Multiple determinants of tobacco use and cessation. In C. T. Orleans & J. Slade (Eds.), *Nicotine addiction: Principles and management* (pp. 59–88). New York: Oxford University Press.

Ford, M. B., Sigurdson, A. J., Petrulis, E. S., Ng, C. S., Kemp, B., Cooksley, C., et al. (2003). Effects of smoking and radiotherapy on lung carcinoma in breast carcinoma survivors. *Cancer, 98*(7), 1457–1464.

Frank, S. H., & Jaen, C. R. (1993). Office evaluation and treatment of the dependent smoker. *Primary Care, 20*(1), 251–268.

Garces, Y. I., Yang, P., Parkinson, J., Zhao, X., Wampfler, J. A., Ebbert, J. O., et al. (2004). The relationship between cigarette smoking and quality of life after lung cancer diagnosis. *Chest, 126*(6), 1733–1741.

Garvey, A. J., Bliss, R. E., Hitchcock, J. L., Heinhold, J. W., & Rosner, B. (1992). Predictors of smoking relapse among self-quitters: A report from the normative aging study. *Addictive Behavior, 17*(4), 367–377.

Griebal, B., Wewers, M. E., & Baker, C. A. (1998). The effectiveness of a nurse-managed minimal smoking cessation intervention for hospitalized patients with cancer. *Oncology Nursing Forum, 25*(5), 897–902.

Gritz, E. R., Fingeret, M. C., Vidrine, D. J., Lazev, A. B., Mehta, N. V., & Reece, G. (2005). Successes and failure of the teachable moment: Smoking cessation in cancer patients. *Cancer, 106*(1), 17–27.

Gritz, E. R., Nisenbaum, R., Elashoff, R. E., & Holmes, E. C. (1991). Smoking behavior following diagnosis in patients with stage 1 non-small cell lung cancer. *Cancer Causes Control, 2*(2), 105–112.

Hatsukami, D. K., Hughes, J. R., & Pickens, R. W. (1985). Blood nicotine, smoke exposure and tobacco withdrawal symptoms. *Addictive Behavior, 10*(4), 413–417.

Hays, J. T. (2000). Tobacco dependence treatment in patients with heart and lung disease: Implications for intervention and review of pharmacological therapy. *Journal of Cardiopulmonary Rehabilitation, 20*(4), 215–223.

Hays, J. T., Hurt, R. D., Rigotti, N. A., Niaura, R., Gonzales, D., Durcan, M. J., et al. (2001). Sustained release bupropion for pharmacologic relapse prevention after smoking cessation: A randomized controlled trial. *Annals of Internal Medicine, 135*(6), 423–433.

Heatherton, T. F., Kozlowski, L. T., Frecker, R. C., & Fagerstrom, K. O. (1991). The Fagerstrom Test for Nicotine Dependence: A revision of the Fagerstrom tolerance questionnaire. *British Journal of Addictions, 86*(9), 1119–1127.

Henningfield, J. E., Cohen, C., & Slade, J. D. (1991). Is nicotine more addictive than cocaine? *British Journal of Addiction, 86*(5), 565–569.

Hopwood, P., & Stephens, R. J. (2000). Depression in patients with lung cancer: Prevalence and risk factors derived from quality of life data. *Journal of Clinical Oncology, 18*(4), 893–903.

Hung, R. J., McKay, J. D., Gaborieau, V., Bofetta, P., Hashibe, M., Zaridze, D., et al. (2008). A susceptibility for lung cancer maps to nicotinic acetylcholine receptor subunit genes on 15q25. *Nature, 452*(7187), 633–637.

Jamerson, B. D., Nides, M., Jorenby, D. E., Donahue, R., Garrett, P., Johnston, J. A., et al. (2001). Late term smoking cessation despite initial failure: An evaluation of bupropion sustained release, nicotine patch, combination therapy and placebo. *Clinical Therapeutics, 23*(5), 744–752.

Jorenby, D. E., & Fiore, M. C. (1999). The Agency for Health Care Policy and Research smoking cessation clinical practice guideline: Basics and beyond. *Primary Care, 26*(3), 513–528.

Jorenby, D. E., Leischow, S. J., Nides, M. A., Rennard, S. J., Johnston, J. A., Hughes, A. R., et al. (1999). A controlled trial of sustained release bupropion, a nicotine patch, or both for smoking cessation. *New England Journal of Medicine, 340*(9), 685–691.

Joseph, A. M., Norman, S. M., Ferry, L. H., Prochazka, A. V., Westman, E. C., Steele, B. G., et al. (1996). The safety of transdermal nicotine as an aid to smoking cessation in patients with cardiac disease. *New England Journal of Medicine, 335*(24), 1792–1798.

Karam-Hage, M., & Cinciripini, P. M. (2008). Pharmacotherapy for tobacco cessation: Nicotine agonists, antagonists, and partial agonists. *Cancer Prevention, 9*(6), 509–516.

Kendler, K. S. (2001). The genetic epidemiology of smoking. In R. Clayton (Chair of Section II, Nicotine—individual risk factors for initiation), *Addicted to nicotine: A national research forum.* Retrieved October

31, 2008, from www.nida.nih.gov/meetsum/nicotine/kendler.html

Killen, J. D., Fortmann, S. P., & Telch, M. J. (1988). Are heavy smokers different from light smokers? *Journal of the American Medical Association, 260*(11), 1581–1583.

Knoke, J. D., Burns, D. M., & Thun, M. J. (2008). The change in excess risk of lung cancer attributable to smoking following smoking cessation: An examination of different analytic approaches using CPS-I data. *Cancer Causes Control, 19*(2), 207–219.

Landi, M. T., Dracheva, T., Rotunno, M., Figueroa, J. D., Liu, H., Dasgupta, A., et al. (2008). Gene expression signature of cigarette smoking and its role in lung adenocarcinoma development and survival. *PloS ONE, 3*(2), e1651.

Lerman, C., & Berrettini, W. (2003). Elucidating the role of genetic factors in smoking behavior and nicotine dependence. *American Journal of Medical Genetics, 118B*(1), 48–54.

Lerman, C., Caporaso, N. E., Audrain, J., Main, D., Bowman, E. D., Lockshin, B., et al. (1999). Evidence suggesting the role of specific genetic factors in cigarette smoking. *Health Psychology, 18*(1), 14–20.

Lerman, C., Caporaso, N. E., Audrain, J., Main, D., Boyd, N. R., & Shields, P. G. (2000). Interacting effects of the serotonin transporter gene and neuroticism in smoking practices and nicotine dependence. *Molecular Psychiatry, 5*(2), 189–192.

Lerman, C., Patterson, F., & Berrettini, W. (2005). Treating tobacco dependence: State of the science and new directions. *Journal of Clinical Oncology, 23*(2), 311–323.

Mahon, S. (2005). Review of selected approaches to promoting smoking cessation. *Clinical Journal of Oncology Nursing, 9*(6), 745–747.

McBride, M., & Ostroff, J. S. (2003). Teachable moments for promoting smoking cessation: The context of cancer care and survivorship. *Cancer Control, 10*(4), 325–333.

Meert, A., Mayer, C., Milani, M., Beckers, J., & Razavi, D. (2006). Smoking cessation interventions among cancer patients. *Bulletin du Cancer, 93*(4), 363–369.

Murray, R., Bailey, W., Daniels, K., Bjornson, W., Kurnow, K., Connett, J. E., et. al. (1996). Safety of nicotine polacrilex gum used by 3094 participants in the lung health study. *Chest, 109*(2), 438–445.

Niaura, R., Britt, D. M., Shadel, W. G., Goldstein, M., Abrams, D., & Brown, R. (2001). Symptoms of depression and survival experience among three samples of smokers trying to quit. *Psychology of Addictive Behaviors, 15*(1), 13–17.

Ockene, J. K., Emmons, K. M., Mermelstein, R. J., Perkins, K. A., Bonollo, D. S., & Voorhees, C. C. (2000). Relapse and maintenance issues for smoking cessation. *Health Psychology, 19*(1), (Suppl.), 17–31.

Ostroff, J. S., Jacobsen, P. B., Moadel, A. B., Spiro, R. H., Shah, J. P., Strong, E. W., et al. (1995). Prevalence and predictors of continued tobacco use after treatment of patients with head and neck cancer. *Cancer, 75*(2), 569–576.

Pinto, B. M., Eakin, E., & Maruyama, N. C. (2000). Health behavior changes after a cancer diagnosis: What do we know and where do we go from here? *Annals of Behavioral Medicine, 22*(1), 38–52.

Pizacani, B. A., Martin, D. P., Stark, M. J., Koepsell, T. D., Thompson, B., & Diehr, P. (2008). Longitudinal study of household smoking ban adoption among households with at least one smoker: Associated factors, barriers, and smoker support. *Nicotine & Tobacco Research, 10*(3), 533–540.

Price, J. H., Jordan, T. R., Jeffrey, J. D., Stanley, M. S., & Price, J. A. (2008). Tobacco intervention training in graduate psychiatric nursing education programs. *Journal of American Psychiatric Nurses Association, 14*(2), 117–124.

Prochaska, J. O., Redding, C. A., & Evers, K. E. (1997). The transtheoretical model and stages of change. In K. Glanz, F. M. Lewis, & B. K. Rimer (Eds.), *Health behavior and health education: Theory, research and practice* (pp. 60–84). San Francisco: Jossey-Bass.

Prokhorov, A. V., Hudman, K. S., & Gritz, E. R. (1997). Promoting smoking cessation among cancer patients: A behavioral model. *Oncology, 11*(12), 1807–1814.

Ranney, L., Melvin, C., Lux, L., McClain, E., & Lohr, K. N. (2006). Systematic review: Smoking cessation intervention strategies for adults and adults in special populations. *Annals of Internal Medicine, 145*(11), 845–856.

Rice, V. H., & Stead, L. F. (2008). Nursing interventions for smoking cessation. *Cochrane Database of Systematic Reviews, 1.* (Art. No.: CD001188. DOI: 10.1002/14651858.CD001188.pub3.)

Rossing, M. A. (1998). Genetic influences on smoking: Candidate genes. *Environmental Health Perspectives, 106*(5), 231–238.

Rustin, T. A. (2000). Assessing nicotine dependence. *American Family Physician, 62*(3), 579–584, 591–592.

Schnoll, R. A., James, C., Malstrom, M., Rothman, R. L., Wang, H., Babb, J., et al. (2003). Longitudinal predictors of continued tobacco use among patients diagnosed with cancer. *Annals of Behavioral Medicine, 25*(3), 214–222.

Schwartz, J. S. (1987). *Review and evaluation of smoking cessation methods: The United States and Canada 1978–1985* (Publication No. 87-2940). Washington, DC: US Government Printing Office.

Shiffman, S., Elash, C. A., Paton, S. M., Gwaltney, C. J., Paty, J. A., Clark, D. B., et al. (2000). Comparative efficacy of 24-hour and 16-hour transdermal nicotine patches for relief of morning craving. *Addiction, 95*(8), 1185–1195.

Taylor, K. L., Sanderson Cox, L., Zincke, N., Mehta, L., McGuire, C., & Gelmann, E. (2006). Lung cancer screening as a teachable moment for smoking cessation. *Lung Cancer, 56*(1), 125–134.

Thompson, G. H., & Hunter, D. A. (1998). Nicotine replacement therapy. *Annals of Pharmacotherapy, 32*(10), 1067–1075.

Tsao, A. S., Liu, D., Lee, J. J., Spitz, M., & Hong, W. K. (2006). Smoking affects treatment outcome in patients with advanced nonsmall cell lung cancer. *Cancer, 106*(11), 2428–2436.

Uchitomi, Y., Mikami, I., Kugaya, A., Akizuki, N., Nagai, K., Nishiwaki, Y., et al. (2000). Depression after successful treatment for non-small cell lung carcinoma. *Cancer, 89*(5), 1172–1179.

US Department of Health and Human Services. (2008). Public health advisory: Important information on Chantix (Varenicline). Retrieved December 23, 2008, from http://www.fda.gov/medwAtch/safety/2008/safety 08.htm#Varenicline

US Department of Health and Human Services, Public Health Service. (1988). *The health consequences of smoking: Nicotine addiction: A report of the Surgeon General.* Washington, DC: Center for Health Promotion and Education. Office on Smoking and Health.

Velicer, W. F., Fava, J. L., Prochaska, J. O., Abrams, D. B., Emmons, K. M., & Pierce, J. P. (1995). Distribution of smokers by stage in three representative samples. *Preventive Medicine, 24*(4), 401–411.

Videtic, G. M., Stitt, L. W., Dar, A. R., Kocha, W. I., Tomiak, A. T., Truong, P. T., et al. (2003). Continued cigarette smoking by patients receiving concurrent chemoradiotherapy for limited-stage small-cell lung cancer is associated with decreased survival. *Journal of Clinical Oncology, 21*(8), 1544–1549.

Walton, R., Johnstone, E., Munafo, M., Neville, M., & Griffith, S. (2001). Genetic clues to the molecular basis of tobacco addiction and progress toward personalized therapy. *Trends in Molecular Medicine, 7*(2), 70–76.

Wewers, M. E., Jenkins, L., & Mignery, T. (1997). A nurse-managed smoking cessation intervention during diagnostic testing for lung cancer. *Oncology Nursing Forum, 24*(8), 1419–1422.

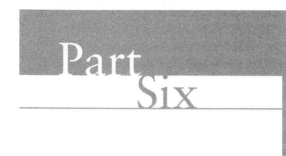

Part Six

Media and Future Research Directions

Chapter 17

Battling Biases: Nursing, Lung Cancer, and the Media

Elisa Becze

Introduction

We live in an age that is dominated by the media. The media is a powerful force, with the ability to shape perceptions and sway opinions. This power stems, in part, from the media's ability to get a message to a large number of people or to key people (i.e., policy makers) (Mason, Dodd, & Glickstein, 2007). Used responsibly, mass media educates the public and heightens awareness about important issues. On the other hand, the media does not always present a balanced view of issues and sometimes presents limited perspectives. The information that the media chooses to cover or not cover is also very powerful. The media often overlooks the nursing perspective.

Even in the 21st century, nurses continue to battle traditional stereotypes regarding roles as healthcare professionals. Newspapers, magazines, books, journals, television, film, and the Internet have influenced the public perception of nursing as a profession and the public's acceptance of nurses as expert sources of health-related information. Likewise, the media's emphasis on health issues is often biased. For example, some cancers, such as breast cancer and prostate cancer, are covered much more frequently in the media than the second most common, yet deadliest, cancer: lung cancer. This chapter describes how cancer information is presented by the media in general, the history of nursing as it is depicted in the media, and opportunities for increasing the use of nurses as health-information resources and comprehensive coverage of cancer-related information.

Presentation of Cancer in the Media

One in three people will receive a diagnosis of cancer in his or her lifetime. Therefore, the predominance of media coverage of cancer should come as no surprise. However, studies have shown that media coverage related to cancer can be biased or may fail to place the information in complete context within the larger picture. For example, potential new cancer treatment drugs may be heralded in the media as the next magic bullet, when in reality the drugs were evaluated only in animal models. At other times the media spreads fear by suggesting that cancer is a death sentence (Redmond, 2007) or that everything causes it (Clarke & Everest, 2006).

Because of the ability of the mass media to shape health behaviors, it is vitally important that nurses recognize areas where additional information would help to place the information presented in a broader context.

Lung Cancer Coverage in US and International Media

Researchers from around the world have observed a media bias against lung cancer. In 2001, Cancer Care, Inc., the Oncology Nursing Society (ONS), and The Wellness Community, in collaboration with the National Cancer Institute, conducted an analysis of media coverage of the four major tumor types (lung, breast, colorectal, and prostate) to determine the prevalence and type of coverage of lung cancer between August 1999 and July 2000 compared with coverage of other cancers during the same time period (Blum, Kennedy, Boerckel, & Rieger, 2001). This was the first major study of its kind to evaluate media coverage of the four major cancers. The findings were shocking: Lung cancer, the number one cause of cancer death, was among the least reported of the four identified tumor types.

More recent studies have had similar findings. In a content analysis of cancer coverage in mass print media in Canada, and more specifically those targeting ethnic minority populations, researchers found that none of the 27 ethnic minority newspapers and only 28 of the 721 mainstream newspapers that were analyzed contained articles on lung cancer (Hoffman-Goetz & Friedman, 2005). The authors said that breast cancer coverage predominated the media at 21%, but coverage was much lower for other cancers that have higher incidences or death rates, including lung (4%), prostate (8%), and

colorectal (4%). Lung cancer is the leading cause of cancer death in Canada, so to have no articles about the disease at all in ethnic minority newspapers is alarming. The results were similar to an earlier study done by Friedman and Hoffman-Goetz (2003), which evaluated cancer coverage in North American newspapers and magazines that target older adults. That study found that only 4 of the 226 articles (2%) were about lung cancer, and none of them contained "mobilizing information" that explained how to prevent or detect the disease.

In 2007, Moriarty and Stryker used a unique perspective to assess the coverage of cancer in the news media. The authors divided news stories into those about highly *preventable* cancers (lung, esophageal, bladder, and skin cancers, according to American Cancer Society [ACS] definitions) and those about highly *detectable* cancers (breast, cervical, prostate, colorectal, and skin cancers, according to ACS). For the preventable cancers, which include lung cancer, they analyzed news stories that contain prevention information; 25% of the stories reviewed in the study discussed tobacco cessation for the prevention of lung cancer, which was second only to diet in quantity of stories about prevention of cancer. However, when the same stories were evaluated for discussing prevention efficacy, the news media paid more attention to diet and sun exposure than to tobacco use.

Some studies that have looked at general cancer coverage in the media have not even mentioned lung cancer, which attests to the media bias. Clarke and Everest (2006) looked at mass English language magazines in the United States and Canada in 1991, 1996, and 2001 to compare cancer coverage across the years. They found that coverage of several types of cancer had increased from 1991 to 1996 and again to 2001;

however, the article did not mention lung cancer coverage for any of those years.

When the media does mention lung cancer, its coverage may contribute to the stereotypes already surrounding patients with the disease. A 2004 study in the United Kingdom by Chapple, Ziebland, and McPherson indicated that press reports and media advertisements contributed to a stigma about patients with lung cancer. Patients reported feeling looked down upon by the public and even healthcare practitioners because they had smoked or were thought to be smokers because they had lung cancer. Patients perceived that the media portrayal and public belief about lung cancer was that the cancer was self-inflicted, although many of the patients had quit smoking years prior or had never smoked.

Celebrities often focus media attention on a disease. With lung cancer, however, few celebrities have stepped up to the spokesperson plate. In recent years, baseball player Cal Ripken, Jr., has been an honorary spokesperson for the Lung Cancer Alliance since 2007, and other celebrities, such as musician Richard Marx and model Christie Turlington, have lent their names to Lung Cancer Awareness Week. Sometimes, however, a celebrity can bring attention to a disease just by being diagnosed with it. In 2005, when the news media announced that news anchor Peter Jennings had died from lung cancer and that Dana Reeve, wife of Christopher Reeve, had been diagnosed with the disease, the *Boston Globe* reported that interest in lung cancer surged (Goldberg, 2005). Nonprofit groups received an influx of calls from people seeking information about lung cancer risk factors and screening options and also saw an increase in donations. Shortly after the Jennings and Reeve announcements, the National Cancer Institute

reported a new 5-year, $80-million initiative to research lung cancer and treatment (Goldberg, 2005).

In the same *Boston Globe* article, a spokesperson for the Lung Cancer Alliance said that "the fight against lung cancer is in the very early stages of a paradigm shift" (Goldberg, 2005). Three years later, this statement still provides both a challenge and an opportunity for the nursing profession to partner with the media and to advocate for a balanced presentation of the management of lung cancer to the public by the media. To seize this opportunity, nurses must have an understanding of how the media has traditionally portrayed the nursing profession and how frequently the media has used nurses as credible sources of information.

The History of Nursing in the Media

Nurses continue to be underrepresented as media resources; this may be based on long-held stereotypes of nurses as healthcare professionals who do not function independently and are merely low-level subordinates to physicians. Clearly, the media has a history of indifference to listening to and quoting nurses as sources of information. On the other hand, nurses also contribute to the lack of their own representation in the media because they are often reluctant to contact reporters, to be interviewed, and to be quoted. Journalists and nursing professionals must work together to change these traditional perceptions. Nurses must learn media skills so that they may interact more effectively with the media. The public can advocate for the use of a variety of sources by journalists, including nursing professionals, for health-related information presented in the media.

The Visibility of Nursing in the Media

Several studies have evaluated the representation of nurses in media coverage of health issues and found it to be startlingly low. Buresh, Gordon, and Bell (1991) analyzed the representation of nurses in the health coverage of three major newspapers. They reviewed the sources of 908 direct quotations by occupation and found that even though nursing represents the largest healthcare profession, nurses accounted for only 1.1% of quotations, falling at the bottom of the list of 11 other professions. Physicians were by far the most frequently quoted group, representing more than 30% of all quotations. The other groups included government officials, patients and families, medical organizations, and an assortment of other professional and nonprofessional healthcare workers. This finding is unsettling for the nursing profession because a profession's public status, legitimacy, and prestige are linked to acknowledgment of its expertise by the journalistic media (Buresh & Gordon, 2006). It is difficult for the public to fully appreciate the value of nursing's role when nurses are so consistently omitted as credible sources of information and, therefore, contributors to health care.

The Woodhull Study

One of the most well recognized studies on the visibility of nursing in the media was published in 1998 by Sigma Theta Tau International, the nursing honor society. Known as the Woodhull Study, it reviewed hundreds of health-related articles from 16 major publications in 1997. On average, nurses were cited only 3% of the time. In the seven newspapers surveyed, nurses and the nursing profession were referenced in only 4% of the articles examined. In the four news magazines, nurses were referenced in 5% of the articles. In the five trade publications, where the full focus was on health care, only 1% of the references were nurses. Most of the references to nursing were fleeting when they did occur. Based on the subject matter in many of the articles, nurses would have served as more appropriate sources of information than the ones selected.

Distortion of the Image of Nursing

Not only is the nursing profession underrepresented in the media as a credible source of healthcare information, its image is frequently distorted by nurse archetypes going back as far as the early 19th century. Common stereotypes include the stern disciplinarian, as portrayed by the character Nurse Ratched in the movie *One Flew Over the Cuckoo's Nest*; the sexpot; the selfless, saintly type; the hero; and the angel of mercy. The news media often focuses on nursing problems or failings but disregards nursing accomplishments. Television, movies, and books suggest that physicians are the only members of the healthcare team or that physicians cure patients whereas nurses only provide care. Decidedly lacking in the media's portrayal of nurses are male nurses and nurses who work as researchers, scientists, teachers, and expert clinicians (Gordon, 2005).

Lusk (2000) analyzed images of nurses in pictorial advertisements from all issues of hospital administration journals published in 1930, 1940, and 1950 (a total of 598 issues). Content analysis of the data was based on Goffman's classic 1979 study on gender advertisements. Lusk found that nurses were portrayed predominantly as young females, eager to please, and lacking apparent wisdom. In group scenes, nurses were portrayed as subordinate to physicians and hospital administrators. In the 1940 advertisements, nurses were shown performing more complex, autonomous activities than in the 1930 and 1950 advertisements. These findings support previous research focused on more recent portrayals of women and nurses in the media. The overt and subtle representations of nurses as subordinates in these advertisements, compared with physicians and administrators, reveal one facet of the historical perspective of nursing as a woman's profession.

Gordon (2005) reported observing that even hospital publications misrepresent nurses in hospital news. Nurses are rarely acknowledged in press releases about research, and the focus of hospital advertising is on medicine, not nursing care. Internal hospital publications also gloss over nursing accomplishments and events in favor of news about physicians.

Nursing on the Internet

In the first study that looked at the image of nursing on the Internet, Kalisch, Begeny, and Neumann (2007) compared the depiction of nursing characteristics on 144 Web sites in 2001 to 152 sites in 2004. Several of the characteristics attributed to nurses remained the same among the three years: educated (71%); intelligent (70%); accountable (63%); respected (61%); trustworthy (59%); warm, kind, and compassionate (47%); and diverse (35%). However, they found that the perception of nurses as attractive, competent, sexually promiscuous, and being "cool" or "with it" increased from

2001 to 2004, whereas the perception of nurses being committed, autonomous, scientific, authoritative, powerful, and creative or innovative decreased among the three years.

Consumer Attitudes About Nursing

In 1999, Sigma Theta Tau International and NurseWeek Publishing, Inc. commissioned Harris Interactive, a worldwide market research and consulting firm best known for the Harris Poll, to conduct a public opinion poll on consumer attitudes about nursing. Overall, the random sample of 1,006 adult US residents was found to have a positive consumer attitude about the nursing profession. When asked about the duties of registered nurses, 91% of those polled realized that nurses monitor patient care, but only 14% knew that some nurses prescribe medications. An overwhelming majority of those polled (92%) reported that they trusted the healthcare information provided by registered nurses, which equaled the percentage that trusted physicians.

The public obviously considers nurses to be trustworthy sources of information on health care, which makes it difficult to understand why nurses are quoted so infrequently by the media. In fact, nurses again topped the Gallup Poll on honesty and ethics in 2006. Approximately 84% of respondents rated nurses as "high" or "very high" in honesty and ethical standards, which was much higher than the number of "high" and "very high" ratings given to the other top five professions: druggists/pharmacists (73%), veterinarians (71%), medical doctors (69%), and dentists (62%) (Saad, 2006). Nurses have been at the top of this list since they were first included in 1999, with the exception of the 2001 poll, in which they were second only to firefighters. The 2001 poll was conducted after the September 11 terrorist attacks.

Opportunity for Change

The public views the nursing profession as credible, moral, and trustworthy but not necessarily as a source of knowledge, power, and influence in the healthcare arena. Although this assessment initially appears to be discouraging, it presents a solid foundation upon which to enact change. The nursing profession can build on the public's view of the profession as credible and trustworthy and can begin to assume a position of authority where matters of health care are concerned.

The Benefits of a Nursing–Media Partnership

One of the most salient reasons for partnering with the media in today's world is simply that nurses have no choice. The media, in its myriad forms, is the platform through which information is transmitted to the general public. Nursing professionals must become comfortable working with the media if they wish to be included in the dissemination of healthcare information. Nurses can then work to ensure that the representation of information related to health in general and cancer in particular is balanced and reflective of the actual need for information (i.e., that important information on major cancers, such as lung, colorectal, breast, and prostate, are covered in proportion to their occurrence in the population).

There are many other compelling reasons why nurses should consider developing a partnership with the media, several of which are outlined in Figure 17–1. Buresh and Gordon

Figure 17–1 Reasons for partnering with the media.

- To shape public policy
- To educate the public
- To enhance the image of nursing
- To help the media present accurate information on issues of concern
- To help the media achieve a balanced perspective on issues
- To advertise new programs
- To aid fund-raising

(2006) envisioned medical practice if nurses assumed more prominent positions as providers of expertise on matters related to health care. They would automatically be placed on the short list of those to interview when health issues arise, the names of nursing experts and professional nursing organizations would be included in journalists' contact lists, and nurses would be included along with other healthcare providers—namely physicians—in all forms of media as expert sources of healthcare information.

The long-term benefits of this new partnership could be extraordinarily powerful. The presence of a nursing perspective in ongoing public discussions about health care would be seen in a broad spectrum of forums, such as state and national politics and town hall meetings, and in a variety of media. Nurses would share equal partnership with other professionals at the tables of power where healthcare policy is formulated. Patients would recognize that the qualifications of the nurses who care for them before, during, and after chemotherapy or radiation therapy and procedures are as important as the qualifications of the physicians. The public would begin to understand exactly what nurses do and the contributions they must make to ensure quality care.

This vision is well within the grasp of nurses who are willing to learn how to use their knowledge and expertise to become more visible to the public at large. They have the numbers—as of 2004, there were approximately 2.9 million registered nurses in the United States—and they clearly have the opportunities to achieve an ongoing partnership with the media.

To begin this partnership, nurses must overcome the barriers that have thus far stifled their working relationship with the media (Buresh & Gordon, 2006). Many of these barriers are personal—for example, a reluctance to be interviewed. Journalists have complained that when they contact nurses to schedule an interview, the nurses often do not return phone calls or are hesitant to provide information. Much of the reluctance is fueled by nurses' common fears, including whether they will be misquoted or that comments will be taken out of context, whether the journalist will be cordial or on the attack during the interview, and whether they will look and sound professional. Although these fears may be well founded, they can all be overcome with practice. It is not within the culture of nursing to seek out the media, as has been the trend among physicians. However, by learning effective strategies for working with the media, nurses can begin to overcome these barriers.

Strategies for Working with the Media

The first step is to decide which form of media to attract—daily and weekly newspapers, books, professional journals, magazines, radio, television, or the Internet—and define the audience. For example, different sources would be selected if the target audience were a group of teenagers

being educated about smoking and its related health risks (e.g., lung cancer) versus a group of senior citizens. Nurses can introduce themselves and their work to the media by pitching newsworthy stories. Look for opportunities to add a nursing angle to current hot-button news items. Don't hesitate to send out well-written press releases; some news media will run entire releases or send out reporters to cover a story. Even phone calls and e-mails may help pique the media's interest in nursing's side of the story (Buresh & Gordon, 2006).

Increasing the Visibility of Nursing in the Media

It is important for nurses to be aware of what is going on in relation to health care locally and nationally. They should pick a particular subject in health care that they have expertise in—for example, lung cancer or symptom management—and pay attention to how stories about that subject are presented. By monitoring the media, nurses can stay abreast of what issues have been addressed, where gaps in cancer coverage have occurred (as has been seen with lung cancer), current hot-button issues, how stories are crafted, and how they as a source can make salient points and enhance reporting to benefit the public's understanding and awareness.

Within their own communities, nurses need to be alert to what is being reported and written and who is doing high-quality reporting on healthcare issues. They should follow the stories, analyze their strengths, and determine why they were published or aired. They need to understand when a hot-button national story or topic can be addressed at the local level in their own communities. Nurses should recognize which reporters in the local media outlets are strong, credible journalists who use a balanced approach when covering controversial issues and how those reporters construct their stories or reports. Nurses who develop relationships with healthcare journalists can yield significant benefits in the long run. They can write or e-mail positive reactions to a journalist whose articles they have read. They can identify themselves as nurses and express their willingness to contribute to future projects that focus on a certain topic. Nurses can propose stories on areas where coverage is lacking or ones that coincide with cancer awareness months.

While gaining a clearer perspective about media coverage on healthcare issues in their communities, nurses need to consider what topics they can appropriately comment on. For example,

nurses have a vast body of knowledge of and experience in symptom management. They need to think about how media pieces could be shaped by their contributions and the contributions of other healthcare professionals, patients, and their caregivers and supporters. Most importantly, nurses at all levels and in all roles should prepare themselves to be poised, knowledgeable, and comfortable sources and spokespersons. Figure 17–2 presents tips on preparing for a media interview.

Nurses do not have to work alone to gain visibility in the media. They can partner with their organization's public relations team, other healthcare providers, and reporters to build mutually beneficial relationships. The public relations team can help nurses gain the expertise

Figure 17–2 Tips for getting ready for a media interview.

Questions to ask yourself:
- Is the interview on a deadline? If yes, how much time do you have to prepare?
- What is the focus of the interview?
- What are the politics around the issue?
- Who is the audience?
- What is the key message you would like to relay to this audience?
- Do you have a quotable quote?
- What do you want the audience to know?
- What are possible questions you may be asked?
- What will be your answers? Rehearse them!

Important dos and don'ts:
- Tell the truth; do not lie or speculate. If you don't know an answer, offer to get it.
- Explain why you may not be able to comment on a particular subject; never say "no comment."
- Be cooperative, accessible, and nonconfrontational.
- Be clear in what you say; avoid using jargon.
- Back up your points with stories. Patient stories can be incredibly powerful in emphasizing key points.
- Remember that nothing you say is ever off the record.
- Learn how to plug the organization—your profession, your hospital, and your professional society.
- Never ask to review the final product.
- Remember that preparation and follow-up are as important, if not more important, than the actual interview.
- Match your message to the medium. Communication strategies will depend on whether the medium is print, radio, or television.

and confidence needed to serve as effective sources and spokespersons. Additionally, the team can work to create media opportunities for nurses and help them pitch story ideas to reporters. Nurses can aid public relations practitioners in their work with the media by translating medical terminology and complex medical issues into information that reporters and the public can grasp.

Nurses also can partner with other healthcare providers to lobby for a media awareness task force within their organization that can identify what information needs to be shared with the public and how that information can best be presented to reporters. Finally, nurses can cultivate partnerships with area reporters by offering to serve as a sounding board and resource. These partnerships will help nurses gain credibility and reliability, and over time, nurses will evolve into a valuable public resource.

Being visible takes planning and thought. Although reporters are always looking for stories within their communities, they may not be particularly excited to cover the "fifth annual lung cancer awareness event" held at their local cancer center. "It's been done already" is the media's common reaction to such repetitive news. However, in preparing for the event, nurses can look at all aspects of the event to develop story ideas. For example, perhaps during a previous event, a patient at high risk for lung cancer received information that led to an early diagnosis and is now willing to talk about the experience. That patient might serve as a special recruiter to get people to attend the event or might be on-site during the event to welcome participants. New twists that give repetitive news a fresh look can help reporters gain a new perspective on how to creatively present a standing topic, and nurses can be instrumental in helping them develop new approaches.

This approach might be very successfully used during Lung Cancer Awareness Month (LCAM) in November by highlighting patients who have survived lung cancer or who have benefited from exciting new advances in detection or treatment modalities. Information about events surrounding LCAM and ways that nurses can get the community (and therefore the media) involved can be found on the Lung Cancer Alliance Web site at www.lungcancer alliance.org. Ongoing lung cancer awareness programs, such as the Caring Ambassadors Lung Cancer Program at www.lungcancercap.org, also provide opportunities for media involvement and attention.

It must be said that the voice of nursing has always been richly informative and comforting. For the most part, the public has benefited from the wealth of knowledge and experience nurses convey through one-on-one contact. Today's nurses can expand the scope and impact of their reach through the communications power offered by print and electronic media. Media relations have become a vital dimension within the largest organization of oncology healthcare professionals in the world, the Oncology Nursing Society (ONS), a group that believes its members should be well prepared to serve as media contacts as part of being nursing leaders. Figure 17–3 lists the resources available from the society to help nurses gain the necessary skills to increase their visibility and value as media contacts. These resources are, for the most part, available in a hard copy version or at www.ons.org. ONS traditionally promotes the availability of these resources to society leaders and its members, as well as to the entire oncology community by way of letters, communiqués, printed and online newsletters, and ads in society journals.

Figure 17–3 Oncology Nursing Society (ONS) resources to help nurses become active and visible leaders in the media.

Press releases	Talking points
Fact sheets	Health policy position papers
Professional backgrounders	Frequently asked questions
Reprints of articles	Bibliographies
PowerPoint presentations	Media and special topic kits
ONS online resources	ONS webcasts and podcasts

To help nurses emerge as strong leaders and vital voices in the media, the society offers the Leadership Development Institute, a year-long experience that combines didactic teaching and the availability of society leaders as mentors. Moreover, nurses can work with the public relations staff at ONS to receive one-on-one coaching to work with the media and to obtain specific background information to aid in media efforts. The public relations staff is committed to raising the profile of nursing in the media and encourages members to become part of the ONS media response team. This group of nursing experts is designed to respond to media inquiries within 24 hours to ensure that the nursing point of view is covered in the media.

Counteracting the Distorted Media View of Nursing

The Center for Nursing Advocacy (www.nursing advocacy.org) was founded in 2001 to increase the public's understanding of the role nurses play in modern health care by promoting accurate portrayal of nurses in the media and encouraging the media to use nurses as expert sources. The center holds ongoing letter-writing campaigns to address misrepresentation of nursing in the media, particularly on television shows such as *ER*, *Grey's Anatomy*, and *House,* as well as in advertising and news articles. The center has successfully stopped numerous advertisers from using "naughty nurses" to promote their products and has petitioned television talk shows such as *Dr. Phil* and *Live with Regis and Kelly* to retract their negative comments about nurses. Groups such as ONS have partnered with The Center for Nursing Advocacy to encourage nurses to participate in these campaigns. By consistently analyzing how nursing is being represented and organizing unified responses from the nursing community, groups like these are working to improve the image of nursing in the media.

Using Media to Address the Nursing Shortage

Sigma Theta Tau International has helped to spearhead the development of a coalition of 43 nursing and healthcare organizations to form Nurses for a Healthier Tomorrow (NHT). The coalition created a Web site (www.nursesource. org), created an advertising campaign, and secured media coverage to spread the word about the nursing shortage and to encourage young people to enter the profession.

Although earlier campaigns focused on educating students about the opportunities and benefits of nursing careers, the current NHT media campaign was designed to increase nurse educator recruitment. The campaign includes a series of print advertisements that feature actual nurse educators as well as an outreach campaign to reach nursing journals and mass media.

Johnson & Johnson introduced the Campaign for Nursing's Future (CNF) in 2002 with the goals of enhancing the image of the nursing profession and attracting and retaining nurses and nurse educators to the profession. The campaign has included a Web site (www.campaign fornursing.com), and national print, television, and interactive advertising. A 2005 study by Donelan, Buerhaus, Ulrich, Norman, and Dittus found that 79% of student nurses, 59% of registered nurses, and 98% of chief nursing officers were aware of CNF activities in 2004. Sixty-seven percent of registered nurses and 92% of chief nursing officers said that the campaign has had a positive impact on the image of nursing careers in the general public.

Nurses in communities around the country can use NHT and CNF as models to create their own campaigns to shatter myths and change perceptions within their clinical and professional arenas. Nurses can also offer to talk with journalists about the nursing shortage and strategies for solving it.

Conclusion

Nursing professionals are now in a clear position to envision a future where they are recognized as important sources of information when matters of health are presented in the media. As part of the mandate of the profession, nursing has an obligation to make certain that information related to health care is reported accurately, to ensure that the information is placed in the proper perspective, and that important information is also presented to the public. The limited coverage of lung cancer, the number one cause of cancer death in the United States, by the media represents one such example. This presents an incredible opportunity for nurses not only to play a leading role in educating the public about lung cancer prevention, detection, and emerging treatment strategies, but to gain recognition of nursing as a vital component of the healthcare delivery system.

References

Blum, D., Kennedy, V. N., Boerckel, W., & Rieger, P. T. (2001). Lung cancer—under-reported in the media. *Proceedings of the American Society of Clinical Oncology, 20*(Part 1) [Abstract #1001]. Cancer Care, The Wellness Community, and Oncology Nursing Society.

Buresh, B., & Gordon, S. (2006). *From silence to voice* (2nd ed.). Ithaca, NY: Cornell University Press.

Buresh, B., Gordon, S., & Bell, N. (1991). Who counts in news coverage of health care? *Nursing Outlook, 39*(5), 204–208.

Chapple, A., Ziebland, S., & McPherson, A. (2004). Stigma, shame, and blame experienced by patients with lung cancer: Qualitative study. *BMJ, 328*(7454), 1470.

Clarke, J. N., & Everest, M. M. (2006). Cancer in the mass print media: Fear, uncertainty and the medical model. *Social Science and Medicine, 62*(10), 2591–2600.

Donelan, K., Buerhaus, P. I., Ulrich, B. T., Norman, L., & Dittus, R. (2005). Awareness and perceptions of the Johnson & Johnson Campaign for Nursing's Future: Views from nursing students, RNs, and CNOs. *Nursing Economic$, 23*(4), 150–156, 180.

Friedman, D. B., & Hoffman-Goetz, L. (2003). Cancer coverage in North American publications targeting seniors. *Journal of Cancer Education, 18*(1), 43–47.

Goldberg, C. (2005, September 26). Changing the face of lung cancer: Long held back by the stigma of smoking, advocacy work and donations gain momentum. *Boston Globe*. Retrieved June 10, 2008, from http://www. boston.com/news/globe/health_science/articles/2005/ 09/26/changing_the_face_of_lung_cancer

Gordon, S. (2005). *Nursing against the odds*. Ithaca, NY: Cornell University Press.

Hoffman-Goetz, L., & Friedman, D. B. (2005). Disparities in the coverage of cancer information in ethnic minority and mainstream mass print media. *Ethnicity and Disease, 15*(2), 332–340.

Kalisch, B. J., Begeny, S., & Neumann, S. (2007). The image of the nurse on the Internet. *Nursing Outlook, 55*(4), 182–188.

Lusk, B. (2000). Pretty and powerless: Nurses in advertisements, 1930–1950. *Research in Nursing and Health, 23*(3), 229–236.

Mason, D. J., Dodd, C. J., & Glickstein, B. (2007). Harnessing the power of the media to influence health policy and politics. In D. J. Mason, J. K. Leavitt, & M. W. Chaffee (Eds.), *Policy and politics in nursing and health care* (3rd ed., pp. 149–168). St. Louis, MO: W.B. Saunders.

Moriarty, C. M., & Stryker, J. E. (2007). Prevention and screening efficacy messages in newspaper accounts of cancer. *Health Education Research, 23*(3), 487–498.

Redmond, K. (2007). Promoting better quality media coverage of cancer [Editorial]. *Nature Clinical Practice Oncology, 4*(11), 613.

Saad, L. (2006). Nurses top list of most honest and ethical professions. Retrieved June 24, 2008, from http:// www.gallup.com/poll/25888/Nurses-Top-List-Most-Honest-Ethical-Professions.aspx

Sigma Theta Tau International. (1998). The Woodhull Study on nursing and the media: Health care's invisible partner. *Revolution, 8*(2), 64–70. Retrieved June 24, 2008, from http://www.nursingsociety.org/Media/ Pages/woodhall.aspx

Chapter 18

Challenges of Conducting Research in Women with Lung Cancer

Sophie Sun

Implementing research on vulnerable populations can present many problems, from the initial conceptualization of the study to the challenges of recruitment and retention. In general, vulnerable populations imply certain sample size requirements due to high attrition rates that result from a subject's day-to-day problems, disability, or death. The various issues related to vulnerability that make data collection include population barriers, changes associated with aging, symptoms, and cultural and socioeconomic factors. This chapter will address the clinical research issues faced when studying women with lung cancer.

Population Barriers

Few cancer nurse researchers have chosen to study women who have lung cancer. This is not surprising, because the majority of patients with lung cancer are diagnosed with advanced-stage disease, presenting with significant physical and psychological distress from the diagnosis, and consequently lung cancer patients are a challenging population to study.

Patients with lung cancer often present with multiple symptoms at diagnosis; thus, symptom control is an important aspect of data collection (Cooley, 2000). Due to the potential for acute medical issues, a serious event protocol (SEP) is often required in research studies. The SEP usually includes diagnoses, signs and symptoms, and interventions for potential problems that are specific to the study population. For example, in lung cancer, the SEP may include superior vena cava syndrome, cardiac tamponade, or suicidal ideation. The implementation of the SEP can increase the time needed for data collection.

Moreover, lung cancer is commonly viewed as a smoker's disease; there is often the perception that the disease is self-induced, and patients often carry the social stigma that they are less deserving of research investigation. Although the majority of lung cancer cases are attributable to tobacco use, it is estimated that 10–15% of females with lung cancer in the United States are never-smokers (Sun, Schiller, Gazdar, & Adi, 2007). Despite having never smoked, these patients can feel ostracized by the public and lack appropriate psychosocial supports.

There is a need for increased efforts for nurse researchers to study women with lung cancer. Better understanding of gender-specific issues among this subgroup will help optimize design and implementation of studies aimed at ultimately improving prevention, diagnosis, and treatment of lung cancer in both men and women.

Changes Associated with Aging

The majority of women with lung cancer are diagnosed at age 65 years or older. Given the older population, challenges of studying this group include decline in cerebral oxygenation (Mehagnoul-Schipper, Vloet, Colier, Hoefnagles, & Jansen, 2000), changes in vision, hearing problems, and comorbidities such as diabetes mellitus, COPD, and cardiovascular disease. Therefore, researchers need to adapt their methodologies to this population by allowing for more time for completing interviews and questionnaires, including larger fonts for written materials, using direct face-to-face communication, and taking age into consideration when defining norms for physiological and laboratory tests (such as pulmonary function tests, renal function) to match specific age groups and gender. The addition of time for data preparation and collection can be a difficult adjustment for researchers and is frequently unrecognized and underacknowledged by funding agencies. Comorbid diseases, lifetime use of tobacco products, the aging process (Sheahan & Musialowski, 2002; Sue, 2000), and functional changes (Grabiner, Biswas, & Grabiner, 2001) demand more physiological time for the body to compensate as well as respond.

Symptoms

Although lung cancer treatment recommendations are similar for men and women, gender differences in reported symptoms have been described (Sarna, 1994, 1998). Common respiratory symptoms that can affect a patient's ability to participate in research include coughing, wheezing, and dyspnea. Symptoms such as fatigue, weight loss, confusion from metastatic disease (most commonly liver, bone, and brain) are frequently present. In addition, serious disruptions in psychological and social aspects of quality of life are common among women with lung cancer, as demonstrated by high rates of self-reported depressed mood, personal and family distress with their diagnosis, and negative conceptualizations of their illness (Sarna, 2005).

Cough

Cough is present in 50–75% of lung cancer patients at diagnosis. Cough frequently occurs in patients in squamous cell and small cell lung carcinomas, which have the tendency to involve the central airways (Hyde & Hyde, 1974; Chute, et al., 1985). Cough can also be associated with COPD, asthma, postnasal drip, or gastroesophageal reflux disease (Carney, et al., 1997). Irritative persistent cough is a complaint of 27% of patients in early disease stages (Vaaler, et al., 1997) and 86–90% of patients in later stages (Vyas, et al., 1998), and it is the chief complaint of younger females with adenocarcinoma (Kuo, Chen, Chao, Tsai, & Perng, 2000). Irritative cancer-related cough can be treated supportively with antitussives; if it is accompanied by dyspnea, it can be treated with bronchodilators, corticosteroids, opioids, oxygen therapy, physiotherapy, inhalation therapy, and/or psychoactive medications (Ripamonti, 1999).

The underlying etiology of cough can be multifactorial in lung cancer patients. Contributing factors include treatment-related effects associated with surgery, radiation, chemotherapy, ongoing tobacco use, medications such as ACE inhibitors, and coexisting lung conditions such as bronchiectasis and tuberculosis. Cough can also be complicated by sleep disturbances, social disruptions, urinary incontinence, headache, syncope, rib fracture, and back pain (Carney, et al., 1997). Although cough is a common symptom, there are no clinical tools specific for its assessment in women with lung cancer, although these are being developed (Chernecky & Sarna, 2001).

Wheezing

Wheezing is a common symptom of lung cancer, as well as an early symptom (Sarna, et al., 2004). However, to date, there have been no cancer-related clinical studies in oncology settings on the symptom of wheezing. Descriptive tools to characterize various aspects of wheezing symptoms among women with lung cancer have been described (Chernecky & Sarna, 2001). These include describing the onset and duration of wheezing (wheeze all the time, wheeze when taking a breath in, wheeze when breathing out), presence of associated shortness of breath, effect of wheezing on sleep and activity, time of day and body position when wheezing is worst, and alleviating factors such as deep breathing or with coughing (which may be indicators of underlying chronic bronchitis).

Dyspnea

Dyspnea is the sensation of difficulty breathing. Approximately 60% of women with non-small cell lung cancer have dyspnea (Chernecky & Sarna, 2001), and it is a persistent symptom (Mercadante, Casuccio, & Fulfaro, 2000). Even though there is no instrument to measure sensitivity for dyspnea (Plat, Bredin, Krishnasamy, & Corner, 2000), it is an early symptom in

10–15% of patients at the time of diagnosis (Ochmanski, 1997), and 65% of patients have the symptom sometime during their illness (Vaaler, et al., 1997). Dyspnea is the most common symptom reported in women with lung cancer (O'Driscoll, Corner, & Bailey, 1999), and it can have a negative impact on the patient's physical, social, and psychological well-being (Gallo-Silver & Pollack, 2000).

Dypsnea does not appear to differ according to histologic subtype, stage, or performance status; it is frequently worse with activity and exertion; it can be exacerbated by anxiety; and it is worse among the elderly (Smith, et al., 2001). There is data showing that nebulized morphine sulfate and fentanyl citrate may significantly improve dyspnea (Coyne, Viswanathan, & Smith, 2002; Bruera, et al., 2006). Nursing interventions that are known to decrease dyspnea in patients with lung cancer include teaching effective ways of coping; training in breathing control techniques, such as progressive muscle relaxation and distraction exercises; and creating opportunities for patients to talk about difficult feelings and concerns (Bredin, et al., 1999).

Dyspnea may not be directly related to extent of disease. In lung cancer, dyspnea is related to an increased mechanical workload on the respiratory system due to tumor load, which results in a need for increased ventilation that adds to the patient's condition of fatigue. In addition, if there is malnutrition, there is a decrease in the force-generating capacity of the diaphragm (Arora & Rochester, 1982) that adds to breathlessness.

In summary, dyspnea is a symptom that frequently has significant physiological and psychological impact on quality of life for women who are living with lung cancer.

Fatigue

Fatigue is a prevalent and distressing symptom among cancer patients, and improved methods of assessment and management are needed (Ahlberg, Ekman, Gaston-Johansson, & Mock, 2003). Sleeplessness and awakening during sleep are common disturbances in the aged (Floyd, Medler, Ager, & Janisse, 2000) as well as in women with lung cancer (Engstrom, Strohl, Rose, Lewandowski, & Stefanek, 1999). Causes of sleeplessness include disease-related symptoms, such as dyspnea and pain; medications, such as steroids given with chemotherapy; and psychosocial issues, including anxiety and depression (Bernhard & Ganz, 1991). The short-term outcome of sleep disturbances is increased fatigue, which adds to symptom distress, and when sleep disturbances are combined with low oxygen saturation and comorbidities, they can significantly affect overall quality of life. Fatigue may also interfere with the patient's ability to complete questionnaires or to participate in focus group sessions.

Interventions to help researchers deal with patient fatigue include giving participants breaks while filling out forms and timing data collection. Nurse researchers should also be aware that they may need to take extra time to help patients complete study forms and documents.

Pain

Pain is a symptom that occurs in 80% of patients with lung cancer (Rhodes, Koshy, Waterfield, Wu, & Grossman, 2001) and can be controlled (Berry, Wilkie, Huang, & Blumenstein, 1999). Although pain can occur anywhere, most frequent symptomatic sites include the chest or shoulder(s), due to intrathoracic disease, and/or the head, spine, abdomen, or pelvis, due to extrathoracic disease. Previous surgery, tumor location, such as with superior sulcus tumors and associated brachial plexopathy, and spinal cord compression may complicate pain management.

A systematic approach to the assessment of pain is required. If a clear history cannot be obtained from the patient, then the caregiver's history can be useful, because it is considered to be similar to the patient's (Lobchuk, Kristjanson, Degner, Blood, & Sloan, 1999). Standard treatments for pain include analgesics, chemotherapy and/or radiotherapy (Langendijk, et al., 2001; Gressen, Werner-Wasik, Cohn, Topham, & Curran, 2000), as well as complementary therapies, such as massage, yoga, acupuncture, or foot reflexology (Stephenson, Weinrich, & Tavakoli, 2000; Distasio, 2008).

In summary, coughing, wheezing, dyspnea, fatigue, and pain are common symptoms experienced by women with lung cancer and consequently provide challenges to study follow-up for nurse researchers.

Cultural and Socioeconomic Factors

Complex socioeconomic factors can have a major impact on patient recruitment and retention for clinical studies. For example, in different geographic areas of the United States, such as in the rural south, cultural and socioeconomic factors, such as general distrust of research, women's roles, family demands, transportation, safety issues, income, and literacy, need to be considered.

To deal with issues of mistrust, the nurse researcher needs to develop a relationship with the patient, which may be facilitated by the patient's clinical care providers (such as their oncologist or clinic nurse). The relationship can be fostered by addressing individual needs and demonstrating genuine interest and concern for the patient's personal and medical issues, maintaining consistency of data collectors, offering patients the opportunity to choose the environment to discuss the research project (home versus hospital), providing flexibility to meet on evenings and weekends, and expressing appreciation for the patient's research contribution. Careful explanation of the informed consent process is necessary with periodic reinforcement to address concerns, such as confidentiality of personal information, that may arise. Moreover, it is important for the nurse researcher to ensure that he or she remains nonjudgmental and unbiased when communicating with patients and their family members.

In addition to issues of mistrust of the clinical research and healthcare community, in many societies women often play multiple roles, such as caregiver, wife, mother, and breadwinner, which can contribute to time and resource constraints and consequently affect their ability to participate in research studies. For example, added child care responsibilities can interfere with women's ability to attend appointments for tests and clinic visits, adding to the physical and emotional stresses due to their lung cancer diagnosis.

For nurse researchers, family demands are additional challenges that can often interfere with research data collection. For example, a routine patient visit may be disrupted by the presence of young children. Researchers must be flexible, available, and mobile to consider family demands; home visits during nonbusi-

ness hours may need to be arranged to accommodate the patient's time and resource constraints.

Transportation, particularly in rural areas, is another major challenge. Patients may have limited access to transportation and may rely on family or friends to drive them to a healthcare facility. In addition, travel distances to major medical centers can be long. Efforts to coordinate travel and maximize efficiency of visits, such as timing office visits, consultations, and laboratory/diagnostic testing on the same day, should be made to accommodate these time and resource limitations.

Another issue that impacts research is personal safety for patients who may live in low income neighborhoods, thus preventing them from going out in the evenings. For home visits, nurse researchers are encouraged to preplan the route and timing of each visit, including determining in advance who will meet them. In addition, accessibility to visit homes may be particularly challenging in remote areas.

Income and literacy can be problematic as well. In rural areas, women's average annual income is approximately $20,000 (US Census Bureau, 2006). Special attention may be required to coordinate resources and transportation. For example, all healthcare visits can be coordinated on the same day. The cost of travel and medications will also need to be considered, and the involvement of social workers may facilitate access to resources, such as compassionate drug access programs, to help minimize the financial burden.

Literacy in cancer patients is a methodological concern, with approximately one-third of patients having less than a high school education.

In some instances, nurse researchers will need to read forms and questionnaires to patients or use interpreters, adding time to data collection. All questionnaires and questions need to be analyzed and words selected at a reading level of eighth grade or below. For some populations, selecting words below the fifth grade reading level may be optimal. There is also the challenge of using language and terminology that is culturally acceptable and understandable.

Summary

Strategies need to be built into all research methodologies that include the study of vulnerable populations, such as women with lung cancer. Particularly, the researcher needs to address the methodological issues of attrition, psychological distress, respiratory symptoms, fatigue, pain, functional decline, aging, and cultural and socioeconomic stresses that are unique to this group.

References

Ahlberg, K., Ekman, T., Gaston-Johansson, F., & Mock, V. (2003). Assessment and management of cancer related fatigue in adults. *Lancet, 362*(9384), 640–650.

Arora, N., & Rochester, D. (1982). Effect of body weight and muscularity on human diaphragm muscle mass, thickness, and area. *Journal of Applied Physiology, 52*(1), 64–70.

Bernhard, J., & Ganz, P. (1991). Psychosocial issues in lung cancer patients. *Chest, 99*(2), 480–485.

Berry, D., Wilkie, D., Huang, H., & Blumenstein, B. (1999). Cancer pain and common pain: A comparison of patient-reported intensities. *Oncology Nursing Forum, 26*(4), 721–726.

Bredin, M., Corner, J., Krishnasamy, M., Plant, H., Bailey, C., & A'Hern, R. (1999). Multicentre randomized controlled trial of nursing intervention for breathlessness in patients with lung cancer. *BMJ, 318*(7188), 901–904.

Bruera, E., Sala, R., Spruyt, O., Palmer, J. L., Zhang, T., & Willey, J. (2006). Nebulized versus subcutaneous morphine for patients with cancer dyspnea: A preliminary study. *Journal of Pain and Symptom Management, 29*(6),613–618.

Carney, I., Gibson, P., Murree-Allen, K., Saltos, N., Olson, L., & Hensley, M. (1997). A systematic evaluation of mechanisms in chronic cough. *American Journal of Respiratory and Critical Care Medicine, 156*(1), 211–216.

Chernecky, C., & Sarna, L. (2001). *The Lung Cancer Cough Questionnaire (LCCQ) and the Lung Cancer Wheezing Questionnaire (LCWQ)*. Poster presentation, ONS Congress, San Diego, CA.

Chute, C. G., Greenberg, E. R., Baron, J., Korson, R., Baker, J., & Yates, J. (1985). Presenting conditions of 1539 population-based lung cancer patients by cell type and stage in New Hampshire and Vermont. *Cancer, 56*(8), 2107–2111.

Cooley, M. (2000). Symptoms in adults with lung cancer. A systematic research review. *Journal of Pain and Symptom Management, 19*(2), 137–153.

Coyne, P. J., Viswanathan, R., & Smith, T. J. (2002). Nebulized fentanyl citrate improves patients' perception of breathing, respiratory rate, and oxygen saturation in dyspnea. *Journal of Pain and Symptom Management, 23*(2), 157–160.

Distasio, S. A. (2008). Integrating yoga into cancer care. *Clinical Journal of Oncology Nursing, 12*(1), 125–130.

Engstrom, C., Strohl, R., Rose, L., Lewandowski, L., & Stefanek, M. (1999). Sleep alterations in cancer patients. *Cancer Nursing, 22*(2), 143–148.

Floyd, J., Medler, S., Ager, J., & Janisse, J. (2000). Age-related changes in initiation and maintenance of sleep: A meta-analysis. *Research in Nursing and Health, 23*(2), 106–117.

Gallo-Silver, L., & Pollack, B. (2000). Behavioral interventions for lung cancer-related breathlessness. *Cancer Practice; A Multidisciplinary Journal of Cancer Care, 8*(6), 268–273.

Grabiner, P., Biswas, S., & Grabiner, M. (2001). Age-related changes in spatial and temporal gait variables. *Archives of Physical Medicine and Rehabilitation, 82*(1), 31–35.

Gressen, E., Werner-Wasik, M., Cohn, J., Topham, A., & Curran, W. (2000). Thoracic reirradiation for symptomatic relief after prior radiotherapeutic management for lung cancer. *American Journal of Clinical Oncology, 23*(2), 160–163.

Hyde, L., & Hyde, C. I. (1974). Clinical manifestations of lung cancer. *Chest, 65*(3), 299–306.

Kuo, C., Chen, Y., Chao, J., Tsai, C., & Perng, R. (2000). Non-small cell lung cancer in very young and very old patients. *Chest, 117*(2), 354–357.

Langendijk, J. A., Aaronson, N. K., de Jong, J., ten Velde, G., Muller, M. J., Lamers, R. J., et al. (2001). Prospective study on quality of life before and after radical radiotherapy in non-small cell lung cancer. *Journal of Clinical Oncology, 19*(8), 2123–2133.

Lobchuk, M., Kristjanson, L., Degner, L., Blood, P., & Sloan, J. (1999). Perception of symptom distress in lung cancer patients: I. Agreement between patients and their caregiving relatives. *Pflege (German), 12*(6), 352–361.

Mehagnoul-Schipper, D., Vloet, L., Colier, W., Hoefnagles, W., & Jansen, R. (2000). Cerebral oxygenation declines in healthy elderly subjects in response to assuming the upright position. *Stroke, 31*(7), 1615–1620.

Mercadante, S., Casuccio, A., & Fulfaro, F. (2000). The course of symptom frequency and intensity in advanced cancer patients followed at home. *Journal of Pain and Symptom Management, 20*(2), 104–112.

Ochmanski, W. (1997). Current capabilities and procedures for diagnosing lung neoplasms. *Przeglad Lekarski (Polish), 54*(2), 126–134.

O'Driscoll, M., Corner, J., & Bailey, C. (1999). The experience of breathlessness in lung cancer. *European Journal of Cancer Care, 8*(1), 37–43.

Plat, H., Bredin, M., Krishnasamy, M., & Corner, J. (2000). Working with resistance, tension and objectivity: Conducting a randomized controlled trial of a nursing intervention for breathlessness. *NT Research, 5*(6), 426–436.

Rhodes, D., Koshy, R., Waterfield, W., Wu, A., & Grossman, S. (2001). Feasibility of quantitative pain assessment in outpatient oncology practice. *Journal of Clinical Oncology, 19*(2), 501–508.

Ripamonti, C. (1999). Management of dyspnea in advanced cancer patients. *Supportive Care Cancer, 7*(1), 233–243.

Sarna, L. (1994). Functional status in women with lung cancer. *Cancer Nursing, 17*(2), 87–93.

Sarna, L. (1998). Effectiveness of structured nursing assessment of symptom distress in advanced lung cancer. *Oncology Nursing Forum, 25*(6), 1041–1048.

Sarna, L. (2005). Quality of life and meaning of illness of women with lung cancer. *Oncology Nursing Forum, 32*(1), E9–E19.

Sarna, L., Evangelista, L., Tashkin, D., Padilla, G., Holmes, C., Brecht, M. L., et al. (2004). Impact of respiratory symptoms and pulmonary function on quality of life of long-term survivors of non-small cell lung cancer. *Chest, 125*(2), 439–445.

Sheahan, S., & Musialowski, R. (2002). Clinical implications of respiratory system changes in aging. *Journal of Gerontological Nursing, 27*(5), 26–34, 48–49.

Smith, E., Hamm, D., Ahles, T., Furstenberg, C., Mitchell, T., Meyer, L., et al. (2001). Dyspnea, anxiety, body consciousness, and quality of life in patients with lung cancer. *Journal of Pain and Symptom Management, 21*(4), 323–329.

Stephenson, S., Weinrich, S., & Tavakoli, A. (2000). The effects of foot reflexology on anxiety and pain in patients with breast and lung cancer. *Oncology Nursing Forum, 27*(1), 67–72.

Sue, D. (2000). Acute respiratory failure in the elderly patient. *Clinical Geriatrics, 8*(12), 37–38, 41–42, 45–46.

Sun, S., Schiller, J. H., Gazdar, A., & Adi, F. (2007). Lung cancer in never smokers—a different disease. *Nature Reviews Cancer, 7*(10), 778–790.

US Census Bureau. (2006). *Historical income tables—People. Table P-5, Regions of People (All Races) by Median Income and Sex.* Retrieved November 17, 2008, from http://www.census.gov/hhes/www/income/histinc/p05ar.html

Vaaler, A., Forrester, J., Lesar, M., Edison, M., Venzon, D., & Johnson, B. (1997). Obstructive atelectasis in patients with small cell lung cancer. Incidence and response to treatment. *Chest, 111*(1), 115–120.

Vyas, R., Suryanarayana, U., Dixit, S., Singhal, S., Bhavsar, D., Neema, J., et al. (1998). Inoperable non-small cell lung cancer: Palliative radiotherapy with two weekly fractions. *Indian Journal of Chest Disease and Allied Sciences, 40*(3), 171–174.

Chapter 19

Evidence-Based Practice and the Healthcare Professional

Janelle M. Tipton

Introduction

The term "evidence-based practice" (EBP) has continued to evolve as a new paradigm in health care. Over the past 15 years, the emergence of evidence-based care or practice has entered the international literature. EBP had its original significance as evidence-based medicine, where the concept was used for decision making for individual patients (Guyatt, et al., 2000; Rutledge & Grant, 2002). EBP also was used to reduce variability in physician practice patterns and to guide the development of research-based clinical protocols and algorithms to improve appropriate use of services. EBP became a foundation for educating medical students on the topic of critical thinking in practice. The utilization of research has been a long-standing model in medicine, with emphasis on randomized controlled trial synthesis as evidence for the basis of care. However, in medicine and nursing alike, EBP also includes evidence sources from observational studies, qualitative studies, and expert opinion (Guyatt, et al., 2000; Haydorn, Baker, Hodges, & Hicks, 1996; Ropka & Spencer-Cisek, 2001).

In 2001, the Committee on Quality of Health Care in America, Institute of Medicine (IOM), advocated that nurses incorporate interventions and outcome measures into our daily work, making it possible to better understand nursing's performance related to quality of care. The quality of patient healthcare outcomes has become a priority and an expectation among several stakeholders: patients and families, healthcare providers, insurance companies, regulatory bodies, and policy makers (Committee on Quality of Health Care in America, 2001; Given & Sherwood, 2005). Public knowledge of standard of care guidelines and outcomes has challenged healthcare professionals to implement "best practice" for conditions such as lung cancer and also to evaluate the impact of the interventions and care on patient outcomes.

Through the use of EBP in the care of lung cancer patients, the goal of improved patient outcomes is desirable and achievable. Lung cancer is a worldwide problem and continues to rank high in both incidence and death rate in patients with cancer (Jemal, et al., 2008). This chapter will provide a background on EBP, discussion of the steps in the EBP process, and examples of use of EBP in caring for patients with lung cancer.

Background

Historically, nursing has answered clinical questions through trial and error, clinical experience, guidance from supervisors and peers, institutional traditions, reasoning, and intuition (Burns & Grove, 1997). Many of these sources are still used; however, increasingly, more nursing practice is based on research and research findings. Nursing can learn much from medicine's efforts to integrate research into practice. Considerable systematic review data exists, including several publications in The Cochrane Collaboration, that shows medicine's efforts to evaluate strategies for changing practice based on research (Beck, 2002). Nursing is in a position to lead EBP efforts in translating research into practice. Utilizing a theoretical base, collaborating with interdisciplinary teams, and creating best practices are some strategies used to look at processes and outcomes of EBP (Rutledge & Bookbinder, 2002; Cook & Grant, 2002).

Helping individuals with lung cancer make decisions involves the integration of research, clinical expertise, and knowledge of the patient's preferences. Although some of the treatment decisions may not result in optimal outcomes, such as the development of metastatic disease or treatment-related complications, it is important to communicate the findings and to continue dialog at every point in the disease continuum. Nurses continue to be knowledgeable and trusted healthcare professionals and can impact patient satisfaction during this process.

Multiple barriers exist as nurses work to implement EBP. Time may be one barrier that seems insurmountable to nurses, when, to the contrary, access to best evidence resources can take only minutes. Larger projects that include searches and analysis of data may require more time and should be discussed early so that time for these activities and meetings are supported. Resources that are necessary in implementing EBP include someone with expertise in leading a team and in evaluating research literature. Access to library and technological resources, databases, and articles may be most available through an academic library, and partnering may be necessary to utilize these resources. Individual and team attitudes and practice patterns may also be barriers. Some nurses may hesitate to deviate from traditional practices because of discomfort with change. Others may have the misperception that EBP is "cookbook nursing" and does not take into consideration individual patient preferences and clinical knowledge. That misperception is unfounded, because key EBP ingredients include not only individual patient preferences and clinical knowledge but also the best available evidence from the literature. Organizational constraints that may impede progress for EBP implementation include lack of administrative support or incentives. EBP may be more successfully implemented when the leadership embraces the concept and is supportive of the staff's involvement (Melnyk, 2002; Hockenberry, Walden, & Brown, 2007). Facilitators of evidence-based practice include ongoing communication, education on the research process/findings, and working with groups with varying levels of expertise (Reavy & Tavernier, 2008).

Evidence-based packages for practice (see Table 19–1) are being developed and can assist nurses in caring for patients with lung cancer. Examples include: (1) practice guidelines and evidence reports, (2) specialty nursing organization clinical guidelines and recommendations, and (3) integrative review reports. In addition,

Table 19–1 Evidence-Based Packages for Practice with Potential Use in Caring for Patients with Lung Cancer

- National Guidelines Clearinghouse
  1. Adjuvant chemotherapy and adjuvant radiation therapy for stages I–IIIA resectable non-small cell lung cancer guideline, Cancer Care Ontario and American Society of Clinical Oncology, December 2007, 13 pages.
  2. Treatment of non-small cell lung cancer—stage IIIA: ACCP evidence-based clinical practice guidelines (2nd ed.), American College of Chest Physicians, January 2003, revised September 2007, 23 pages.
  3. Palliative care in lung cancer: ACCP evidence-based clinical practice guidelines, American Society of Chest Physicians, January 2003, revised September 2007, 36 pages.
  4. Staging of bronchogenic carcinoma, American College of Radiology, 1996, revised 2005, nine pages.
  5. Follow-up of non-small cell lung cancer, American College of Radiology, 1996, revised 2005, six pages.
  6. 18-fluorodeoxyglucose positron emission tomography in the diagnosis and staging of lung cancer: A clinical practice guideline, Cancer Care Ontario, April 2007, 54 pages.

Source: Lung cancer specific guidelines. Retrieved June 23, 2008, from http://www.guideline.gov/index.asp

- US Public Health Service

Treating Tobacco Use and Dependence: 2008 Update http://www.surgeongeneral.gov/tobacco/.

- Miscellaneous professional organizations' guidelines
  1. National Comprehensive Cancer Network (NCCN)
     Clinical Practice Guidelines in Oncology: Non-small cell lung cancer, V.2.2008
     Clinical Practice Guidelines in Oncology: Small cell lung cancer, V.1.2008
     http://www.nccn.org
  2. American College of Chest Physicians (ACCP)
     ACCP evidence-based clinical practice guidelines, 2nd ed., revised September 2007
     http://www.chestnet.org/
  3. American College of Radiology (ACR)
     ACR Appropriateness Criteria, updated 2005.
     http://www.acr.org/

other evidence-based recommendations on topics such as pain management, flushing protocols for central venous catheters, and management of dyspnea can be found in the *Online Journal of Clinical Innovations* (http://www.cinahl.org), the *Online Journal of Knowledge Synthesis for Nursing,* now archived on *Worldviews on Evidence-Based Nursing* (http://www3.interscience.wiley.com/journal/121371704/grouphome/home.html), and the Putting Evidence into Practice resources for nursing practice from the Oncology Nursing Society (ONS) (http://www.ons.org/outcomes). ONS, in its strategic goals, has placed emphasis on the development of evidence-based resources for nurses and education about utilizing evidence-based interventions (Friese & Beck, 2004;

Gobel, Beck, & O'Leary, 2006; Given & Sherwood, 2005).

The number of related guidelines has increased in the past several years. Many of the guidelines are related to treatment; however, there are guidelines that relate to symptoms, rehabilitation, screening, chemoprevention, and palliative care (Smith & Berg, 2008; Rutledge & Kuebler, 2005). This data can be synthesized by an individual or a group and may be incorporated into an institutional practice change using the evidence. Implementation will take time and may have barriers. Change can be difficult and may be facilitated by having relevant members of the healthcare team involved at the outset.

Definition

According to DePalma, EBP is:

> *a total process beginning with knowing what clinical questions to ask, how to find the best practice, and how to critically appraise the evidence for validity and applicability to the particular care situation. The best evidence then must be applied by a clinician with expertise in considering the patient's unique values and needs. The final aspect of the process is evaluation of the effectiveness of care and the continual improvement of the process (DePalma, 2000, p. 115).*

EBP can be viewed as a process and a product, whereby the product is the translation of evidence into an innovative practice change (Rutledge & Bookbinder, 2002).

EBP Process

There are many available resources available to clinicians who are interested in learning more about the EBP process. There are several steps involved in this process, and in clinical practice it is not surprising that the steps may not always be completed linearly, because there may be times when you take a step or two backwards before moving forward. The more experience you have working with this process, the more comfortable you may become in utilizing the concepts and eventually making a practice change.

According to the Oncology Nursing Society (2008), there are six steps in the EBP process: (1) problem identification, (2) finding the evidence, (3) critique, (4) summarize the evidence, (5) application to practice, and (6) evaluation. Each step is described in the following paragraphs.

Problem Identification

The problem emerges from a clinical situation in which there is a knowledge gap or uncertainty. It is important to clearly phrase the problem to direct the search for the answer. It may also be helpful to utilize a team to come up with the clinical question. The appropriate allotment of time to begin the EBP will help to guide the work and process and assist in prioritizing the most important clinical issues at hand. The clinical question should include the following components:

- Patient or problem being addressed
- Phenomenon or intervention being considered
- Comparison intervention, when relevant
- Clinical outcomes of interest

Examples of questions related to lung cancer may be issues of prevention and screening methods, selection and interpretation of diagnostic tests for diagnosis, questions regarding the most beneficial therapies, prognosis of a patient's outcome related to a specific treatment, and the best education strategies for colleagues, patients, or family members. An example of a question that a staff nurse might ask is, "What types of smoking cessation strategies work best for patients who are hospitalized for lung cancer and want to stop smoking?" An advanced practice nurse may ask, "Should CT scans be used to screen high-risk patients for lung cancer?"

Finding the Evidence

The evidence needed in an EBP effort may be found in a variety of sources, from computerized bibliographical databases to your own quality improvement department. In trying to find evidence, nurses are urged to get help. For one reason, finding evidence is very time consuming even when done with maximum efficiency, and (theoretically) the more persons involved, the less any one person has to do. Second, those who are familiar with a certain search method may find better sources of information.

The Oncology Nursing Society EBP Resource Center provides an overview in the search for evidence. There is a step-by-step description of doing a literature search and links to several computerized bibliography databases. This is also a good time to get to know your librarian, if one is available. Some of your searches will be successful while others may not. You may need to carefully identify your search terms to obtain precise information in your search. Table 19–2

Table 19–2 Web References for Health Professionals Caring for Patients with Lung Cancer

Site	URL	Description
Oncology Nursing Society (ONS)	http://www.ons.org	The ONS site is not lung cancer-specific, but it does include a lung cancer clinical resource area with disease overview, diagnosis, treatment, education, and resources.
Lungcancer.org (sponsored by Cancer*Care* and the Oncology Nursing Society)	http://www.lungcancer.org/	Lung Cancer 101 provides information on lung cancer diagnosis and treatment, frequently asked questions, and clinical trials information.
Lung Cancer Alliance	http://www.lungcanceralliance.org/	This site provides information on lung cancer news and a lung cancer survivors' community.
National Cancer Institute (NCI) of the US National Institutes of Health (NIH)	http://www.nci.nih.gov/cancer_information/cancer_type/lung/	The NCI Web site provides statistics, treatment, and clinical trial information.
Caring Ambassadors Program (CAP)	http://www.lungcancercap.org	CAP provides information on lung cancer news and facts and figures.

provides a listing of Web references that include educational materials for healthcare professionals who are caring for patients with lung cancer.

Critique

Critiquing evidence leads to its evaluation. Evaluation of the evidence includes determination of its merit, feasibility, and utility as a basis for making a practice change. The goal is to evaluate the scientific merit and potential clinical applicability of each study's findings, and with a group of studies that cover similar problem areas, to determine what findings have a strong enough basis to be used in practice. The original research studies or integrative reviews/meta-analyses may be evaluated.

A team approach is best, and the work can be divided in many ways. This is a good time to collaborate with researchers or advanced practice nurses, which will encourage mentorship and integration of nurses with different backgrounds.

The Oncology Nursing Society EBP Resource Center provides several sets of critiquing criteria and tools that may be used to organize the data. There are recommendations on the critiques of abstracts, integrated reviews, clinical practice guidelines, quality improvement reports, and Web site credibility.

Summarize the Evidence

Nurses must synthesize the evidence and combine the knowledge components to form a new product. This is a challenging job that involves a move from the literature search and critique phase into the synthesis phase. The research evidence is combined with other evidence to make concrete practice recommendations. The ONS EBP Resource Center provides some of the how-tos related to summarizing evidence. A triad model for performing a research synthesis uti-lizing an advanced practice nurse, a nurse researcher, and an educator (Rutledge, DePalma, & Cunningham, 2004) is very successful. Again, it is important to explore assistance resources at this stage of the EBP process.

One of the supportive care issues for some patients with lung cancer is the rash associated with some of the small molecule-targeted agents. Developing guidelines for evidence-based interventions for the management of the rash would involve reviewing the available literature and packaging the new information based on the current evidence.

Application to Practice

Before a practice change can be implemented, it is important to apply the three stages of adopting a practice innovation (Rogers, 1995): knowledge, persuasion, and adoption. Educating involved staff members about EBP and the purpose of the practice change will assist with understanding this phase of the process. In addition, it is important to outline the expected outcomes of changes. These may be clinical outcomes, financial outcomes, and process-related outcomes. Planning for the changes and the associated barriers and bridges is crucial in the process leading up to the implementation phase. When those components are completed, it is then important to implement a trial or pilot program. This will enable staff members to adjust and will be an important time for communication about the practice change. Last, the adoption phase provides relevant evaluation data that can be used to accept or reject the practice change.

Evaluation

The evaluation plan is the last, but equally important, step of the process to determine if the change occurred. The outcomes and benchmarks need to be reviewed for comparison both pre- and postpractice change.

The process and outcomes that need to be evaluated include: (1) correct utilization of new practice, (2) identification of any unforeseen barriers, adequacy of education, and availability of support, (3) effects of practice changes on patient outcomes and staff for at least two consecutive quarters after implementation, and (4) the staff's level of knowledge about the new practice and determination of ongoing educational needs so that educational updates can be planned periodically.

This is also a time to promote staff input. An example includes maintaining a visible presence for staff members to be able to communicate concerns or questions via a hotline, e-mail, posters, or to an EBP planning group that is making rounds. Providing ongoing support, information, and results of data will also continue the feedback that is necessary to show communication. If possible, it can also be a time for celebration and reward, drawing attention to quality performance and involvement in the process.

Examples of Using Evidence-Based Practice with Lung Cancer Patients

Care of the patient with lung cancer crosses an entire care continuum. Nurses who are interested in utilizing EBP can use the process at many different points in this continuum. Patients with lung cancer are definitely at high risk for the development of multiple symptom problems, and evidence-based interventions should be explored for supportive care (Joyce, Schwartz, & Huhmann, 2008). As early as 2001, there was recognition of the need for guidelines for management of breathlessness or dyspnea in cancer patients (Krishnasamy, Corner, Bredin,

Plant, & Bailey, 2001). The ONS Web site includes data for dyspnea interventions (DiSalvo, Joyce, Tyson, Culkin, & Mackay, 2008), and currently there is a plan for update of the data. It is important to review the data periodically, because new information is published frequently (Ben-Aharon, Gafter-Gvili, Leibovisi, & Stemmer, 2008). Unfortunately, for some clinical problems there is little data on evidence-based interventions. This is also a challenge for nursing to begin to do more research where the data is sparse and where there is opportunity to show improvement in patient outcomes. Table 19–3 shows clinical areas during the care continuum and possible questions that might be explored.

To explore the topic in more depth, take the question previously posed by the staff nurse, "What types of smoking cessation strategies work best for patients who are hospitalized for lung cancer and want to quit smoking?" A nurse might begin to find evidence on this topic by talking to colleagues who are local within the institution, in the region, and nationally, if possible. A search could also be done on PubMed (http://www.pubmed.com), CINAHL (http://www.ebscohost.com/cinahl/), and The Cochrane Library (http://www.cochrane.org). A search on PubMed using the search terms "smoking cessation and lung cancer" resulted in 208 references. Using "smoking cessation and lung cancer and evidence-based practice" resulted in four additional references. Some articles were applicable, while others were not. The CINAHL search required a subscription and identified nine references using the search terms. The Cochrane Library search located 71 articles, not all specific to patients who were already diagnosed with lung cancer. Figure 19–1 highlights several articles chosen from a PubMed search on June 23, 2008, to begin addressing the question.

Table 19–3 Lung Cancer Clinical Problems and Questions: Evidence-Based Care for Lung Cancer Through the Care Continuum

Clinical Problem	Possible Question
Prevention: Smoking cessation strategies	What types of smoking cessation strategies work best for individuals who want to quit smoking?
Early detection: Screening for lung cancer, role of CT scanning	Should CT scans be used in high-risk patients to screen for lung cancer?
Diagnostic strategies: PET scanning	Is the PET scan a good radiologic exam to assist in the diagnosis and staging of lung cancer?
Treatment: Evidence-based guidelines	What is an appropriate therapy for a patient with non-small cell lung cancer, metastatic to one site (adrenal)?
Supportive care: Patient education	What are appropriate education materials for lung cancer patients?
Supportive care: Management of symptoms	What is the best treatment for erlotinib toxicities rash?
Survivorship issues	What are the late effects of radiation therapy?
Palliative care	What are the most effective interventions to minimize dyspnea?

Many hospitals across the nation are implementing smoke-free campuses, and it is important for oncology nurses to be aware of and be included in the policy development. Smoking cessation strategies may be discussed with lung cancer patients in a variety of inpatient and outpatient settings (Cooley, Sipples, Murphy, & Sarna, 2008). These guidelines can provide nurses with information and allow them to give better patient care. Patients who are underserved may lack resources to quit smoking and are often diagnosed at later stages (Ward, et al., 2008). Nurses are in a unique position to identify problems in their regional areas and utilize evidence-based resources for patients. This is an example of a clinical problem that involves the evaluation of scientific data, clinical expertise, and recognition of patient preferences for possible interventions.

Specific Problems in Lung Cancer

When caring for patients with lung cancer, some specific problems have begun to warrant clinical study. Care of elderly patients with lung cancer can be challenging due to preexisting comorbidities, toxicity of therapies, and supportive care needs. Elderly patients may experience a cluster of symptom problems at any stage of lung cancer; however, patients who are diagnosed with advanced disease are more likely to

---

Figure 19–1 PubMed articles.

This figure lists selected articles from PubMed to begin addressing the question: What types of smoking cessation strategies work best with hospitalized lung cancer patients who want to quit smoking?

Review Articles

Browning, K. K., & Wewers, M. E. (2003). Smoking cessation and cancer. *Seminars in Oncology Nursing, 19*(4), 268–275.

Carter, C. L., Key, J., Marsh, L., & Graves, K. (2001). Contemporary perspectives in tobacco cessation: What oncologists need to know. *Oncologist, 6*(6), 496–505.

Cooley, M. E., Sipples, R. L., Murphy, M., & Sarna, L. (2008). Smoking cessation and lung cancer: Oncology nurses can make a difference. *Seminars in Oncology Nursing, 24*(1), 16–26.

Ebbert, J. O., Sood, A., Hays, J. T., Dale, L. C., & Hurt, R. D. (2007). Treating tobacco dependence: Review of the best and latest treatment options. *Journal of Thoracic Oncology, 2*(3), 249–256.

Henningfield, J. E., Fant, R. V., Buchhalter, A. R., & Stitzer, M. L. (2005). Pharmacotherapy for nicotine dependence. *CA: A Cancer Journal for Clinicians, 55*(5), 281–299.

Westmaas, J. L., & Brandon, T. H. (2004). Reducing risk in smokers. *Current Opinion in Pulmonary Medicine, 10*(4), 284–288.

Nonreview Articles

Baser, S., Shannon, V. R., Eapen, G. A., Jimenez, C. A., Onn, A., Lin, E., et al. (2006). Smoking cessation after diagnosis of lung cancer is associated with a beneficial effect on performance status. *Chest, 130*(6), 1784–1790.

Sanderson Cox, L., Patten, C. A., Ebbert, J. O., Drews, A. A., Croghan, G. A., Clark, M. M., et al. (2002). Tobacco use outcomes among patients with lung cancer treated for nicotine dependence. *Journal of Clinical Oncology, 20*(16), 3461–3469.

Schnoll, R. A., Rothman, R. L., Newman, H., Lerman, C., Miller, S. M., Movsas, B., et al. (2004). Characteristics of cancer patients entering a smoking cessation program and correlates of quit motivation: Implications for the development of tobacco control programs for cancer patients. *Psychooncology, 13*(5), 346–358.

Schnoll, R. A., Zhang, B., Rue, M., Krook, J. E., Spears, W. T., Marcus, A. C., et al. (2003). Brief physician-initiated quit-smoking strategies for clinical oncology settings: A trial coordinated by the Eastern Cooperative Oncology Group. *Journal of Clinical Oncology, 21*(2), 355–365.

---

experience multiple symptoms. Common symptom clusters reported by patients with lung cancer at the time of diagnosis include fatigue, weakness, weight loss, appetite loss, nausea, vomiting, and altered taste (Gift, Jablonski, Stommel, & Given, 2004; Gift, Stommel, Jablonski, & Given, 2003; Fox & Lyon, 2006).

Continued research on symptom clusters in lung cancer patients will likely yield clinically relevant information that can impact patient outcomes. These studies have the potential to provide further information to help develop appropriate nursing interventions. Studies on symptom clusters will provide valuable links between symptom management research and clinical practice (Miaskowski, 2006). Recent literature has also examined the Human Response to Illness Model to further understand the additional stressor that many lung cancer patients may experience: the societal stigmatization of their illness related to cigarette smoking. A better understanding of the stressors that are experienced by lung cancer patients will also drive the development and implementation of interventions to prevent or alleviate the effects of this stress response (Hansen & Sawatzky, 2008).

Opportunities for Further Research

Further evidence is needed in the literature to support patients who receive multimodal therapy and concurrent therapies for lung cancer. Depending on the stage at diagnosis and performance status factors, patients may be treated very aggressively with several types of cancer treatment, including surgery, radiation therapy, chemotherapy, and biological therapy. The sequence of the therapies is dependent on several factors, but they can be very grueling for patients and challenging for caregivers to provide support. Little data is available for interventions that may improve patient outcomes through these phases of therapy; thus, it is very important to identify the patients at highest risk through systematic assessment (Ropka, Padilla, & Gillespie, 2005). Additionally, nursing's role has yet to be measured in improving patient outcomes in patients with lung cancer. Descriptive articles exist for nurses in navigator-like roles, but few articles discuss the measurement of patient outcomes (Seek & Hogle, 2007; London and South East Lung Cancer Forum for Nurses, 2004). A few studies have documented the role of the specialized and advanced practice nurse in caring for patients with lung cancer (McCorkle, et al., 1989; Moore, et al., 2002). These studies provide beginning evidence to document improvement in patient quality of life as well as fiscal outcomes.

References

Beck, S. L. (2002). Strategies to translate research into practice. *Seminars in Oncology Nursing, 18*(1), 11–19.

Ben-Aharon, I., Gafter-Gvili, A., Leibovici, P. M., & Stemmer, S. M. (2008). Interventions for alleviating cancer-related dyspnea: A systematic review. *Journal of Clinical Oncology, 26*(14), 2396–2404.

Burns, N., & Grove, S. K. (1997). *The practice of nursing research. Conduct, critique, and utilization.* Philadelphia: W. B. Saunders.

Committee on Quality of Health Care in America, Institute of Medicine. (2001). *Crossing the quality chasm: A new health system for the 21st century.* Washington, DC: National Academies Press.

Cook, L., & Grant, M. (2002). Support for evidence-based practice. *Seminars in Oncology Nursing, 18*(1), 71–78.

Cooley, M. E., Sipples, R. L., Murphy, M., & Sarna, L. (2008). Smoking cessation and lung cancer: Oncology nurses can make a difference. *Seminars in Oncology Nursing, 24*(1), 16–26.

DePalma, J. (2000). Evidence-based clinical practice guidelines. Seminars in Perioperative Nursing, 9(3), 115–120.

DiSalvo, W. M., Joyce, M. M., Tyson, L. B., Culkin, A. E., & Mackay, K. (2008). Putting evidence into practice: Evidence-based interventions for cancer-related dyspnea. *Clinical Journal of Oncology Nursing, 12*(2), 341–352.

Friese, C. R., & Beck, S. L. (2004). Advancing practice and research: Creating evidence-based summaries on measuring nursing-sensitive patient outcomes. *Clinical Journal of Oncology Nursing, 8*(6), 675–677.

Fox, S. W., & Lyon, D. E. (2006). Symptom clusters and quality of life in survivors of lung cancer. *Oncology Nursing Forum, 33*(5), 931–936.

Gift, A. G., Jablonski, A., Stommel, M., & Given, W. (2004). Symptom clusters in elderly patients with lung cancer. *Oncology Nursing Forum, 31*(2), 203–210.

Gift, A. G., Stommel, M., Jablonski, A., & Given, W. (2003). A cluster of symptoms over time in patients with lung cancer. *Nursing Research, 52*(6), 393–400.

Given, B. A., & Sherwood, P. (2005). Nursing-sensitive patient outcomes: A white paper. *Oncology Nursing Forum, 32*(4), 773–784.

Gobel, B. H., Beck, S. L., & O'Leary, C. (2006). Nursing-sensitive patient outcomes: The development of the putting evidence into practice resources for nursing practice. *Clinical Journal of Oncology Nursing, 10*(5), 621–624.

Guyatt, G. H., Haynes, R. B., Jaeschke, R. Z., Cook, D. J., Green, L., Naylor, C. D., et al. (2000). Users' guides to the medical literature: XXV. Evidence-based medicine: Principles for applying the users' guides to patient care. *Journal of the American Medical Association, 284*(10), 1290–1296.

Hansen, F., & Sawatzky, J. V. (2008). Stress in patients with lung cancer: A human response to illness. *Oncology Nursing Forum, 35*(2), 217–223.

Haydorn, D. C., Baker, D., Hodges, J. S., & Hicks, N. (1996). Rating the quality of evidence for clinical practice guidelines. *Journal of Epidemiology, 49*(7), 749–754.

Hockenberry, M., Walden, M., & Brown, T. (2007). Creating an evidence-based practice environment: One hospital's journey. *Journal of Nursing Care Quality, 22*(3), 222–231.

Jemal, A., Siegel, R., Ward, E., Hao, Y., Xu, J., Murray, T., et al. (2008). Cancer statistics, 2008. *CA: A Cancer Journal for Clinicians, 58*(2), 71–96.

Joyce, M., Schwartz, S., & Huhmann, M. (2008). Supportive care in lung cancer. *Seminars in Oncology Nursing, 24*(1), 57–67.

Krishnasamy, M., Corner, J., Bredin, M., Plant, H., & Bailey, C. (2001). Cancer nursing practice development: Understanding breathlessness. *Journal of Clinical Nursing, 10*(1), 103–108.

London and South East Lung Cancer Forum for Nurses. (2004). Guidelines on the role of the specialist nurse in supporting patients with lung cancer. *European Journal of Cancer Care, 13*(4), 344–348.

McCorkle, R., Benoliel, J., Donaldson, G., Georiadou, F., Moinpour, C., & Goodall, B. (1989). A randomized clinical trial of home nursing care for lung cancer patients. *Cancer, 64*(6), 1375–1382.

Melnyk, B. M. (2002). Strategies for overcoming barriers in implementing evidence-based practice. *Pediatric Nursing, 28*(2), 159–161.

Miaskowski, C. (2006). Symptom clusters: Establishing the link between clinical practice and symptom management research. *Supportive Care in Cancer, 14*(8), 792–794.

Moore, S. J., Corner, J., Haviland, M., Wells, E., Salmon, C., Normand, M., et al. (2002). Nurse-led follow-up and conventional medical follow-up in management of patients with lung cancer: Randomised trial. *British Medical Journal, 325*(7373), 1145–1147.

Oncology Nursing Society. (2008). *EBP process.* Retrieved on October 1, 2008, from http://onsopcontent.ons.org/toolkits/evidence/Process/index.shtml

Reavy, K., & Tavernier, S. (2008). Nurses reclaiming ownership of their practice: Implementation of an evidence-based practice model and process. *The Journal of Continuing Education in Nursing, 39*(4), 166–172.

Rogers, E. M. (1995). *Diffusion of innovations* (4th ed.). New York: Free Press.

Ropka, M. E., Padilla, G., & Gillespie, T. W. (2005). Risk modeling: Applying evidence-based risk assessment in oncology nursing practice. *Oncology Nursing Forum, 32*(1), 49–56.

Ropka, M. E., & Spencer-Cisek, P. (2001). PRISM: Priority symptom management project phase 1: Assessment. *Oncology Nursing Forum, 28*(10), 1585–1594.

Rutledge, D. N., & Bookbinder, M. (2002). Processes and outcomes of evidence-based practice. *Seminars in Oncology Nursing, 18*(1), 3–10.

Rutledge, D. N., DePalma, J. A., & Cunningham, M. (2004). A process model for evidence-based literature syntheses. *Oncology Nursing Forum, 31*(3), 543–550.

Rutledge, D. N., & Grant, M. (2002). Introduction. *Seminars in Oncology Nursing, 18*(1), 1–2.

Rutledge, D. N., & Kuebler, K. K. (2005). Applying evidence to palliative care. *Seminars in Oncology Nursing, 21*(1), 36–43.

Seek, A. J., & Hogle, W. P. (2007). Modeling a better way: Navigating the healthcare system for patients with lung cancer. *Clinical Journal of Oncology Nursing, 11*(1), 81–85.

Smith, J. J., & Berg, C. D. (2008). Lung cancer screening: Promise and pitfalls. *Seminars in Oncology Nursing, 24*(1), 9–15.

Ward, E., Halpern, M., Schrag, N., Cokkinides, V., DeSantis, C., Bandi, P., et al. (2008). Association of insurance with cancer care utilization and outcomes. *CA: A Cancer Journal for Clinicians, 58*(1), 9–31.

Chapter 20

When Lung Cancer Consumers Seek Evidence

Julie M. Bowman

Marilyn L. Haas

Just as health care continually evolves, so does individuals' involvement in their healthcare choices. Even as far back as 1978, the World Health Organization (WHO) stated, "The people have the right and duty to participate individually and collectively in the planning and implementation of their health care" (WHO, 2006). Individuals who are coping with lung cancer certainly are not an exception to this affirmation. Certainly, the Internet has changed how cancer patients and their caregivers participate in their care (Eysenbach, 2003). Such patients think of themselves as "purchasers of medical care" and can demand the right to make choices along with adherence to quality standards of care (Hines, 2001).

Newly diagnosed patients with cancer often have complex informational and educational needs related to diagnosis and treatment (Anderson & Klemm, 2008). Now with easy access to health-related information via the Internet, patients can make decisions about their care without difficulty. Or can they? With so much information available online, how can consumers determine the validity of the source? This chapter provides guidance for individuals with lung cancer as they seek evidence-based practice for their treatment. Also, this chapter will identify current and reliable consumer resources and support related to living with lung cancer.

Print and Video/Audio Materials for Consumers

Individuals with lung cancer may seek various resources for specific aspects of their treatment or condition. Lung cancer individuals may secure patient education booklets or pamphlets, textbooks, fact sheets, and other print materials from national organizations, such as the American Cancer Society (ACS) or the National Cancer Institute (NCI). Individuals may seek information from healthcare professionals, and oncology nurses are excellent resources for a newly diagnosed lung cancer patient. Oncology nurses use printed materials to supplement their initial teaching session. Institutions or agencies often develop their own printed materials to supplement generic materials.

Written materials are just one of the excellent tools that can be used in the teaching and learning process. Effective patient educators from all disciplines understand the overall purpose of patient and family education and follow through with all aspects of the educational process. In selecting resources for patient education, the educator should keep in mind that education needs to be adapted to the appropriate age, developmental need, culture, and language for the specific patient or significant other (Sarna & Ganley, 1995; Rutledge, Donaldson, & Pravikoff, 1999). According to the 2003 National Assessment of Adult Literacy, only 13% of individuals had proficient literacy rates or processing skills to perform more complex and challenging literacy activities (National Center for Education Statistics, 2003). Forty-four percent of persons were at an intermediate literacy level or had skills necessary to perform moderately challenging literacy activities. Fourteen percent of this population were below a basic level or had no more than the most simple and concrete literacy skills.

It is vitally important that printed materials chosen for lung cancer patients and families be evaluated for appropriateness of reading level. Reviewing samples of written content and performing readability statistics will prove to be beneficial. Recent word-processing programs have this capacity; for example, the spelling and grammar function in Word 2007 can assist in performing this function. Written resources for lung cancer patients that may be helpful to patients and families are provided in Table 20–1.

Use of the Internet

The Internet enables patients to access greater amounts of health information than ever before. In fact, in 2007, 71% of American adults accessed the Internet, and 80% of Internet users searched for health information online (Internet

Activities, 2008). According to the Pew Internet & American Life Project, 73% of adults use the Internet. Females and males use the Internet almost equally (71% of women and 74% of men). Individuals who earn less than $30,000 (53%) use the Internet, even though they have fewer resources. According to Internet World Stats (2008), the dominant language on the Internet is English.

Two of the most common uses of the Internet are to obtain information and communicate using e-mail. It is estimated that 80% of Internet users research information about health/medical information (Internet Activities, 2008). Two researchers conducted a study regarding the usage of the Internet in a lung cancer clinic (Peterson & Fretz, 2003). A total of 184 patients from a multidisciplinary thoracic oncology clinic were surveyed over a 3-month period. Data was analyzed on 139 (75%) of the patients. Not surprisingly, the Internet was the most common nonphysician source of information. Sixty percent expressed interest in searching the Internet, whereas 16% actually performed searches. These users held a higher socioeconomic status, and older adult users were increasing in numbers. While e-mail is a quick method to communicate, it is available for patient-to-patient correspondence, but it is not commonly implemented between physicians and patients due to the security of information.

While patients can have information at their fingertips via the Internet, individuals still report the following barriers: lack of access (44% reported they would use the Internet if they had access), age (older patients use computers less often than younger patients), and level of education (formally educated people use the Internet more frequently) (Helft, Eckles, Johnson-Calley,

Table 20–1 Written Resources for Patients with Lung Cancer

Organization	Contact Information	E-mail/Web Site	Written Resource(s)
Lung Cancer Alliance	Phone: 202-463-2080 Lung Cancer Information Line: 800-298-2436 (9:00 a.m. to 5:00 p.m. Eastern Time)	http://www.lungcanceralliance.org[1]	Available free: PDF downloads *Lung Cancer Alliance Times* Spirit and Breath Newsletter LCA Clinical Trials Education Frankly Speaking About Lung Cancer
American Cancer Society	Phone: 1-800-ACS-2345	www.cancer.org	For purchase: "QuickFACTS on Lung Cancer" Available free: Lung Cancer Treatment Guidelines for Patients The Staging of Cancer, 7th edition (Lung) Set Yourself Free: A Smoker's Guide The Decision Is Yours The Smoke Around You Living Smoke Free for You and Baby Tobacco and LGBT Community (Some materials are also available in Spanish.)
American Lung Association	61 Broadway, 6th Floor New York, NY 10006 Phone: 1-800-LUNG-USA; 1-800-548-8252	www.lungusa.org	Available free: Fact sheets on smoking cessation, tobacco control, lung cancer, and air quality

continues

Table 20–1 Written Resources for Patients with Lung Cancer (continued)

Organization	Contact Information	E-mail/Web Site	Written Resource(s)
Caring Ambassadors (CAP Lung Cancer)	604 E. 16th St., Suite 201 Vancouver, WA 98663	www.lungcancercap.org	For purchase: *With Every Breath: A Lung Cancer Guidebook*
Lungcancer.org (a program of Cancer*Care*)	Floor 22 275 Seventh Ave. New York, NY 10001 Phone: 1-800-813-HOPE Fax: 212-712-8495	info@cancercare.org http://www.lungcancer.org	Available free: Lung Cancer: Caring for Your Bones When You Have Lung Cancer Lung Cancer: Treatment Update Multiple non-lung-cancer specific publications: Coping with a Cancer Diagnosis Care giving Cancer*Care* for Kids Finding Financial Help and Resources Managing Treatment and Side Effects Prevention and Early Detection Research and Clinical Trials Coping with Grief and Bereavement Publications in Spanish and Russian A Helping Hand: The Resource Guide for People with Cancer

Organization	Contact	Internet	Resources
Hospice Education Institute	3 Unity Square P. O. Box 98 Machiasport, ME 04655-0098 Hospicelink: 1-800-331-1620 Phone: 207-255-8800 Telefax: 207-255-8008	info@hospiceworld.org www.hospiceworld.org	For purchase: *Notes On Symptom Control In Hospice & Palliative Care* by Dr. Peter Kaye
Hospice Foundation of America	Phone: 1-800-854-3402	info@hospicefoundation.org www.hospicefoundation.org	Available free: *Journeys* newsletter Multiple brochures on grief, support for family/friends (some available in Spanish) For purchase: *A Guide for Recalling and Telling Your Life Story* *Living with Grief* (book series)
National Cancer Institute	6116 Executive Boulevard, Room 3036A Bethesda, MD 20892-8322 Phone: 1-800-4-CANCER TTY: 1-800-332-8615	cancergovstaf@mail.nih.gov www.cancer.gov	Available free: What You Need To Know About Lung Cancer Multiple non-lung cancer-specific publications on treatment options, clinical trials, nutrition, genetics, coping with cancer, risk factors/causes, prevention, tobacco/smoking, testing for cancer
National Comprehensive Cancer Network	275 Commerce Dr., Suite 300 Fort Washington, PA 19034 Phone: 215-690-0300 Fax: 215-690-0280	www.nccn.org	Available free on-line: Lung Cancer: Treatment Guidelines for Patients

continues

Table 20–1 Written Resources for Patients with Lung Cancer (continued)

Organization	Contact Information	E-mail/Web Site	Written Resource(s)
National Coalition for Cancer Survivorship	1010 Wayne Ave., Suite 770 Silver Spring, MD 20910 Phone: 301-650-9127; 888-650-9127 Fax: 301-565-9670	info@canceradvocacy.org; www.canceradvocacy.org; www.canceradvocacy.org/toolbox	Available free: What Cancer Survivors Need to Know About Health Insurance Working It Out: Your Employment Rights As a Cancer Survivor Self-Advocacy: A Cancer Survivor's Handbook Teamwork: The Cancer Patient's Guide to Talking with Your Doctor You Have the Right To Be Hopeful A Cancer Survivor's Almanac: Charting Your Journey The Cancer Survival Toolbox (some materials also available in Spanish)
National Lung Cancer Partnership	222 N. Midvale Blvd., Suite 6 Madison, WI 53705 Phone: 608-233-7905 Fax: 608-233-7893	www.nationallungcancerpartnership.org	Available free: Living with a Diagnosis of Lung Cancer

& Daugherty, 2005). Race and income are not barriers. As healthcare providers, recognizing these barriers is important when helping patients surf the Internet for information.

Online Evidence-Based Searching for Consumers

When counseling information-seeking consumers, the major concern for healthcare providers is the validity and quality of the information that is given or found regarding lung cancer. Although patients report that physicians are their most highly trusted source of healthcare information, only 10.9% contacted their physicians initially for information, whereas 48.6% chose online sources first (Anderson & Klemm, 2008). The sheer size of the information base available on the World Wide Web is a concern.

A self-directed approach implies that patients are informed about their health care. Although information technology may help consumers make better choices about health care, using the Internet to access health-related information can be challenging (Anderson & Klemm, 2008). Internet searches may not provide information that is personally relevant to patients (Anderson & Klemm, 2008). Excessive information can challenge patients emotionally and psychologically. People who encounter multiple choices for treatment online may expect too much (i.e., to find the perfect choice for them), discover that they are unable to act upon the information (indecision), or have difficulty discerning the differences among their choices (Shaller, et al., 2005; Woolf, Krist, Johnson, & Stenborg, 2005).

Most patients use a search engine to find information on the Internet. On an average day, nearly 60 million people use search engines (Internet Activities, 2008). Search engines have become an increasingly important part of the online experience of American Internet users. They enable individuals to quickly find Web sites that are related to a specific topic of interest. The latest data from comScore shows that Google is the most heavily used search engine, followed by Yahoo! Search, MSN Search, Ask Jeeves, and AOL Search (Internet Activities, 2008). Because search engines have been developed in different ways, each may direct patients to different sites given identical key words or search terms. In general, they "pull" or find Web site pages that have the key word or search term anywhere on the page. Table 20–2 illustrates how the search terms "lung cancer" and "nutrition" resulted in hits on Google. For advanced or more scientific search engines, refer to Table 20–3.

Other evidence-based searches can be located on The Cochrane Collaboration Consumer Network. At this site, a search request for cancer, then lung cancer, resulted in several hits (http://www.cochrane.org/docs/newcomersguide.htm on July 12, 2008). There were many multiple reviews, abstracts, summaries, and articles that may or may not be interpretable to consumers. A sample of some of the hits follows:

- Steroids, radiotherapy, chemotherapy, and stents for superior vena cava syndrome
- Chemotherapy for brain metastases from small cell lung cancer
- Surgery for early stage non-small cell lung cancer
- Palliative radiotherapy regimens for non-small cell lung cancer
- Second line chemotherapy for non-small cell lung cancer

The Cochrane Collaboration is an international nonprofit organization that aims to help people make informed decisions about health care by reviewing and promoting the best available ev-

Table 20–2 Annotated Descriptions (Finding and Links) of First Eight Web Pages in a Search for "Lung Cancer" and "Nutrition" Using Google*

Nutrition in Cancer Care—National Cancer Institute	How to lower everyone's lung cancer risk—Nutrition Notes—msnbc.com	Therapeutic Nutrition and Lung Disease—Cancer Prevention . . .	Lung Cancer Diet and Nutrition Manual	Cancer Community & Resource Center for People Living With Cancer	Complementary and Alternative Medicines Used to Help Treat Lung . . .	Roswell Park Cancer Institute—Nutrition for Lung Cancer Patients . . .	Chapter 12 Nutrition Lung Cancer
Lung Cancer Prostate Cancer Breast Cancer Colon Cancer Esophageal and Gastric Cancer. Advanced Cancer. Nutrition-related side effects may occur or become . . . www.cancer.gov/cancertopics/pdq/supportivecare/nutrition/Patient/page6	Sep 30, 2005 . . . After the death of anchorman Peter Jennings from lung cancer and the diagnosis of Dana Reeves, widow of Christopher Reeves, . . . www.msnbc.msn.com/id/9530903/	Some lung diseases can be prevented through good lifestyle choices, such as proper nutrition and exercise. If you've already been diagnosed with a lung . . . lungdiseases.about.com/od/nutrition/od/nutrition/Therapeutic_Nutrition.htm	Lung Cancer Diet and Nutrition Manual: what to eat for lung cancer? Discuss lung cancer diet helping alleviate symptoms such as taste change and sore mouth . . . www.healthcastle.com/lung_cancer_diet.shtml	Personalized Web Page; Latest Cancer & Nutrition News . . . Lung Cancer—Oat Cell, Lung Cancer—Small Cell, Lung Cancer—Squamous Cell, Lymphoma, Melanoma . . . www.cancercompass.com/	Discover cancer hospitals for patients who believe in conventional lung cancer . . . nutrition, acupuncture, mind-body medicine or spiritual support, . . . www.cancercenter.com/lung-cancer/complementary-therapies.cfm	Weight loss in lung cancer patients can be serious. Poor nutrition can lead to loss of protein stores, in the body, which can cause muscle wasting, . . . www.roswellpark.org/.../Lung_Cancer/Support_for_Lung_Cancer_Patients/Nutrition_for_Lung_Cancer_Patients \	File Format: PDF/Adobe Acrobat—View as HTML be challenging as some symptoms of lung cancer and side effects of treatment can interfere with eating and nutrition. This chapter reviews the basic . . . www.lungcancerguidebook.org/lungcancerguidebook/LCGuidebook%20Aug05/Ch12_0605.pdf

*Note: This search led to 369,000 hits for lung cancer and nutrition in 0.18 seconds with SafeSearch on.

Table 20–3 Medical Web Sites for Searching Medical-Related Information

Name	URL
Google Scholar Beta	http://scholar.google.com/
SearchMedica	http://www.searchmedica.com/
PubMed	http://www.ncbi.nlm.nih.gov/pubmed/
UpToDate	http://www.uptodate.com
The Cochrane Collaboration	http://www.cochrane.org
Oncology Nursing Society	http://www.ons.org/research/
OncoLink	http://www.oncolink.com/

idence on the effects of interventions and treatments. It is a charity registered in the United Kingdom. Its governing body is the Steering Group, with a secretariat based in Oxford, England.

Credibility of Web Page Information

When consumers begin to read through the Web pages they have found, they need guidelines to evaluate the solidity of their finds. Consumers often trust search engines to be fair and unbiased when posting search results. However, most individuals know little about the operation of search engines, how searches are conducted, or the criteria for presenting the results (Lorence & Greenberg, 2006). The Health on the Net Foundation Code of Conduct (HONcode) helps identify credible, reliable medical and health Web sites (see Figure 20-1). The Oncology Nursing Society Web site (accessed July 12, 2008) directs the user to the HON Code of Conduct Web site (http://www.hon.ch/HONcode/Conduct.html). The NCI Web site directs users to the following Web site: *Is Information on the Web Reliable?* (http://understandingrisk.cancer.gov/media/internet.cfm).

Readers should be attentive to content, site ownership, sponsors, quality of material, peer review, updates, links to other sites, advertising, and privacy statements provided on Web pages (see Figure 20-2).

The Oncology Nursing Society has determined that the three most critical criteria in evaluating health-oriented Web sites are credibility of the information provider, disclosure of sponsorship, and privacy of any data that is collected from consumers (Clark & Gomez, 2001).

1. The credibility of the information provider can be determined in several ways. While not always true, Web sites that are sponsored by government agencies, such as the National Cancer Institute, or nonprofit organizations, such as the American Cancer Society, usually can be relied upon to have credible information, while those sponsored by for-profit organizations may need to be judged more carefully. Hopefully, the credentials and places of employment for the authors are given as well.

   Other support for site credibility is a list of members of a medical/nursing advisory board who would have previewed

Figure 20–1 Symbol for Health on the Net Foundation Code of Conduct.

Source: http://www.hon.ch/HONcode

content prior to its being available on the Web site. This information is often available by clicking on the link to "About us" or "About this site." Contact information may also be given for someone who is responsible for the Web site so that readers/users can contact someone for clarification of ongoing questions. These public disclosures about the nature and authors of the

Figure 20–2 Suggested criteria for evaluating health-related resources found online.

Authors	Authors are listed. Credentials, educational background, and affiliations of the author(s) are provided. Author contact information is available.
Information	The information is: Accurate Comprehensive Current Easy to read
References	References are: Listed Appropriate Recent
Sponsor	Sponsor is identified and is a reliable source, for example, government agencies (.gov), medical schools (.edu), and nonprofit groups that focus on disease research and education (.org). Commercial sites (.com) may or may not be helpful, depending on whether they are providing a consumer service or trying to sell a product.
Electronic media	Links are appropriate. Graphics are useful. Web pages load quickly. Web site is easy to navigate.

Privacy and security	Privacy statement explains clearly what the site owner will do with any personal information it asks for. If joining a chat room or online discussion, the site states the terms of using the service.
	  Security software information is evident.
	  Encryption protocols are disclosed.

Evaluation	Visitors can contact the Web site administrator with problems, questions, or feedback.

Source: Courtesy of *Clinical Journal of Oncology* (Anderson & Klemm, 2008, p. 60, permission granted from Jones and Bartlett).

Web site create some sense of quality control (Eng, 2001). Also very important for information that affects the treatment and care of patients is the date of the latest Web site posting. Out-of-date information is much less useful to consumers. As with print information, credibility is enhanced when information is supported by references—either print materials or Web site URLs.

2. Sponsorship disclosure may include reporting of any commercial and noncommercial support for the Web site. Advertisements presented on the site should be clearly presented as such and should not be potentially confused with the content.

3. When a Web site seeks information from a Web site user, the privacy of this data should be ensured by the sponsoring organization. Thus, confidentiality of data, including the identity of a user, should be respected, and a statement to this effect on the Web site is important. Several organizations (e.g., Health on the Net Foundation) have made recommendations about security and consumers (Clark & Gomez, 2001). A statement such as, "We subscribe to the HONcode principles of the Health on the Net Foundation" assists the user in knowing that the site is ethical.

Accuracy of Internet Content

Although the provision of inaccurate information to a potential audience is not a new phenomenon, the Internet is unique. Information posted online has the potential for reaching a very wide audience. Medical misinformation (e.g., incomplete, out of context, incorrect, outdated) is available online and coexists with reliable material posted by credible sources. The lay public may not have the skills necessary to discriminate between sites that provide nonbiased, well-researched information and those that do not (this may not apply to some educational sites). Just as information obtained from family and friends may not be accurate, online discussion groups that are not reviewed or facilitated by healthcare professionals also may disseminate incorrect information (Anderson & Klemm, 2008). Providers are encouraged to refer patients to specific sites that they believe have highly accurate information (such as the Web site for the Lung Cancer Alliance, Caring Ambassadors Program (CAP), and others mentioned in Table 20-4).

Online Support for Consumers

Persons with lung cancer who are Internet users may desire to communicate with other patients who have lung cancer or family members of patients with lung cancer. In 1986, Listservs were popular, and they were the first electronic mailing software applications. A Listserv is an e-mail group to which people subscribe based upon common interests. Individuals can join or leave a list without the need for human administration. Listservs automatically deliver e-mail to subscribers of a mailing list that has been organized around a specific topic or interest group. The interested person should be warned that Listserv membership can lead to receipt of many more e-mails than desired, so let the user beware!

Another method to communicate is the Internet forum. Early Web-based forums began around 1996 and were commonly referred to as

Table 20–4 List of Lung Cancer-Related Web Sites Judged Reliable in Terms of Authorship, Sponsorship, and Content

Organization*	Web Site	Description
Non-Lung Cancer-Specific American Cancer Society (ACS)	www.cancer.org	Includes a multitude of informative links, including types of treatments, treatment centers, treatment decision tools, Living with Cancer, Cancer Survivors Network, complementary and alternative methods, local resource information, and books and resources. Some information is available in Spanish.
National Cancer Institute (NCI)	http://www.cancer.gov/	This site links to all NCI sites, including Cancer Net (wide range of cancer information), Cancer Trials (clinical trial information), Cancer Information Service (national information and education network), and CancerNet en Español (cancer-related information in Spanish).
Oncology Nursing Society (ONS)	www.ons.org (go to Patient Education link)	Available topics include: prevention and detection, diagnosis, treatment, symptom management, psychosocial, and disease-specific information.
CancerCare	www.cancercare.org	CancerCare provides information about sexuality, workplace issues, caregivers, clinical trials, end-of-life concerns, fatigue, novel treatments, pain, patient-to-patient network, and policy/advocacy. Services are provided by oncology social workers in person, over the phone, or through the Web site.

continues

Table 20–4 List of Lung Cancer-Related Web Sites Judged Reliable in Terms of Authorship, Sponsorship, and Content (continued)

Organization*	Web Site	Description
Cancer Hope Network	www.cancerhopenetwork.org	Free, confidential, one-on-one support to people with cancer and their families.
Cancer Information and Counseling Line (CICL)	www.amc.org/contact.html	This site is a service of the AMC Cancer Research Center. It provides a national toll-free telephone information line designed to help people with cancer and their families and provides medical information and emotional support through short-term counseling and resource referrals.
National Hospice and Palliative Care Organization (NHPCO)	www.nhpco.org	NHPCO offers information about hospice care and finding a hospice program.
Mayo Clinic	www.mayohealth.org	Mayo Clinic's Health Lifestyle Planners provides assistance in building healthy habits related to weight, exercise, stress reduction, and smoking cessation.
CenterWatch OncoLink	www.centerwatch.com www.oncolink.upenn.edu	CenterWatch is a publishing and information services company. Information is geared toward patients and pharmaceutical, biotechnology, and medical device companies and research centers that are involved in clinical research around the world. Their Web site includes a list of IRB-approved clinical trials that are being conducted internationally.

continues

Table 20–4 List of Lung Cancer-Related Web Sites Judged Reliable in Terms of Authorship, Sponsorship, and Content (continued)

Organization*	Web Site	Description
		OncoLink's Web site's mission is to help cancer patients, families, healthcare professionals, and the general public get accurate cancer-related information at no charge. Both non-lung cancer and lung cancer-specific information is provided by University of Pennsylvania cancer specialists.
Lung Cancer-Specific Lung Cancer Alliance	www.alcase.org	Lung Cancer Alliance provides information about lung cancer, psychosocial support, early detection and diagnostic imaging, and advocacy about issues that concern lung cancer survivors.
Macmillan Cancer Support	www.cancerbackup.org.uk/ Cancertype/Lung	This is a United Kingdom national cancer information service provided by oncology nurses and physicians. It provides up-to-date information, practice advice, and support to cancer patients. Both non-lung cancer and lung cancer-specific information is available.
Caring Ambassadors Program (CAP)	www.lungcancer.org	CAP is a nonprofit organization with a mission to better the lives of people who are living with lung cancer and their loved ones through state-of-the-art information, awareness efforts, advocacy, and support.
YourSurgery	www.yoursurgery.com (click on Chest then Thoracotomy)	This link provides details about thoracotomy surgical procedures. It describes the anatomy of the lungs, pathologies, symptoms, and complications, including helpful graphics.

continues

Table 20–4 List of Lung Cancer-Related Web Sites Judged Reliable in Terms of Authorship, Sponsorship, and Content (continued)

Organization*	Web Site	Description
New York Online Access to Health	www.noah-health.org (click on Index A to Z then Lung Cancer)	This site provides links to information about types of lung cancer, diagnosis and treatment, risk factors and prevention, statistics, women with lung cancer, advanced lung cancer, chemotherapy, radiotherapy, surgery, clinical trials, living with lung cancer, and additional resources.
Lungcancer.org	www.lungcancer.org	This Web site has a special section for patients and families that addresses the basics of lung cancer, from screening to treatment and clinical trials.
Revolution Health	http://www.revolutionhealth.com/ conditions/cancer/lung-cancer/ ?s kwcid=lung%20cancer%20 online|1126532304	This Web site offers support, information about risk factors, treatments, and links to other resources.

*Note: Many of the organizations that sponsor these Web sites have print materials that can be accessed via an online request.

newsgroups, message boards, bulletin boards, or discussion groups. Messages are posted in chronological order or as a threaded discussion. Typically, there are forum administrators that can edit, delete, move, or otherwise modify any thread on the forum (http://en.wikipedia.org/ wiki/Internet_forum). Individuals need to be aware that some forums are anonymous and offer full anonymity or pseudonymity, so users should beware.

Some Internet resources connect patients with counselors or use one-on-one communication to ease emotional burdens. Four Web sites that may assist patients who need emotional support are: Cancer Hope Network, Cancer Information and Counseling Line (CICL), Caring Ambassadors Program (CAP), and Revolution Health (see Table 20-4). Cancer Hope Network matches one-on-one volunteers who have had similar experiences with lung and other cancers. CICL is a national toll-free information line. CAP has an Ask the Doc service where general questions can be submitted, and the response will be posted with a detailed response (specific individualized recommendations cannot be accommodated). Revolution Health has three support groups: face-to-face, Internet, and telephone support by buddies.

A blog is another Internet communication resource. The term is a contraction for Web log.

Blogs are Web sites that are typically maintained by an individual with regular entries of commentary descriptions or experiences. These sites can contain graphics or videos. Blogs can be personal, corporate, or media based. As reported in *ONS Connect* (July 8, 2006), ONS expects to launch a blog–possibly on YouTube–to connect its membership. One example of a blog can be found on the Lance Armstrong Foundation and NexCura Web site at http://www.livestrong. org/site/c.khLXK1PxHmF/b.4012249 (retrieved July 25, 2008).

There are several Web sites (see Table 20-4) that have e-news, navigator programs, links to related Internet resources, supportive care information, as well as many other options for the consumer with lung cancer. For example, Lungcancer.org has a free monthly e-mail newsletter (Cancer*Care* E-News) that individuals can sign up for. This newsletter gives up-to-date information on Cancer*Care* programs and services, as well as tips for people who are coping with cancer. New York Online Access to Health has multiple links to related lung cancer Web sites, and Lungcancer.org has support services through education, counseling, and financial assistance.

Risks to Consumer Use of Internet Information

The use of poor quality resources and gathering of misinformation are two major risks that persons with lung cancer face when they seek information on the Internet. The oncology nurse acts as a patient advocate and should warn patients of potential problems. Patient counseling and assistance will help validate information found by patients before making major treatment decisions or self-care practice changes. For example, Donald, a 58-year-old patient with stage III adenocarcinoma of

the lung, tells the nurse who is administering his chemotherapy that he is concerned about his recent 10-pound weight loss. He mentions wanting to try a liquid dietary supplement he found out about on the Internet. The nurse encourages him to bring the information with him to his next visit or fax it to her so she can assess the validity of the product. In the meantime, she might want to gather some evidence-based information about nutritional supplements and have it ready to discuss with Donald.

Resources to Recommend to Consumers

Table 20-4 includes a variety of Internet resources that have been evaluated according to the criteria previously described and determined to be credible sites. The table includes non-lung cancer and general sites. Consumers can be directed to specific sites according to their information needs. For example, the patient in the previous example discussed having trouble with his weight and wanting some information about nutrition. The oncology nurse might recommend the following specific sites: Revolution Health, NCI, or ACS.

Summary

The Internet has a plethora of Web sites that claim to have all of the answers—on topics ranging from health care to clinical conditions—and sometimes emotional support. Many persons who have lung cancer will want to use the Internet for information gathering on lung cancer-specific information and more general knowledge. Nurses and healthcare professionals can counsel them and warn them to be aware of the potential pitfalls of such information. Patients should be urged to do their research systematically, evaluating their finds as to credibility, disclosure of sponsorship, and confidentiality of information shared. Specific Internet sites are available that contain accurate, comprehensive information about lung cancer and related issues that are important to lung cancer patients and their families.

References

Anderson, A. S., & Klemm, P. (2008). The Internet: Friend or foe when providing patient education? *Clinical Journal of Oncology Nursing, 12*(1), 55–63.

Clark, P. M., & Gomez, E. G. (2001). Details on demand: Consumers, cancer information and the Internet. *Clinical Journal of Oncology Nursing, 5*(1), 19–24.

Eng, T. R. (2001). *The eHealthLandscape: A terrain map of emerging information and communication technologies in health and health care.* Princeton, NJ: Robert Wood Johnson Foundation.

Eysenbach, G. (2003). The impact of Internet on cancer outcomes. *CA: A Cancer Journal for Clinicians, 53*(6), 356–371.

Helft, P., Eckles, R., Johnson-Calley, C., & Daugherty, C. (2005). Use of the Internet to obtain cancer information among cancer patients as an urban county hospital. *Journal of Clinical Oncology, 23*(22), 4954–4962.

Hines, S. E. (2001). Sharing decision making with patients. *Patient Care (35)*7, 21–31.

Internet Activities. (2008). *Pew Internet & American Life Project.* Retrieved June 16, 2008, from http://www.pewinternet.org/trends/Internet_Activities_2.15.08.htm

Internet World Stats. (2008). *Internet world users by language: Top 10 languages.* Retrieved November 17, 2008, from http://www.internetworldstats.com/stats7.htm

Lorence, D. P., & Greenberg, L. (2006). The zeitgeist of online health search: Implications for a consumer-centric health system. *Journal of General Internal Medicine, 21*(2), 134–139.

National Center for Education Statistics. (2003). *National assessment of adult literacy.* Retrieved June 27, 2008, from http://nces.ed.gov/naal/kf_demographics.asp

Peterson, M., & Fretz, P. (2003). Patient use of the Internet for information in a lung cancer clinic. *Chest, 123*(2), 452–457.

Rutledge, D. N., Donaldson, N. E., & Pravikoff, D. S. (1999, October 15). Principles of effective adult-focused patient education in nursing. *The Online Journal of Clinical Innovations, 2*(Article 2), 1–22.

Sarna, L., & Ganley, B. (1995). A survey of lung cancer patient education materials. *Oncology Nursing Forum, 22*(10), 1545–1550.

Shaller, D., Rybowski, L., Stepnick, L., Sofaer, S., Hibbard, J., Kanouse, D., et al. (2005). Consumers in health care: The burden of choice. *California Health Care Foundation.* Retrieved January 1, 2008, from http://www.chcf.org:80/topics/view.cfm?itemID=115327

Woolf, S. H., Krist, A. H., Johnson, R. E., & Stenborg, P. S. (2005). Unwanted control: How patients in the primary care setting decide about screening for prostate cancer. *Patient Education and Counseling, 56*(1), 116–124.

World Health Organization (WHO). (2006). *Declaration of Alma-Ata, International Conference on Primary Health Care, Alma-Ata, USSR, 6-12 September, 1978; Declaration IV.* Retrieved June 24, 2008, from http://www.euro.who.int/AboutWHO/Policy/20010827_1

Index

A

accuracy of Internet resources, 345

ACS. *See* American Cancer Society

acupressure, 62

acupuncture, 61–62, 143–144, 144

adenocarcinoma, 6–7, 29. *See also* non-small cell lung cancer (NSCLC)
    biology of, 29
    increased incidence of, 28

adhesion. *See* cellular adhesion

advance directives, 145–146

advocacy groups. *See* patient navigation; support groups

aesthetics, for dyspnea, 137

affective factors
    breathlessness and, 198, 201, 202
    hope. *See* living with hope
    nutritional status, 159–161
    smoking (tobacco), 285–286

African Americans, 5, 17

age (patient), 162
    appropriateness of printed materials, 336
    care of elderly patients, 330–331
    chemotherapy for elderly patients, 85–86, 146
    incidence of lung cancer and, 5–6
    surgical therapy outcome and, 51, 57
    women with lung cancer, 316

air (pushed), for dyspnea, 208

air pollutants, 10–11, 12

AJCC Cancer Staging Manual, TNM staging, 8, 11–12

albumin, 180–181

ALCASE (now Lung Cancer Alliance), 13, 276, 327, 337, 348

Alimta. *See* pemetrexed

Alliance for Lung Cancer Advocacy, Support, and Education. *See* ALCASE

alopecia, 251

alternative therapies. *See* complementary and alternative therapies

American Cancer Society (ACS), 337, 346
    CT screening recommendations, 37
    PN (patient navigator) program, 261–262, 262–263, 265, 271–272

American College of Surgeons, CT screening recommendations, 37

American Lung Association, 337

ANA (American Nurses Association), on assisted suicide, 149

anemia, fatigue and, 125

anesthetics, 137

angiogenesis, sustained, 25–26

anorexia, 159
    pharmacologic strategies for, 189
    symptom management strategies, 182, 186, 189–190

antianxiety medications, for dyspnea, 207

anticholinergics
    for dyspnea, 135–136
    for fatigue, 126

antidepressants
    for anxiety, 139
    for appetite, 190
    for fatigue, 125, 126

antiemetics, 93, 96

antipsychotic drugs, 140–141

anxiety, 138–140
    breathlessness and, 198, 201, 202
    common worries of patients, 249–251
    with dyspnea, 134
    nutritional status and, 159
    during treatment, 250–252

anxiolytic therapy for dyspnea, 207–208

apoptosis avoidance, 21–23

application to practice (EBP), 328

asbestos, 11

ASCO (American Society of Clinical Oncology)
    on advanced or unresectable NSCLC, 82
    antiemetic recommendations, 96
    on neoadjuvant treatment of NSCLC, 83–85

Ask the Doc service, 349

assessment, diagnostic. *See* detection of lung cancer

assistance for individuals with lung cancer. *See* education (patient); emotional support and counseling; patient navigation; support groups

assisted suicide, 148–149

atmospheric radon. *See* indoor radon exposure

atrial fibrillation, postoperative, 56

attitudes toward nursing, 307–308

autocrine stimulation, 18, 21

autofluorescence bronchoscopy, 40

Avastin. *See* bevacizumab

axillary thoracotomy, 51–53
    wound infection, 56